HEALTH TRANSITIONS IN ARCTIC POPULATIONS

Edited by T. Kue Young and Peter Bjerregaard

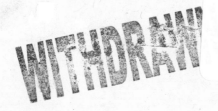

The Arctic regions are inhabited by diverse populations, both indigenous and non-indigenous. *Health Transitions in Arctic Populations* describes and explains changing health patterns in these areas, how particular patterns came about, and what can be done to improve the health of Arctic peoples.

This collaborative study correlates changes in health status with major environmental, social, economic, and political changes in the Arctic. Together the contributors explore commonalities in the experiences of different peoples while recognizing their considerable diversity. The volume focuses on five Arctic regions – Greenland, Northern Canada, Alaska, Arctic Russia, and Northern Fennoscandia. A general overview of the geography, history, economy, population characteristics, health status, and health services of each region is provided, followed by discussion of specific indigenous populations, major health determinants and outcomes, and, finally, an integrative examination of what can be done to improve the health of circumpolar peoples.

Health Transitions in Arctic Populations offers both a detailed examination of key health issues in the North and a vision for the future well-being of Arctic inhabitants.

T. KUE YOUNG is a professor in the Department of Public Health Sciences at the University of Toronto.

PETER BJERREGAARD is a research professor in the National Institute of Public Health at the University of Southern Denmark.

Health Transitions in Arctic Populations

Edited by T. Kue Young and Peter Bjerregaard

A Contribution to International Polar Year
by the International Network for Circumpolar Health Research

UNIVERSITY OF TORONTO PRESS
Toronto   Buffalo   London

ISBN 978-0-8020-9109-3 (cloth)
ISBN 978-0-8020-9401-8 (paper)

Printed on acid-free paper

Library and Archives Canada Cataloguing in Publication

Health transitions in arctic populations / edited by T. Kue Young and Peter
Bjerregaard.

Includes bibliographical references.
ISBN 978-0-8020-9109-3 (bound) ISBN 978-0-8020-9401-8 (pbk.)

1. Health transition – Arctic regions.   2. Arctic peoples – Health and
hygiene.   3. Public health – Arctic regions.   I. Young, T. Kue
II. Bjerregaard, Peter, 1947–.

RC957.H43 2008   362.10911'3   C2007-907217-8

University of Toronto Press acknowledges the financial assistance to its
publishing program of the Canada Council for the Arts and the Ontario Arts
Council.

University of Toronto Press acknowledges the financial support for its
publishing activities of the Government of Canada through the
Book Publishing Industry Development Program (BPIDP).

Contents

Tables

Figures

Maps

Colour plates follow page 170.

Preface

This book is a contribution to the International Polar Year (IPY) by the International Network for Circumpolar Health Research. Unlike the last IPY some fifty years ago, which focused mostly on the physical sciences, the IPY of 2007–9 recognizes the importance of the human dimension in the Arctic and promotes knowledge creation, dissemination and translation in health research. Our book aims to summarize the state of existing knowledge on human health in the Arctic, stimulate further research, and provide relevant information to policymakers and health care providers. We have deliberately recruited a majority of contributors from the younger generation of new researchers in this field, with the hope that they will continue to sustain the solid foundations that have been laid in circumpolar health research in the past several decades.

· The idea of this book was first born shortly after our last book collaboration, *The Circumpolar Inuit*, was published in 1998. We were invited to develop a teaching module on health and health care for a course on contemporary issues in the circumpolar world offered by the University of the Arctic. Another assignment was to contribute an entry on health and disease in the Arctic to the *Encyclopedia of the Arctic* (2005). In both instances we found that we knew a lot about the health of only one major population group in the Arctic, namely the Inuit, and very little about the other groups, both indigenous and non-indigenous. There was no ready-made, single source of information that we could consult to fulfill these two tasks. The challenge was on – why couldn't we fill this important gap ourselves?

· Our task was made easier by the launching of the International Network for Circumpolar Health Research (INCHR) in 2004. INCHR links researchers, trainees, and those who support health research from Canada, the Nordic countries, Russia, and the United States. While an informal network has existed since the early days of the 'circumpolar health movement' in the 1960s and 1970s, facilitated by the international health congresses, INCHR takes a step further to formalize international collaboration and cooperation. We did not envisage INCHR to be just another organizer of meetings and conferences. We knew a published book would be a concrete project that involved a large number of INCHR members and that would also fulfill the objectives of the network.

We would not have been able to complete this book project without the assistance of many individuals and organizations. Several individuals reviewed parts of the manuscript and provided helpful comments: from Canada were Catherine Carrie of the National Aboriginal Health Organization, Laurie Chan of the University of Northern British Columbia, André Corriveau of the Northwest Territories Department of Health and Social Services, and Keren Rice of the University of Toronto's Aboriginal Studies Program; from Denmark, Tine Curtis of the National Institute of Public Health; from Finland, Juhani Hassi of the University of Oulu; and from the United States, Brian Saylor of the University of Alaska Anchorage Institute of Circumpolar Health Studies. The staff of statistical agencies provided data requested by us, notably Helena Korpi of Statistics Finland, Mika Gissler of STAKES, and Keun Hwang of Statistics Greenland. Winfried Dallmann of the Norwegian Polar Institute prepared most of the colour maps. Katherine Minich, research officer at the University of Toronto, helped organize the bibliography. At the University of Toronto Press, executive editor Virgil Duff and managing editor Anne Laughlin have been most encouraging and helpful throughout the production of the book, from conception to realization. Beth McAuley was most thorough in copy-editing the manuscript and improved it considerably.

Editing a book is no fun – it is certainly harder than writing one. Our task has been lightened by the dedication and commitment of our contributors. Despite being incredibly busy people, they have, by and large, been prompt in producing and subsequently revising the manuscripts. The electronic age has certainly helped us in communicating with one another and in accessing information through the internet. Producing this book together has cemented friendships and enhanced collaborations, both new and old. There is truly an international network of like-minded individuals who share similar views of academic scholarship, scientific research, and knowledge dissemination.

Finally, we acknowledge the financial support of the Canadian Institutes of Health Research, through its award of a team grant (CTP-79853) on circumpolar health research to Kue Young. The knowledge dissemination component of this five-year grant supported background research associated with the book project, meetings among contributors and editors, and also a publication subsidy to the University of Toronto Press. The support from the Directorate of Health in Greenland and the Karen Elise Jensen Foundation allowed Peter Bjerregaard to continue his studies of health in the Arctic and to dedicate much of his time to the dissemination of the knowledge thus obtained.

HEALTH TRANSITIONS IN ARCTIC POPULATIONS

1 Introduction

KUE YOUNG AND PETER BJERREGAARD

This is a book about the health of the diverse populations who inhabit the circumpolar regions in the northern hemisphere. It describes and explains their changing patterns of health, how these came about, and what can be done to improve the health of these populations. We utilize the concept of 'health transitions' and apply it to the circumpolar world. We correlate changes in health status with major environmental, social, economic, and political changes in the regions. We seek commonalities in the experience of Arctic populations, while recognizing their immense diversity.

A circumpolar approach to identifying common issues and developing solutions that transcends national borders has increasingly been adopted by national and subnational governments, indigenous peoples' organizations, as well as professional and scientific associations. Examples include the Inuit Circumpolar Conference (established in 1977, now known as the Inuit Circumpolar Council), the International Union for Circumpolar Health (established in 1981), the International Arctic Science Committee (established in 1990), the Northern Forum (established in 1993), and the Arctic Council (established in 1996), among others.[1] By producing this book, we hope to consolidate and disseminate the burgeoning body of knowledge on circumpolar health and to promote international collaboration and cooperation in health research, health policy, and health care.

Defining the Arctic

In this book, we use the terms 'circumpolar' and 'Arctic' interchangeably, although, strictly speaking, 'circumpolar' also refers to the

Table 1.1   Northern administrative regions within Arctic countries: Land area, population, and population density

Country/ Northern regions	Population Total	Indigenous	% indigenous	Area[a] (sq. kms.)	Population density[b]
United States[c]	288,378,100	4,154,700	1.4	9.5 m	30.4
State of Alaska	641,700	122,140	19.0	1,530,700	0.4
Canada[d]	31,613,000	1,391,970	4.4	9.98 m	3.3
Yukon Territory	30,400	7,390	24.3	483,450	0.06
Northwest Territories	41,500	21,080	50.8	1,171,920	0.04
Nunavut Territory	29,500	25,200	85.5	2,121,100	0.01
Denmark[e]	5,427,500	7,000	0.1	43,098	125.9
Greenland[f]	56,900	50,400	88.6	2,184,700	0.03
Faroe Islands[g]	48,200	-	-	1,400	34.4
Iceland[h]	299,400	-	-	103,000	2.9
Norway[h]	4,640,200	60,000	1.1	323,802	14.3
Finnmark	72,900	⎫		48,618	1.5
Troms	153,600	⎬ 57,000	12.3	25,877	5.9
Nordland	236,300	⎭		38,456	6.1
Sweden[h]	9,047,800	36,000	0.4	441,370	20.5
Norrbotten	251,700	18,000	7.2	106,012	2.4
Västerbotten	257,700	6,000	2.3	59,284	4.3
Finland[h]	5,255,600	10,000	0.2	338,145	15.5
Lappi	185,800	8,000	4.3	98,947	1.9
Russian Federation[i]	145,166,700	252,200	0.2	17,075,400	8.5
Murmansk Oblast	892,500	2,120	0.2	144,900	6.2
Kareliya Republic	716,300	4,900	0.7	172,400	4.2
Arkhangelsk Oblast	1,336,500	8,460	0.6	587,400	2.3
[Nenets AO]	41,500	7,780	18.7	176,700	0.2
Komi Republic	1,018,700	920	0.1	415,900	2.4
Yamalo-Nenets AO	507,000	37,280	7.4	750,300	0.7
Khanty-Mansi AO	1,428,000	28,500	2.0	523,100	2.7
Taymyr AO	39,800	9,880	24.8	862,100	0.05
Evenki AO	17,700	4,080	23.1	767,600	0.02
Sakha Republic	949,300	32,540	3.4	3,103,200	0.3
Magadan Oblast	182,700	4,990	2.7	461,400	0.4
Koryak AO	25,200	10,240	40.6	301,500	0.1
Chukotka AO	53,800	16,860	31.3	737,700	0.1

[a]Area data obtained from the Encyclopedia of the Arctic (Nuttall 2005).
[b]Population density (persons per square kilometre) and % indigenous were calculated from data as reported in the table.
[c]U.S. population data are from the 2005 American Community Survey available from the U.S. Census Bureau's American FactFinder website (http://factfinder.census.gov);

Table 1.1   (*continued*)

indigenous people refer to American Indians and Alaska Natives, including those reporting one race only and in combination with other races.

[d]Canadian population data are from the 2006 Census available from the Statistics Canada website (www12.statcan.ca/English/census06/data); indigenous people refer to First Nations, Inuit, and Métis, including those with multiple origins – their numbers are extrapolated from their proportions in the 2001 Census.

[e]Data for Denmark do not include Greenland or the Faroe Islands, both part of the Danish monarchy under Home Rule. Danish population on 1 January 2006 is from Statistics Denmark (www.statbank.dk); estimate of Inuit residents in Denmark based on Togeby (2002) and Bjerregaard et al. (2003a).

[f]Greenland population on 1 January 2006 is from Statistics Greenland (www.statgreen.gl); indigenous people refer to Inuit, identifiable as 'persons born in Greenland'

[g]Faroe Islands population on 1 January 2006 is from Hagstova Føroya, the statistical agency of the territory (www.hagstova.fo).

[h]Nordic countries data are derived from national population registries as on 1 January 2006 for Norway (http://statbank.ssb.no)and 31 December 2005 for Sweden (www.ssd.scb.se), Finland (www.stat.fi), and Iceland (www.statice.is). Indigenous people refer to the Sami. Sami population estimates for Sweden and its two northern regions are made by Hassler based on the Sami population cohort as described in Hassler et al. (2005) and also in chapter 9. Other Sami populations are the upper end of ranges provided by various Sami parliaments.

[i]Russian data are from the 2002 Census (www.gks.ru). Indigenous people refer to the forty officially recognized 'indigenous, numerically small peoples of the North, Far East, and Siberia' (see chapter 5 for further explanation); AO = autonomous *okrug*.

Antarctic. We are interested in the vast geographical region that stretches across the 'top' of the world. Its precise borders, however, are difficult to define. The Arctic Circle, at 66°32′ N, is an imaginary line on the map and, apart from being a marker of solar radiation (encircling the 'land of the midnight sun'), has little meaning on the ground. Geographers have used a variety of markers to delimit the extent of the Arctic region, including the treeline, the 10° Celsius July isotherm, and the line of continuous permafrost. These do not coincide in all areas, and at various points they deviate north and south of the Arctic Circle, often substantially.[2]

It is important to recognize that, in addition to its physical environmental attributes, the Arctic is also a geopolitical and sociocultural construct. Various international bodies and publications have attempted to define it, for example the Arctic Monitoring and Assessment Program (AMAP) or the *Arctic Human Development Report* (AHDR).[3] As often as health statistics are collected by government agencies, they are usually aggregated by administrative divisions. For the purposes of this book, we have defined our boundaries based on such administrative divisions (see table 1.1, map 1). Iceland and the Faroe Islands will not be covered individually but some statistics are included for comparison. The whole of Alaska and Greenland are included. The northernmost counties in Norway (*fylke*), Sweden (*län*), and Finland (*lääni*) constitute the northern regions of those countries. While northern Canada traditionally comprises only the three northern territories, all located above 60° N latitude, our discussion of Canadian Inuit will also include those residing in the Nunavik region in northern Quebec and in Labrador. The definition of a northern region for Russia is complex and is further discussed in chapter 5.

In all, the Arctic regions included in table 1.1 encompass 17 million square kilometres, sustaining a sparsely distributed population of just under 10 million inhabitants, about 5 per cent of whom are indigenous.

The Arctic Environment

That the Arctic is cold is immediately obvious. The mean annual temperature is below freezing, and the mean July temperature is around 10°C. The line joining places with such a mean temperature (isotherm) is sometimes used to define the Arctic. Climatic variation exists as a result of mountain barriers, proximity to open waters, extent of surface snow and ice cover, and the duration of daylight and darkness. Despite the image of a white expanse, precipitation is generally low: the high Arctic is, in fact, a polar desert. While pack sea ice is found year round between the high Arctic islands, elsewhere the Arctic coast is ice-free for several months of the year. Coastal areas of Alaska and Greenland enjoy warmer temperatures due to the moderating influence of the waters of the Pacific and Atlantic Oceans. Indeed, in southwestern Greenland, the coast is ice-free throughout the year.[4]

The physical features of the land are varied – plains, plateaus, mountains, hills and valleys are traversed by rivers and dotted with lakes, and a long coast line is indented by fjords and majestic glaciers (see map 2). The arctic soil is dry, thin and poor; permafrost – perennially frozen ground – can be found widely at varying depths, preventing adequate drainage. Except in the high Arctic islands, where there is only bare rock and gravel, some vegetation – mostly lichens, moss, grass, and sedges – covers large areas, much of it under snowcover during most of the year. In the short summer growing season, when there is continuous daylight, blooming flowers enrich the landscape with a variety of colours. Plant life is an important food source for the herbivores, which form a critical link in the Arctic's food chain. The treeline demarcating the treeless tundra from the boreal forest, or taiga, is not so much a line as a transitional zone where low shrubs turn into trees, and trees grow increasingly taller and denser, as the Arctic merges into the subarctic.

The relatively low biodiversity in the Arctic decreases progressively from the tundra-taiga border northwards towards the Pole. The major marine and terrestrial mammals include different species of seals and whales, polar bears, muskoxen, caribou, walruses, and furbearers such as arctic foxes, hares, and wolves. Reindeer, the domesticated variety of caribou, are widely distributed and have been husbanded by indigenous peoples in northern Eurasia for centuries. Avian species include ptarmigan, snowy owl, ducks, geese, guillemot, and raven, most of which are migratory. Fish such as lake trout and whitefish can be found in rivers and lakes, and species such as arctic char move seasonally from the sea into freshwater areas. Marine species include salmon, cod, halibut, capelin, and herring found off the coasts of Alaska and Greenland. Shrimps and crabs also abound. While the number of species is small, individual species may be present in large numbers, and there are seasonal bursts of high productivity. Within any given locality, there is also considerable year-to-year fluctuation.

Arctic Peoples

Table 1.2 presents various demographic indicators of the Arctic regions covered in this book. The various regions differ from the larger nation states of which they are a part in terms of fertility and age structure. The differences are most profound in northern Canada, Alaska, and Greenland, primarily because of the relatively high proportion of indigenous people, and are least in the Nordic countries. The population was on the increase during the 1950s across the circumpolar north. It peaked at different times in different places – in northern Finland in the 1960s, northern Norway in the 1980s, northern Sweden and Russia in the 1990s – while in northern Canada, Alaska, and Greenland the population continues to grow.[5]

A major concern of this book is the health of the indigenous peoples. The term 'indigenous' appears to be the most accepted internationally

Table 1.2   Selected demographic indicators of northern regions

Country/ Northern regions	Age distribution		Crude birth rate[a]	Total fertility rate[b]	Life expectancy[c]	
	% <15	% 65+			M	F
United States[d]	*21.0*	*12.1*	*14.1*	*2.04*	*74.8*	*80.1*
State of Alaska	24.1	6.6	15.7	2.41	74.2	79.1
Canada[e]	*18.9*	*13.0*	*10.4*	*1.51*	*77.0*	*82.0*
Yukon Territory	21.0	6.0	11.1	1.58	74.1	79.6
Northwest Territories	27.1	4.4	16.2	1.96	73.7	78.8
Nunavut Territory	37.1	2.2	25.9	3.06	67.2	70.2
Denmark[f]	*18.7*	*15.2*	*12.1*	*1.76*	*74.9*	*79.6*
Greenland[g]	24.8	5.7	16.1	2.41	64.6	70.4
Faroe Islands[h]	22.8	13.5	14.7	2.51	77.1	81.5
Iceland[f]	*21.8*	*11.7*	*14.5*	*2.00*	*79.0*	*82.6*
Norway[f]	*19.5*	*14.7*	*12.6*	*1.80*	*76.6*	*81.7*
Finnmark	20.5	13.6	11.8	1.90	74.6	80.6
Troms	19.7	13.8	11.6	1.79	76.5	81.5
Nordland	19.3	16.3	10.2	1.83	76.7	82.0
Sweden[f]	*17.3*	*17.3*	*10.7*	*1.64*	*77.8*	*82.3*
Norrbotten	16.2	19.1	9.3	1.70	76.6	81.6
Västerbotten	16.7	17.7	9.8	1.56	77.6	82.1
Finland[f]	*17.3*	*16.0*	*10.9*	*1.75*	*74.8*	*81.6*
Lappi	16.6	17.2	9.7	1.86	73.7	81.1
Russian Federation[i]	*16.4*	*13.0*	*9.7*	*1.27*	*58.8*	*72.0*
Murmansk Oblast	16.2	7.1	9.5	1.29	56.9	70.3
Kareliya Republic	16.1	12.2	9.7	1.31	53.9	69.3
Arkhangelsk Oblast	16.8	11.5	10.1	1.40	55.6	70.0
[Nenets AO]	23.1	6.5	14.5	1.88	51.8	67.9
Komi Republic	17.7	8.1	10.6	1.40	55.5	69.1
Yamalo-Nenets AO	22.6	1.6	13.3	1.64	61.9	72.3
Khanty-Mansi AO	20.6	3.0	13.1	1.59	62.2	73.0
Taymyr AO	23.4	2.9	14.7	2.00	55.2	68.6
Evenki AO	24.3	4.2	15.0	2.12	55.5	67.4
Sakha Republic	24.3	5.3	14.5	1.91	58.1	70.6
Magadan Oblast	17.1	4.6	10.6	1.44	57.4	69.8
Koryak AO	22.3	4.2	11.9	2.16	46.5	63.2
Chukotka AO	21.0	1.9	13.2	2.17	55.0	64.5

[a]Crude birth rate (CBR): number of livebirths per 1,000 population.
[b]Total fertility rate (TFR): number of livebirths per woman.
[c]Life expectancy (LE) at birth in years.
[d]United States 2000–4 data on TFR and CBR are from the National Center for Health Statistics (NCHS) VitalStats website (www.cdc.gov/nchs/datawh/vitalstats.htm); age-distribution is from the 2005 *American Community Survey* (U.S. Census Bureau http://factfinder.census.gov); LE data for Alaska 2000 and U.S.A. 2003 are from NCHS.

Table 1.2 (*continued*)

---

[e]Canadian data are from Statistics Canada's Canadian Vital Statistics Birth Database CANSIM Table 102-4501: mean 2000–4 for CBR and TFR; mean 2000–2 for life expectancy; age distribution is from the 2001 Census (www12.statcan.ca/english/census01/home/index.cfm).

[f]Age distribution data for the Nordic countries are derived from national population registries as on 1 January 2006 for Norway and Denmark and 31 December 2005 for Sweden, Finland and Iceland obtained from the respective national statistical agencies; mean 2000–4 CBR, TFR, and life expectancy are obtained from EUROSTAT (http://epp.eurostat.ec.europa.eu) for national data and the respective national statistical agencies for northern regional data (for URL addresses see notes to table 1.1).

[g]Greenland data are from Statistics Greenland (www.statgreen.gl); age distribution as on 1 January 2006; CBR, TFR, and life expectancy are for mean of 2000–4.

[h]Faroe Islands data are from Hagstova Føroya, the statistical agency of the territory (www.hagstova.fo); age distribution is as on 1 January 2006; CBR, TFR, and LE data are mean of 2000–4.

[i]Russia: age distribution for the country and regions are based on the 2002 Census; national and regional CBR data are mean of 2000–4, from Federal State Statistics Service (www.gks.ru); TFR for Russia (2000–4) and the regions (2004) are from *Demographic Yearbook of Russia* (Federal State Statistics Service 2006a); LE data are for 2000–4, from *Regions of Russia* (Federal State Statistics Service 2006b).

and will be used in this book, except in referring to groups in specific countries where terms such as 'Aboriginal' and 'Native' are acceptable. Many indigenous peoples occupy the northern reaches of the Eurasian landmass, from the Sami in Scandinavia to the Chukchi in the easternmost tip of Russia. The Inuit, who today live under four national flags, can be found in Chukotka, Alaska, northern Canada, and Greenland. An all-encompassing definition of indigenous peoples is elusive; indeed, a definition is conspicuously absent from the *United Nations Declaration on the Rights of Indigenous Peoples*. Some United Nations agencies, the International Labour Office, the World Bank, and international law generally apply four criteria to distinguish indigenous peoples:

1 indigenous peoples usually live within (or maintain attachments to) geographically distinct ancestral territories;
2 they tend to maintain distinct social, economic, and political institutions within their territories;
3 they typically aspire to remain distinct culturally, geographically, and institutionally rather than assimilate fully into national society; and
4 they self-identify as indigenous or tribal.[6]

Figure 1.1   Genetic tree of 16 Arctic populations in Eurasia and North America

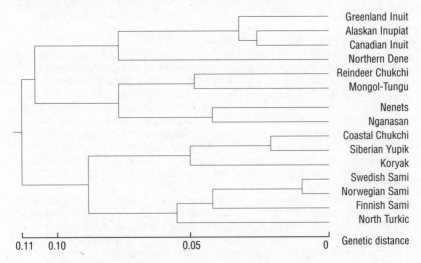

		Greenland Inuit
		Alaskan Inupiat
		Canadian Inuit
		Northern Dene
		Reindeer Chukchi
		Mongol-Tungu
		Nenets
		Nganasan
		Coastal Chukchi
		Siberian Yupik
		Koryak
		Swedish Sami
		Norwegian Sami
		Finnish Sami
		North Turkic

0.11   0.10   0.05   0   Genetic distance

Source: Redrawn from Cavalli-Sforza, Menozzi, and Piazza (1994:227).

Some countries have legislation that defines and recognizes specific groups as indigenous. The constitution of Canada, for example, identifies First Nations (or 'Indians'), Inuit, and Métis as 'Aboriginal.' In the United States, a variety of treaties and agreements define 'American Indians and Alaska Natives.' Beginning in the 1920s, the Soviet government accorded various ethnic groups the status of 'numerically small peoples of the North, Siberia and the Far East.' At the dissolution of the Soviet Union, there were twenty-six such groups in Russia. By 2005 the number had grown to forty-one. Excluded are non-Slavic national minorities such as the Turkic-speaking Yakuts (Sakha), the Buryats (close kins of the Mongols), and the Komi in European Russia, who speak an Uralic language close to Finnish. These are sizable groups that number in the hundreds of thousands and have their own republics.[7] The distinction between 'national minorities' and 'indigenous peoples' is also made in countries such as Norway, where the Finnish-speaking Kvens are considered a minority but not indigenous. As the table of contents of this book indicates, not all regions and peoples within the Arctic are reviewed in the same detail.

Among the diverse peoples in the Arctic, some are more closely related genetically and culturally than others. Based on statistical analyses of various genetic markers, genetic 'trees' can be constructed which show the genetic distance between population groups.[8] One such tree, based on sixty genes, shows the relationship between sixteen Eurasian and North American Arctic groups (fig. 1.1). Small sample sizes necessitated the pooling of linguistically close groups – hence the 'Mongol-Tungu' group pooled samples of Evens, Evenki, and Buryat, while the 'North Turkic' groups included the Yakut, Dolgan, Tuva, and Altai. It should be noted that different trees will result if a different mix of populations and/or different sets of genetic markers are studied. Genetic relationships among present-day culturally and linguistically defined ethnic groups can be obscured by heavy intermarriage with, or adoption of the language and cultural practices of, neighbouring groups in historic times.[8]

The genetic tree shown in figure 1.1 is based on so-called classical markers such as blood groups, red cell enzymes, serum proteins, white cell antigens, and immunoglobulins. The modern era of genomics has allowed polymorphisms at the DNA level (variation in genetic sequences) to be studied, which has added considerably to our understanding of genetic affinities between populations. By focusing on the rates and patterns of mutations on mitochondrial DNA (mtDNA, which is inherited from mother to all children) and the non-recombinant region of the y-chromosome (NRY, passed on from father to son), much new insight is gained in reconstructing human evolution, especially the prehistoric migrations of populations. As discussed further in chapter 9, mtDNA and NRY studies indicated that the Sami had received little genetic flow from Asiatic Siberian peoples.

For indigenous peoples of North America, their Asiatic origin is widely accepted, based on the accumulated genetic evidence from living and past Siberian and North American populations. However, there is still considerable debate on the number and timing of the waves of migrations and their likely routes.[9]

Arctic peoples also belong to many different language families (map 3). Linguists and anthropologists do not completely agree on the classification and nomenclature, especially with regards to larger aggregations of 'super-families.' In Arctic North America, the Eskimo-Aleut family extends from Greenland to Alaska, and has about 3,000 members in Chukotka. The Na-Dene family comprises the Athabascan languages spoken in Alaska and northern Canada, as well as Haida and Tlingit. (This particular grouping is controversial – see chapter 8.) In Asiatic Russia, at the easternmost is the Chukotko-Kamchatkan family, with two branches, one of which comprises Chuckchi and Koryak, and the other Itelmen, spoken in Kamchatka. The Altaic family covers much of the Far East and Central Asia, and is divided into a Turkic branch, which is a large conglomerate of some thirty languages across the steppes, from Turkey to the Arctic, including Yakut and Dolgan, a Mongolian branch (which includes Buryat), and a Tungusic branch (to which the Evens and Evenki belong). Situated astride the Ural Mountains, dividing Europe from Asia, is the Uralic family. It can be further divided into Samoyed (which includes Nenets, Enets, Nganasan, and Selkups), Finnic (to which Finnish, Sami, Komi, Udmurt, and also Estonian belong), and Ugric (which includes Khanty and Mansi, and also Hungarian). Russian and the Scandinavian languages are all members of the vast Indo-European family of languages, which also include English and French, two of the colonizing languages of Arctic North America. Given the extensive immigration and trend towards multiculturalism, especially in North America, one can surmise that many of the world's languages not mentioned above are most likely represented in Arctic communities today.[10]

Arctic Prehistory

The settlement of the Arctic is part of the story of the migration of modern *Homo sapiens* 'out of Africa' some 60,000 years ago. By 45,000 years ago, they had reached Europe. During the next 20,000 years much of Eurasia was colonized, as far north as 60° N in Siberia and the Urals. Successful occupation of the Arctic required anatomical and physiological adaptation, dietary changes, and technological innovation, particularly in clothing and shelter. The archaeological evidence suggests that the colonization process was characterized by a series of thrusts and retreats coinciding with climatic oscillations during the Pleistocene period (the Ice Age), which opened and closed habitats.[11]

Around 20,000 years ago, with the end of the cold peak of the Last Glacial Maximum (when the world's ice cover was at its maximum, from about 24,000 to 21,000 years ago), humans were able to maintain a sustained presence above the Arctic Circle. In the west, as the massive Fennoscandia icesheet began to retreat around 12,000 years ago, people moved into southern Scandinavia. By 10,000 years ago, the coasts of western Norway and southern Sweden were occupied up to

63° N. Between 10,000 and 7,000 years ago, the Komsa culture thrived on the coast of Finnmark above 70° N and extended eastward to the Kola Peninsula.

In Siberia, the Dyuktai culture flourished about 15,000 years ago around the middle Lena Basin, associated with the distinctive 'microblade' technology. Using wedge-shaped microblade cores, small and sharp stone blades were produced in large numbers, which could be fixed into grooves of a bone or antler and used as weapons or tools. This unique adaptation to the northern environment was widely disseminated in northeast Asia and was later carried into the Americas. Around 12,000 years ago, the Sumnagan culture appeared, which quickly spread across Siberia and into the tundra. By 10,000 years ago, human settlement extended from Chukotka in the east to the Taymyr Peninsula in the west.

From about 60,000 years ago, the sea level at the Bering Sea was as much as 120 metres below today's level, exposing the Beringia land bridge between Chuktoka and Alaska. The term 'land bridge' projects an image of a narrow strip of land, but in fact, Beringia was an ecologically heterogeneous land mass that extended from the Kolyma River in Siberia to the Mackenzie River in the Northwest Territories, over 3,000 kilometres in length, and some 1,500 kilometres at its widest.[12]

Humans likely occupied Beringia around 15,000 years ago and migrated into North America, together with fellow travellers such as animals and plants (and perhaps also parasites and microbes). It is difficult to pinpoint the 'date' of entry. Much earlier migrations (by tens of thousands of years) have been proposed, dependent on the acceptance of the antiquity of various South American archaeological sites indicating human occupation. The oldest confirmed site of human occupation in Alaska is Swan Point, near Fairbanks, containing artifacts such as microblades, which have been dated to some 12,000 years ago. While some claim that the animal bones with signs of human modification that have been found in Old Crow Flats and Bluefish Caves in the Yukon are 25,000 to 42,000 years old, such claims have not been generally accepted.[13] (Chapters 3 and 4 discuss further the archaeology of Alaska and northern Canada.)

From Beringia, further movement to the east was blocked by the Cordilleran and Laurentide icesheets, which were coalesced until around 12,000 years ago, when an ice-free corridor between them became open and allowed movement southward, which led to the initial peopling of the Americas. An alternative scenario, that of a coastal route, was feasible even earlier, perhaps 17,000 years ago. From 12,000 years ago, increasing warming and rising sea level erased Beringia and severed the land link with Asia. From time to time new cultures emerged in Alaska which would 'seed' the rest of the North American Arctic.

In the mid-1980s, the three-migration model was proposed for the peopling of the Americas. It postulated an earliest wave of migrants who eventually occupied the whole hemisphere and were the ancestors of all North, Central, and South American Indians. This was followed by the Na-Dene wave, and lastly, the Eskimo-Aleut. Originally based on data from linguistics, archaeology and classical genetic markers, the model received some support from later mtDNA studies, which attached dates of 36,000 to 18,000 years ago for the first, 10,000 to 5,000 years ago to the second, and 7,000 to 5,000 years ago to the third migration. However, a competing and more parsimonious model, based on the same body of mtDNA and also NRY data, argued for a single migration.[14] (Further details on the genetics of Inuit and Dene people are provided in chapters 7 and 8.)

Global warming 7,000 years ago ushered in the Neolithic period (Late Stone Age) in Eurasia, which saw the development of a marine-based subsistence that promoted the colonization of the Arctic from Norway to Chukotka. Around 2,000 years ago northern Europe entered the Iron Age. Reindeer herding and plant cultivation were practised. Culturally the ethnic identity of the local populations became recognizable, for example as Sami (from northern Norway to the Kola Peninsula) and Nenets (along the coast of the White Sea and Barents Sea). In Alaska, a maritime-based economy emerged in the northwest coast around 4,500 years ago – the Arctic Small Tool tradition – and reached as far east as Pearyland in northern Greenland. It was replaced by the Dorset culture, which thrived between 3,000 and 1,000 years ago, at which time it came to an abrupt end, to be replaced by yet another culture that had sprung up from the Bering Sea coast. The Thule, the direct forebears of today's Inuit, successfully adapted to arctic living.

The movements of people and the rise and demise of cultures and ethnic groups in the Arctic over the course of tens of thousands of years demonstrated the strong impact of the physical environment, especially climate change, and the various physiological, behavioural, social, and cultural changes that allow the people to adapt to, and survive in, one of the most challenging habitats on the planet.

Demographic and Health Transitions

In the time since humans settled in the Arctic, their health has undergone many changes. Changes in fertility and mortality in populations have generally followed certain patterns, often referred to as *demographic transition* by demographers. In general, populations move from a stage of high fertility and high mortality to one of low fertility and low mortality. During the transition, the mortality rate falls first, to be followed by fertility. For most western European countries, the transition from stage one (high mortality, high fertility) to stage two probably began around the mid-eighteenth century when death rates began to fall, while fertility remained high. Stage three began about a century later, when fertility began to decline. The low mortality-low fertility of stage four was achieved by the mid-twentieth century. It is a useful descriptive tool, although there is disagreement on the model's ability to explain and predict demographic change.[15]

There is a companion theory to that of demographic transition, which describes and explains the long-term temporal changes in the pattern of health and disease in populations. It is called *health transition* or *epidemiologic transition*. As originally formulated in the 1970s, there are three stages: the age of pestilence and famines, the age of receding pandemics, and the age of degenerative and human-made diseases. The concept has gained currency in the population health literature, and its application in health planning and policy in developing countries are recognized by many international development agencies.[16]

The decline in mortality experienced by most developed countries over the last two centuries has been the subject of much inquiry. Some scholars, for example, Thomas McKeown, attributed the decline primarily to an improvement in standards of living and nutritional status and discounted the role of medical care and public health interventions, as the decline generally preceded the introduction of such innovations as antibiotics and vaccines. Since its appearance in the 1970s, the McKeown thesis has generated considerable controversy, and others have reinterpreted the data and assigned a more prominent role to specific public health measures. The role of health care, however, does not lie primarily in reducing mortality, but in relieving pain and suffering, preventing disability, and improving quality of life.[17]

We believe health transition to be a useful framework to describe and explain the changes in the pattern of health and disease that Arctic populations, especially indigenous peoples, have experienced. The pattern, especially of emerging chronic diseases and injuries and the decline of infectious diseases, has been widely observed in other populations undergoing rapid social, cultural, and economic change around the world. Such an approach would permit some speculation into future developments and provide a guide to potentially effective interventions.

We will demonstrate that Arctic populations differ in the burden of disease and distribution of health determinants from their respective national populations. Within the North itself, there are disparities between indigenous and non-indigenous peoples; and among indigenous peoples, between different ethnocultural groups. In addition to a comprehensive literature review, we have collected extensive health, demographic, and socio-economic data from the circumpolar countries and their northern regions. To facilitate international comparisons, we created a circumpolar mortality database from existing national and regional mortality statistics and used a common standard population in computing age-standardized rates. [18]

Organization of the Book

This book is divided into five parts, entitled Regions, Peoples, Determinants, Consequences, and Strategies. Part One focuses on five Arctic regions – Greenland, Northern Canada, Alaska, arctic Russia, and northern Fennoscandia. It provides a general overview of the geographic features, historical development, economic conditions, population characteristics, health status, and health services for each of these regions. Where possible, comparisons are made between these northern regions and their respective national data; and within the 'north,' between the indigenous and non-indigenous residents, to the extent that they can be identified. Much of the information is obtained from official sources where regional breakdown is available.

Part Two discusses three specific indigenous populations whose homelands cross modern national boundaries – the Inuit in Greenland, Canada, Alaska, and Russia; the Dene in Canada and Alaska; and the Sami in Norway, Sweden, Finland, and Russia. In investigating health patterns of these peoples, it is important to recognize and understand their geographical, historical, and cultural background. Much of the information is obtained from the published literature on specific populations and communities.

Part Three covers the major groups of health determinants, their distribution, and how they are causally associated with specific diseases and health conditions. Each chapter gives a general circumpolar perspective, explains key concepts for the non-specialist readers, and provides more-detailed case studies of the health determinant in one or more region or population for which research data are available. While there are many ways to classify health determinants (or risk factors), in this book they are grouped under the following categories: the environment and living conditions; diet, nutrition, and physical activity; smoking, alcohol, and substance use; genetic susceptibility; and cold exposure, adaptation, and performance.

Part Four is about diseases or health outcomes, which are 'consequences' of the population's exposure to the determinants described in Part Three. Several groups of such consequences are analysed, including infectious diseases; cardiovascular diseases, diabetes, and obesity; cancer; injuries and violence; mental health and suicide; and maternal and child health. As in Part Three, there is a general circumpolar perspective and discussion of key concepts, followed by detailed case studies of the burden and distribution of the health problem in the population, risk factors, and methods for prevention, and control in one or more region or population.

Part Five provides an integrative examination of what can be done to improve the health of circumpolar peoples and includes a discussion of key issues affecting the existing systems of health care, especially public health, and a vision for the future.

NOTES

1 Further information about these organizations can be found on www.inuit.org (Inuit Circumpolar Conference), www.iuch.org (International Union for Circumpolar Health), www.iasc.no (International Arctic Science Committee), www.northernforum.org (Northern Forum), and www.artic-council.org (Arctic Council). Links to these and other arctic scientific organizations and health agencies are provided in the website of the International Network for Circumpolar Health Research (www.inchr.org).

2 For a comprehensive discussion on boundary issues, see Nuttall and Callaghan (2000:xxxix–xxxi), and the entry 'Arctic: Definitions and Boundaries' in the *Encyclopedia of the Arctic* (Nuttall 2005:117–21).

3 See maps in Arctic Monitoring and Assessment Program (AMAP) (1997:6) and the *Arctic Human Development Report* (*AHDR*) (2004:18), showing their Arctic boundaries.

4 For further details on the Arctic environment, consult AMAP (1997, 2003), *AHDR* (2004), and the encyclopedic *Arctic Climate Impact Assessment* (*ACIA*) (2005).

5 For a detailed demographic analysis, see the chapter by Bogoyavlenskiy and Siggner in *AHDR* (2004:27–41).

6 These criteria can be found in the document 'Who Are Indigenous Peoples,' posted on the United Nations Development Program's Civil Society Organizations Division website (http://www.undp.org/cso/ip/faq.html). Coates (2004) provides a thorough review of the issues of definitions. The UN Declaration remained a draft from 1995 to 2006, when it was adopted by the Human Rights Council (the resolution was voted against by both Canada and Russia), which recommended it to the General Assembly (www.ohchr.org/english/issues/indigenous/declaration.htm). The International Labour Office's Convention 169, 'concerning indigenous and tribal peoples in independent countries,' can be found on www.ilo.org/ilolex/english/convdisp1.htm.

7 The English-language website of the Arctic Network for the Support of the Indigenous Peoples of the Russian Arctic based at the Norwegian Polar Institute (www.npolar.no/ansipra) provides a comprehensive listing and description of these groups. Visit also the website of the Russian Association of Indigenous Peoples of the North (www.raipon.org).

8 For a discussion of the statistical methods, the underlying assumptions, their limitations, and data sources, see Cavalli-Sforza, Menozzi, and Piazza (1994:25–41, 226–9). Genetic distances are quantitative measures of the degree to which populations share genetic variation.

9 For an introduction to the vast literature on the peopling of the Americas, see Szathmary (1993), Schurr (2004), Mulligan et al. (2004), and Eshleman, Malhi, and Smith (2003).

10 The classification and names of the language families are primarily based on those in the 15th edition of *Ethnologue: Languages of the World* (Gordon 2005), available on line at www.ethnologue.com/family_index.asp.

11 Hoffecker (2005) provided a succinct summary of the archaeological evidence of the prehistory of the Arctic.

12 See Hoffecker and Elias (2003) for a discussion of the interplay of environmental factors in Beringia and its impact on human settlement. The Bering land bridge was originally proposed by botanist Hultén in the 1930s, and included only the continental shelf. Its boundaries have been expanded since the 1960s.

13 See volume 3 of the Smithsonian Institution's *Handbook on North American Indians* on archaeology of Beringia and northwestern North America (Dixon 2006).

14 The original three-migration theory was proposed by Greenberg, Turner, and Zegura (1986). Wallace, Garrison, and Knowler (1985) were the first to test the model with mtDNA data and supported it, followed by more extensive analyses (Torroni et al. 1992, Shields et al. 1993, and Starikovskaya et al. 1998). Merriwether, Rothhammer, and Ferrell (1995) countered with the one-migration theory, which was also supported by Zegura et al. (2004), using NRY data.

15 Chesnais (1992) provided a comprehensive cross-national survey of demographic transition patterns. For a recent critique of the theory, see Sreter (2003).

16 See Omran (1971). Olshansky and Ault (1986) suggested adding a fourth stage – the age of delayed degenerative diseases – to account for the decline in mortality in the industrialized countries of such diseases as heart diseases and the postponement of the age of death among the elderly. For its planning and policy implications, especially for developing countries, see Gribble and Preston (1993), Jamison et al. (1993), and Phillips (1994).

17 McKeown's ideas can be found in his books, notably *The Role of Medicine: Dream, Mirage or Nemesis* (2d ed., 1979), and *The Origins of Human Disease* (1988). See Sreter (1988) and Colgrove (2002) for critiques and reinterpretation. Bunker et al. (1994) and Mackenbach (1996) calculated reductions in mortality attributed to specific interventions.

18 We chose the European standard population as used in EUROSTAT, the statistical agency of the European Commission out of convenience, as age-standardization has already been done for the Nordic countries and their northern regions. The age distribution is as follows: 0–14, 22,000; 15–19, 7,000; 20–24, 7,000; 25–29, 7,000; 30–34, 7,000; 35–39, 7,000; 40–44, 7,000; 45–49, 7,000; 50–54, 7,000; 55–59, 6,000; 60–64, 5,000; 65–69, 4,000; 70–74, 3,000; 75–79, 2,000; 80–84, 1,000; 85+, 1,000.

PART ONE

Regions

2 Greenland

PETER BJERREGAARD AND THOMAS STENSGAARD

Although Greenland – or Kalaallit Nunaat in Greenlandic – is the world's largest island, only a narrow coastal strip is inhabited (map 4). The population in 2006 was 57,000, of which almost 90 per cent were Inuit. This Inuit majority is by far the largest of any indigenous people in any jurisdiction of the circumpolar region. Greenland has, since 1979, had its own Home Rule government with extensive powers, and negotiations for self-determination are in progress. However, half of the national income still consists of subsidies from Denmark, the former colonial master.[1]

The Inuit of Greenland refer to themselves collectively as Greenlanders (*kalaallit*) and reserve the word Inuit for occasions where an international (Pan-Eskimo) connotation is appropriate. Inhabitants of Greenland who are not *kalaallit* are referred to by their country of origin – for instance, Danes. Greenland and Denmark are both integral parts of the Kingdom of Denmark. Although there have been attempts to refer to them as 'North Denmark' and 'South Denmark,' respectively, such usage is ill-advised and has not been widely accepted.

Geographical Features

The total area of Greenland is 2,184,700 square kilometres, similar in size to Mexico, twice that of the Canadian province of Ontario, and three times that of the American state of Texas, but 82 per cent of it is covered by an ice cap, which, at its maximum, reaches a thickness of 3,500 metres. The country is mountainous, with the highest peaks in east Greenland. Precipitation decreases from south to north; the northern area, Pearyland, is an arctic desert. While the climate is arctic throughout, it varies considerably. The capital, Nuuk, at 64° N, is on roughly the same latitude as Fairbanks (Alaska), Iqaluit (Nunavut), Reykjavik (Iceland), Trondheim (Norway), Umeå (Sweden), Vaasa (Finland), and Yakutsk (Russia). It has cool summers and relatively warm winters, with mean temperatures in August and January of +7° C and –9° C, respectively. Due to the warm Irming Current, a branch of the Gulf Stream, the water is open all year round as far north as Sisimiut, at 67° N. North of Sisimiut, the sun disappears for some time during the winter, and for as long as three months in Upernavik.[2]

Historical Development

Greenland has been populated several times from both the west (Canada) and the east (Scandinavia). The first people to populate Greenland came from the Canadian Arctic around 2500–2000 BC, and are referred to as Paleo-Eskimos. Archaeologists have identified the Independence culture, named after the fjord in northeastern Greenland, and the Saqqaq culture in southwestern Greenland, which were contemporaneous and belonged to the Arctic Small Tool Tradition that originated in Alaska and spanned the North American Arctic. It is believed that these pre-Dorset cultures developed into the Dorset culture after 1000 BC without new immigrants. The Dorset people appeared to have abandoned Greenland for the first 700 years of the first century AD, when the country was empty, only to reappear later, initiating the Late Dorset Period.[3]

The first immigration from the east took place in AD 985 when the Icelander Eirík the Red and his followers landed in south Greenland. The Norse (Vikings) had themselves settled in Iceland only a little over 100 years earlier. They established two main settlements on the west coast of Greenland, one near present-day Nuuk, called 'Western Settlement,' and the other one, to the southeast near present-day Nanortalik, called 'Eastern Settlement.' These averaged about 1,400 people each.

Around AD 1200, the ancestors of the present-day Inuit crossed the strait between Canada and Greenland. These people are sometimes referred to as the Neo-Eskimos, who belonged to the Thule culture, which had originated in the Bering Sea coast in Alaska (see chapter 7). They soon spread across the whole island, and for a few years Greenland was home to the Dorset people, the Inuit, and the Norse. The Inuit were technologically more advanced – they were particularly adept at hunting marine mammals – than either the Dorset people or the Norse, and they outlasted both. The Norse settlements lost contact with Iceland during the early fifteenth century, and it is believed that the colony had died out by AD 1500. The disappearance of the Norse remains an enigma, the subject of much debate and speculation. Likely the onset of the Little Ice Age around 1450–1500 put tremendous stress on what was still a medieval European farming-based society.[4]

In 1721 the Norwegian missionary Hans Egede started Danish-Norwegian settlement in Greenland, which has lasted until today. European whalers had visited Greenland for several hundred years, but Egede came with the intent to convert the presumed Catholic Norse inhabitants of Greenland to the Lutheran version of Christianity. However, as he would soon discover, the Norse had perished while the Inuit flourished. This was the start of the Danish colonization of Greenland, which brought Christianity, literacy, smallpox, tobacco, alcohol, and European food, guns, and cloth, and took away whale oil, furs, and minerals. The Danish colonization is said to have been a benign one, but Greenland managed to generate a net profit for Denmark until 1950.[5]

Egede settled among the Inuit and established a colony named Godthåb (Good Hope), at the site of present-day Nuuk. During the rest of the eighteenth century, colonies were established throughout the Greenlandic west coast south of the 75th parallel. Denmark adopted a protectionist, not to say paternalistic, attitude towards the Greenlanders and quite efficiently controlled all traffic between the outside world and the Greenland colonies until the Second World War. The Moravian missionaries were allowed to establish a few settlements in southern and central Greenland. By the end of the eighteenth century the Greenlanders of the west coast were by and large Christianized.

The number of Danes in Greenland remained at a few hundred, that is, around 2 per cent of the total population, and consisted of employees of the Royal Greenland Trade Department (*Den Kongelige Grønlanske Handel*) and the clergy. Eventually some intermarriage occurred: many Greenlandic families can trace their origins back to Danes or Norwegians employed in the colonial service. Some Greenlanders were sent to Denmark for training as coopers, carpenters, and teachers. East Greenland (Tunu) was not colonized until the late nineteenth century, and north Greenland (Avannaarsua) not until the beginning of the twentieth century. After some dispute with Norway over northeast Greenland, which was used as hunting grounds by Norwegian fur hunters, but otherwise uninhabited, the International Tribunal in The Hague granted Denmark full sovereignty over all of Greenland.

The Second World War changed Greenland's character irrevocably. The Americans built air bases at Kangerlussuaq (Søndre Strømfjord) and Narsarsuaq, and the long isolation of Greenland came to an end. After the war, a commission was established to suggest reforms and new ways of development. In 1953 Greenland became an integral part of the Kingdom of Denmark when the island was given the status of a county. Extensive infrastructural development occurred during the 1950s, 1960s, and 1970s, transforming Greenland from a traditional hunting society into a modern society where most people relied on earning wages. The social and cultural changes were profound with the influx of Danes, whose share of the population increased from less than 3 per cent in the 1940s to almost 20 per cent in the 1970s. The concentration of the Inuit in fewer and larger towns on the central part of the west coast accelerated.

In the 1970s many young Greenlanders began to voice their wish for Home Rule or outright independence. Popular discontent with Greenland's status became the dominant political issue. Home Rule, which was formally introduced in 1979, initiated a gradual transfer of responsibility for most public sectors, excluding foreign affairs, defence, and finance. The last sectors to be transferred were health and social services in 1992. Greenlandic Home Rule has been a success in spite of financial problems due to diminishing revenue from fishing, and a desire for outright independence is heard only infrequently. It must be kept in mind that the Greenlandic economy is heavily subsidized by Denmark. However, Danish subsidies are transferred as a lump sum so that the Home Rule government can allocate resources according to its own priorities. Greenland joined the European Community as part of Denmark in 1973 but left it in 1985, although it retained some associate status as an overseas territory. It has a renewable fishing agreement with the European Union and continues to maintain close relationships with the other Nordic countries.[6]

Population, Language, and Culture

The increase in Greenland's population since the early twentieth century is shown in figure 2.1. The proportion of the population not born in Greenland has declined from a peak of almost 20 per cent in 1975 to around 12 per cent since the late 1990s. The 57,000 inhabitants

Figure 2.1   Growth in Greenland's population since 1901

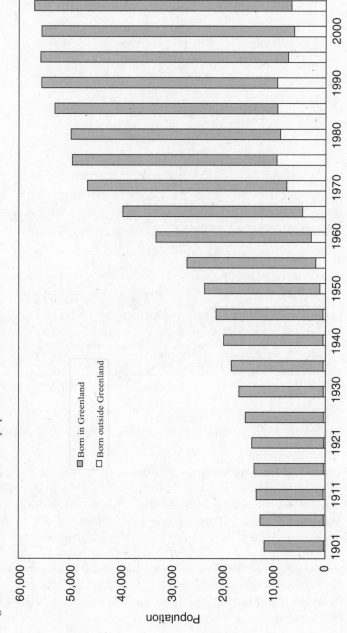

Source: Updated from Bjerregaard and Young (1998).

Figure 2.2   Age–sex distribution of Greenland's population

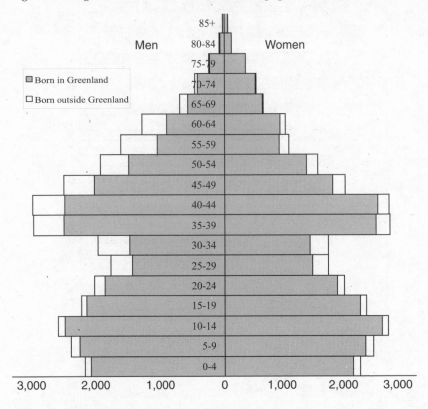

Source: Statistics Greenland (www.statgreen.gl).

are concentrated on the south-central west coast, with only 3,500 (6 per cent) living on the east coast and less than 1,000 (1.5 per cent) in the far north. There are seventeen small towns and approximately sixty villages or settlements. Towns vary in size from almost 15,000 in the capital, Nuuk, to less than 700 in the three smallest towns. It is not the size that determines the status of a town but the presence of the municipality headquarters, a hospital or health centre, and a school. In 1945, 61 per cent of the population lived in the villages; by 1995 the proportion was down to 19 per cent. It has continued to decline slightly, to 17 per cent in 2005.

Figure 2.2 shows the population structure of Greenland. It is composed of a broad-based upper half similar to the shape of the population pyramid in developing countries, positioned on top of a more barrel-shaped column similar to the population pyramid in industrialized countries. The shift between the two portions takes place around the age of forty-five, equivalent to the birth cohorts of 1965–70. In the late 1960s the crude birth rate also decreased sharply, from 45 to 22 per 1,000 over a ten-year period. During these few years, a countrywide birth-control campaign was carried out with the insertion of intrauterine devices in approximately half of the female population of reproductive age. In the early years of the twenty-first century, the crude birth declined further to 16 per 1,000, and Greenlandic women would on average give birth to 2.4 children over their lifetimes.

Another notable feature of the population pyramid is the surplus of males in the age groups 20–69. This is caused partly by the fact that more women than men migrate to Denmark, a result of the relatively large number of Danish men in the country who return to Denmark with their Greenlandic wives.

The population is a relatively young one but nevertheless ageing. In 2005, 25 per cent were below fifteen years of age and 5.5 per cent were sixty-five years or older; a projection for 2015 gives estimates of 22 per cent and 8 per cent, respectively.

The Inuit in Greenland have a distinct culture, which is the result of several hundred years of cultural exchange with Danish, European, and global societies. Cultural items that are today seen as traditionally Greenlandic – for instance Christian hymns, the women's pearl embroidery, and hunting tools – were all imported from Europe during the nineteenth century.[7]

Language and diet are central markers of Greenlandic culture. The Greenlandic language is an Inuit language closely related to Inuktitut in Canada and Inupiat in Alaska. Results from genetic analyses involving mitochondrial DNA concur with linguistic and archaeological evidence that present-day Greenlanders are descended from Alaskan Neo-Eskimos. Interestingly, there is no evidence from analyses of mtDNA that the Norse had contributed to the gene pool on the maternal side. On the other hand, a study of Y-chromosomes showed a high degree of Scandinavian admixture, as much as 60 per cent, most likely with Danish colonists rather than the Norse.[8]

Greenlandic has three major dialects – West Greenlandic, which is spoken by the majority and which forms the basis for the written language, East Greenlandic, and North Greenlandic or Inughuit. The script was invented by the Moravian missionary Samuel Kleinschmidt in the mid-nineteenth century. It uses the Latin alphabet. Danes, and Greenlanders who grow up in Denmark with Danish as their first language, have trouble learning Greenlandic because the language is fundamentally different from Indo-European languages, and because the incentives to learn Greenlandic are limited. Although Greenlandic is the majority language in Greenland, both Greenlandic and Danish are official languages, and Danish is used in government and in higher education. Unilingual speakers of Greenlandic are thus at a considerable disadvantage in modern society, yet it is the policy of the government to strengthen the Greenlandic language in the schools.

The traditional Greenlandic diet was based on marine mammals and fish with the addition of what little plant food could be found, for example, kelp, berries, and stomach contents of herbivores. While local food today still makes up approximately 20 per cent of the diet, the spectrum of food items is much narrower, usually consisting of meat and blubber of marine mammals – seals in particular – game birds, fish, caribou, and musk ox. The dietary transition started already in the early twentieth century; in 1902, 18 per cent of calories were imported; by 1932, it was as much as 62 per cent. The cultural importance of *kalaalimernit* (Greenlandic food) is larger than its dietary impact. *Kalaalimernit* is perceived as healthy, satisfying, and giving strength and warmth to a much larger extent than imported food. It is eaten as a snack with friends and colleagues, as a main meal throughout the day – often at irregular hours – and is always regarded as something special and as part of a social event. Not eating *kalaalimernit* and not preferring it to imported food is unthinkable for a Greenlander. The degree to which an outsider eats and likes for instance muktuk, seal, and dried fish is a measure of his/her willingness to be a part of Greenland society.[9]

Socio-economic Conditions

In 2003, the gross domestic product of Greenland was 172,497 Danish kroner per person, equivalent to U.S.$24,356, compared to U.S.$31,465 for Denmark and U.S.$30,677 for Canada.[10] The economy is by and large based on subsidies from Denmark, which amount to almost half of the public expenses, and the export of shrimps and other fish products. This creates a rather fragile economy that is vulnerable to political changes in Denmark (not a serious threat) and to fluctuation in world market prices for a limited number of export items (a real threat). It should furthermore be kept in mind that the costs of running a country with Greenland's climate and infrastructure are very high.

Because of the importance of traditional subsistence activities in the villages, Statistics Greenland defines labour force as the number of adults aged 15–62 living in towns. During 2000–4, the size of the labour force averaged 33,300 persons, or 83 per cent of the total population of the country in that age group. The average unemployment rate during this period was 6.8 per cent (7.1 per cent among men and 5.8 per cent among women). These figures are lower than in the mid-1990s when unemployment was 13 per cent among men and 10 per cent among women.

In terms of income, there are both regional disparities and disparities between individuals born outside the country and native Greenlanders. Nuuk reported the highest taxable income for single individuals and couples born in Greenland, and also for couples born outside Greenland. For singles born outside Greenland, the highest income was reported from the remote northern municipalities of Upernavik and Uummannaq. The ratio between the highest and lowest income municipalities was only about 2. Individuals born outside Greenland reported higher incomes than those born in Greenland in all municipalities, and among singles and couples. The ratio ranged from 1.3 to as high as 5.4.

Education levels continue to improve. In the five-year period since 1998–9, the number of individuals with post-secondary education, including vocational, teacher's training, and university education, has tripled.

Health Status

Life expectancy increased significantly in Greenland during the 1950s, but the increase has slowed markedly since 1960. In 1950, life expectancy in Greenland was at a level with countries such as Thailand and somewhat higher than in China, but both countries overtook Greenland around 1970. In the beginning of the twenty-first century, life expectancy in Greenland was at the level of countries like India, Mongolia, Bolivia, Russia, and Indonesia.

Generally, in countries of the world, life expectancy correlates with wealth. There is a significant association between life expectancy and

Figure 2.3   Trends in infant mortality rates in Greenland and Denmark

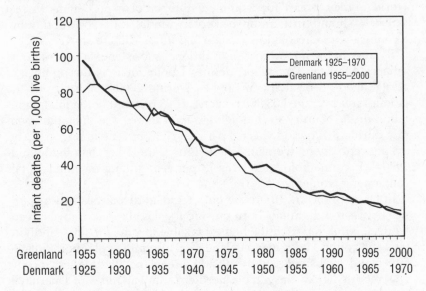

Sources: Statistics Greenland (www.statgreen.gl) and Statistics Denmark (www.statbank.dk).

the logarithm of the gross national product. A few countries, among which is Greenland, do not follow this rule. The GNP of Greenland was more than U.S.$20,000 per capita, but life expectancy was similar to that of countries with GNPs in the range of U.S.$3,000 to $6,000 per capita.

Infant mortality is another measure of general health in a population. In Greenland, infant mortality has been steadily decreasing for at least fifty years, from almost 120 in 1950 to around 10/1,000 in 2000–4 (fig. 2.3). However, this is still high and far from the 4.7/1,000 in Denmark. For a long time, the curves for infant mortality in Greenland and Denmark followed each other, but with Greenland lagging thirty years behind Denmark. There was a pronounced regional variation in infant mortality in the 1980s, but this inequity has successively become reduced as a result of improved living conditions and health care.[11]

Besides infant mortality, the causes of death that are responsible for most potential years of life lost and for keeping life expectancy low are suicide and tobacco-related diseases. If these were removed as causes

Figure 2.4   Age-standardized mortality rates (ASMR) by cause in Greenland

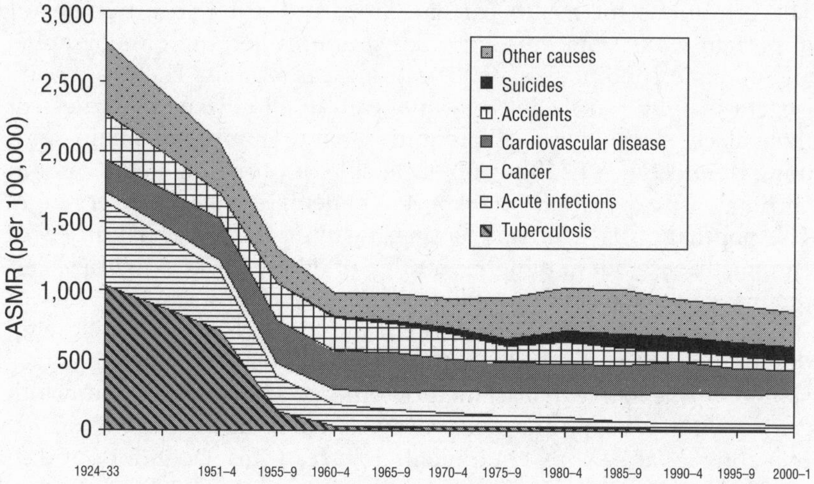

Note: ASMR – age standardized mortality rate per 100,000, standardized to the Greenland population of 2000 by the direct method.
Source: Updated from Bjerregaard and Young (1998).

of death, life expectancy in Greenland would increase from 63 to 71 years for men and from 68 to 74 years for women.

Greenland experienced a major health transition during the twentieth century and especially during the latter half of the century (fig 2.4). In 1950, mortality was high and the main causes of death were tuberculosis and acute infectious diseases. During the 1950s, the importance of these diseases as causes of death diminished sharply and total mortality decreased. However, as mortality from infections, heart diseases, and accidents continued to decrease, new causes of death gained importance, particularly cancer and suicide.

It must be kept in mind that discussing the health conditions in Greenland is equivalent to discussing the health conditions of the Greenland Inuit who presently make up almost 90 per cent of the population. Besides, few studies have been made of the health of the immigrant (Danish) population in Greenland, because a substantial proportion of this small population group consists of transient workers who return to Denmark in cases of illness or disability.

Health Services

The conditions for health care in Greenland differ in a number of important ways from those in other countries because of geographic and climatic conditions as well as historical reasons. The health care system is obligated to deliver equal care to all citizens regardless of their place of residence. This requires a large number of small – and not cost-effective – health centres capable of providing acute care; in addition, the expenses for transport of patients and staff are very high. The population is relatively young, resulting in a lower burden of chronic disease but in a higher burden of other diseases, injuries, and pregnancy-related conditions than in Denmark, for instance.

Greenland is divided into sixteen health districts roughly following the municipalities. Each district has a small hospital or health centre staffed by one to five district medical officers. The hospitals and health centres offer primary and emergency care and are equipped with an operating theatre, X-ray equipment, delivery ward, laboratory, and so on. The district medical officers handle uncomplicated deliveries, legal abortions, common internal diseases, and psychiatric cases, but under unfavourable weather conditions they must be prepared to handle complicated cases that can include major, life-saving surgery. For example, most operations for extrauterine pregnancy, appendicitis, and trauma are performed in the districts. Patients with complicated non-acute diseases are referred to visiting specialists, to the central hospital in Nuuk, or to a university hospital in Denmark.

All districts have a dental clinic, which is usually located in the hospital or in the school. In villages with a population of more than 300, there is a nursing station with a few beds. In villages with a population of more than seventy, there is a small clinic staffed by a health aide. The clinic is often just an extra room in the house of the health aide. In the smallest villages, a locally trained health worker has a medicine chest to be used according to the directions of the district medical officers. All villages are visited regularly by staff from the district hospital who offer primary health care, preventive care, and vaccinations.

In Nuuk, primary health care is separated from secondary care, the latter being offered by Queen Ingrid's Hospital, which is both the local hospital for Nuuk and the referral hospital for all of Greenland. The hospital has 156 beds in medical, surgical, and psychiatric wards and is staffed by specialists who cover a number of medical specialities: psychiatry, internal medicine, orthopedic surgery, gynecology, obstet-

Table 2.1   Per capita health care expenditures in the Nordic countries, 2004 (in euros)

	Public financing	Private financing	Total expenditures	Per cent of GDP
Greenland	2,118	5	2,123	9.1
Denmark	2,605	505	3,110	8.9
Faroe Islands	2,057	252	2,309	8.5
Finland	1,647	503	2,150	7.5
Iceland	2,963	591	3,554	9.9
Norway	3,633	719	4,352	9.7
Sweden	2,416	429	2,845	9.1

Source: NOMESCO (2006).

rics, general surgery, pediatrics, dermatology, anaesthesiology, and radiology. The specialists visit the health districts outside Nuuk on a regular basis. Primary care and emergency care are offered by a primary health clinic, which also serves the villages in the district. Dental care focuses on systematic preventive care and treatment of children, including orthodontics. Adults are offered basic treatment, including fillings, extractions, and dentures.

Health aides, and recently nurses, are trained in Greenland while physicians and dentists are trained abroad, usually in Denmark. There is an increasing proportion of Greenlanders among nurses and physicians, but the fact that most physicians and nurses are still Danes with a very limited knowledge of the Greenlandic language sets a natural limit to their interaction with the patients, the majority of whom have little knowledge of the Danish language. A large proportion of outsiders work at the higher levels of health care, making improvements in communication difficult since many choose to stay for only a few years or for even a shorter time.

All health care, including drugs, contraceptives, and dental care, is financed by the government and is free of charge for the residents. The total expenses for health care amounted to 2,123 euros in 2004 (table 2.1). This is similar to the other Nordic countries despite the fact that it is relatively more expensive to offer health care in a geographically and climatically challenged country like Greenland than in Europe. Approximately 12 per cent of the total expenditures were used for the transport of patients, staff, and supplies.

When the responsibility for the health care sector was taken over by the Home Rule government in January 1992, it was accompanied by a grant of approximately 600 million Danish kroner (about U.S.$100 million). Since then, the annual grant has been regularly adjusted upwards and exceeded a billion Danish kroner (about U.S.$167 million) in 2006.

Throughout the 1990s there was considerable discussion of the organization of the health care sector over such issues as the inefficiency of small hospitals and the difficulties in recruiting qualified professional staff. Despite these discussions, no substantial changes were introduced to this structure. The division of Greenland into municipalities meant that each municipality has been reluctant to give up its hospital, its emergency room service, and the associated jobs for the local economy. The small, sparse, and scattered population poses immense challenges to the health care system, and the considerable subsidy from Denmark will continue to be needed for the foreseeable future. There have been pilot projects in telemedicine and in electronic patient records, but neither has made any significant impact on the organization and delivery of health services. The organization of health services in Greenland has changed little since Home Rule, but in fact, has remained essentially the same as when its foundation was laid in the 1920s. There have been proposals for reducing the number of municipalities, certainly a politically sensitive issue, but if and when such changes are implemented, there will need to be a positive impact on health care delivery also.

When describing the future of the Greenlandic health care system, a number of factors must be considered. The changing disease pattern will have an influence on the organization and content of the services offered. The demand for treatment services at a high professional level will not diminish but will increase. Greenland has engaged in this development as well, with increased centralization of some services in Nuuk and the acquisition of high-tech equipment. A number of Greenlanders have received heart and liver transplants, paid for by the Greenlandic health care system but, of course, performed outside Greenland. At the same time, it is clear that the changes in disease patterns (e.g., the increase in prevalence of diabetes) point to the need for an increased effort in health promotion.

There is a shortage of nearly all categories of health professionals in Greenland. Since 1996, nurses have been trained locally but are insufficient to meet the demand. Physicians and other staff are still imported from Denmark, but the supply cannot always be assured, since there are also shortages within Denmark. Each year, only one or two Greenlandic physicians are being trained in Denmark. Since the late 1990s, it has been possible for medical graduates to undertake their specialist training in general practice in Greenland.

Not only is there economical dependence on Denmark to sustain the health care system in Greenland, the culture of the system is influenced by Danish norms. It is a system created by Danes and staffed by Danes who are trained within a Danish framework. While both the Danish and Greenlandic languages are used in the health care system, all record keeping is done in Danish. It is a recurrent topic of discussion, when speaking of how Greenland is run and administered, that there is a wish for a more Greenlandic and less Danish way of doing things. This is certainly one of the great challenges of the future, to establish a new and separate culture and identity in the health care system. The task is daunting, but the years ahead promise to be exciting.

NOTES

1   Much of the general information about Greenland in this chapter was updated from Bjerregaard and Young (1998). Current information (available also in English) about Greenland can be obtained from the homepage of the Greenland Home Rule government (www.nanoq.gl).
2   All statistical data in this chapter, unless otherwise specified, were obtained from Grønlands Statistik (Statistics Greenland) at www.statgreen.gl. A short pamphlet *Greenland in Figures* is published annually in English.
3   For an overview of recent research into archaeology in Greenland, see Grønnow and Pind (1996). Hoffecker (2005) provided a non-technical introduction to the prehistory of the Arctic. McGhee (1996) focused on the Paleo-Eskimos.
4   The rise and fall of the Norse settlements, together with other 'failed' cultures such as the Maya, Anasazi, and Easter Islanders, was discussed in *Collapse*, the popular book by Jared Diamond (2004). Lynnerup and Nørby (2004) summarized recent research on demographic modelling of the Norse based on analyses of skeletal remains and on the Norse diet from isotope studies.
5   The definitive history of Greenland available in English is the three-volume work by Gad (1971–82).

6 For a critique of the persistence of colonialism under Home Rule, see Petersen (1995). Caulfield (1997) examined the impact of world systems on contemporary Greenland society and the sustainability of traditional activities such as whaling.

7 For descriptions of traditional Greenlandic culture, see the various chapters in the *Arctic* volume of the Smithsonian Institution's *Handbook of North American Indians* (Gilberg 1984; Kleivan 1984; Petersen 1984). Nuttall (1992) reported on his ethnographic research in Upernavik region.

8 See Saillard et al. (2000) for mitochondrial DNA studies and Bosch et al. (2003) for studies on y-chromosomes. For general discussion on the genetics of the peopling of North America, see Schurr (2004), Schurr and Sherry (2004), Eshleman, Malhi, and Smith (2003). Genetic data from the 1960s, based on the GM system, estimated 40 per cent admixture among the people of west Greenland, compared with only 6 per cent in Igloolik, Canada (Szathmary 1993).

9 See Pars (2001) on contemporary use of traditional and imported food in Greenland.

10 GDP per capita figures (in U.S.$) can be found in the UNDP's *Human Development Report 2005*, available online from http://hdr.undp.org/reports/global/2005/pdf/HDR05_HDI.pdf.

11 See Bjerrgaard and Misfeldt (1992) for regional variation in infant mortality rates during the 1980s.

3 Northern Canada

KUE YOUNG

As stated in the introduction, northern Canada is defined in this book administratively to include Yukon, the Northwest Territories, and Nunavut. These three territories, which are sometimes referred to as the Territorial North by Canadian geographers, share the latitude 60° N as their southern land border (map 5). The region, with its 4 million square kilometres, constitutes some 40 per cent of Canada's land mass and is among the world's most sparsely populated areas. (See chapter 7 for information on the Inuit living in the northern parts of Quebec [Nunavik region] and in Labrador.)

Northern Canada is a frontier (or hinterland) of the modern Canadian state and its dominant culture, but it is also a homeland for indigenous peoples – the Inuit, First Nations (or 'Indians'), and Métis. As a frontier, it promises wealth to be extracted by outsiders, from the Klondike gold rush in the Yukon in the late nineteenth century to the modern resource-development megaprojects undertaken by multinational corporations. As a homeland, it signifies a deep commitment by the indigenous peoples to preserving, protecting, and promoting their cultural heritage, physical environment, and natural resources. The tensions between these two visions of the North have characterized much of its history and are still evident today.

Geographic Features

Northern Canada can be divided into several major physiographic regions: the Canadian Shield, the Interior Plains, the Cordillera, and the Arctic Islands (map 2). The Canadian Shield consists of ancient Precambrian rocks that were smoothed and moulded by glacial erosions and that cover much of Nunavut and the eastern Northwest Territories. The Interior Plains is the northward extension, through the Mackenzie River Valley, of the Great Plains of the western American states and Canadian provinces. The Cordillera, a complex of mountains, plateaus, and valleys, is the northward extension of the Rockies through much of the Yukon and into Alaska. The Arctic archipelago contains coastal plains, plateaus, and mountains. Several major rivers course through the region, such as the Mackenzie and Coppermine which drain into the Arctic Ocean, and the waters of the Yukon River's tributaries which eventually empty into the Pacific. The landscape is dotted by wetlands and several large lakes, notably Great Bear and Great Slave, which are part of the chain of lakes that extends southeastward to the Great Lakes.[1]

The climate is cold, with a long winter and a brief, cool summer. The major climatic factor is the low level of solar energy, resulting in cooling of the land and the building of frigid air masses. The dry cold air, which surges southward, is the source of many winter blizzards in the rest of Canada. Precipitation is low in the polar desert of the high latitudes but increases as the Arctic merges into the subarctic climatic zone in the south, and especially in the mountainous Cordillera to the south-west.

The vegetation cover is varied and ranges from boreal forest (of spruce, pines, fir, birch, aspen, and others) in the south-west to mosses and lichens in the tundra to the barenness of the polar desert in the high Arctic.

Historical Development

The Asian origin of the original inhabitants of the North American continent is generally accepted by archaeologists and anthropologists. Humans moved westward into the Americas via a now-submerged Bering land bridge, Beringia (see chapter 1).

The 'discovery' of the Americas by Christopher Columbus in 1492 ushered in a new era of European exploration. Beginning in the late sixteenth century, English explorers sailed into the Arctic Ocean in search of the Northwest Passage. A host of explorers with names such as Frobisher, Davis, Hudson, and Baffin are today remembered by various bays, straits, islands, and other geographical features in the Arctic.[2]

The Hudson's Bay Company (HBC) was established in London in

1670 by royal charter, granting it exclusive trading rights in the vast hinterland draining into Hudson and James Bays. In the late eighteenth century, traders such as Samuel Hearne and Alexander Mackenzie covered on foot much of the present-day Northwest Territories. The disappearance of British naval officer John Franklin in the late 1840s spurred an unprecedented search effort. While it did not find Franklin, it generated much valuable knowledge of the Arctic. It was not until the early twentieth century that the Northwest Passage was finally navigated by Norwegian explorer Roald Amundsen.

The era of Arctic exploration was followed by one of colonization. Initially, the hunting life remained largely intact despite the introduction of items of European material culture, such as iron tools, firearms, and fabrics. Christianity in its various forms began to replace traditional beliefs and shamans disappeared from the people's life, at least overtly.

The present-day northern territories were part of the vast expanse of Rupert's Land, granted to the Hudson's Bay Company by the British Crown. Soon after the modern federal state of Canada was born, the HBC sold its land holdings to the Canadian government in 1870, and they became known as the Northwest Territories. The British government retained jurisdiction over the Arctic Islands, but these were transferred to Canada a decade later. The Northwest Territories shrunk in size in subsequent years as new provinces were carved out of it. Yukon became a territory in 1898 with a federally appointed commissioner and council located in Dawson City. Until the Second World War, the Northwest Territories was governed by an appointed commissioner and a council of senior civil servants in Ottawa. It was not until 1967 that the seat of territorial government was moved to Yellowknife. The council became fully elected by 1975. The most recent boundary change occurred with the passage of the *Nunavut Act* in 1993. In 1999 the Nunavut Legislative Assembly was sworn in at the territorial capital of Iqaluit (formerly Frobisher Bay). *Nunavut* means 'our land.' (Note that Nunavut is similar to, but should not be confused with, *Nunavik* for the Ungava region in northern Quebec or with *Nunivak* Island in Alaska.)

In Canada, territorial governments exercise only the powers assigned to them by the federal government, such as education, social services, wildlife management, and so on. In many ways, the territories are 'not-yet provinces.' Because of their small population, territories have a low tax base, and much of their operating budget is in the form of 'transfer payments' from the federal government. However, some tax revenues from natural resources also go to Ottawa, an increasingly contentious issue.

Until the outbreak of the Second World War, the North was very much neglected and forgotten. Southerners regarded it as not much more than a barren wasteland with little economic potential. The indigenous peoples were left to the traders and missionaries, who offered assistance in times of distress. The federal government's presence was usually in the form of widely scattered detachments of the Royal Canadian Mounted Police. (The name of Canada's national police was kept for historical and romantic reasons – horses were not used in the Arctic patrols!) During the war, the North acquired strategic importance. It provided a transportation link between the United States and Europe, with a chain of landing strips for airplane refuelling, and the Alaska Highway was built through southern Yukon.

In the 1950s, the pace of change intensified. New townsites were developed, and the Canadian government actively encouraged sedentary settlement where health, education, and welfare services could be conveniently administered and delivered. The beginning of mining activities in the 1950s and later (for gold, silver, lead, zinc, copper, and diamond) further consolidated the local population as well as introduced large numbers of migrant workers from southern Canada. The Cold War hastened the modernization of the northern frontiers with the construction of radar stations and airstrips (the Distant Early Warning or DEW line along the 70th parallel).

Throughout the Canadian Arctic, many noticeable changes occurred. These included prefabricated houses; manufactured clothes; store-bought food; a decline in hunting and its replacement by wage labour, the cottage industry in handicrafts (soapstone carving, silkscreen prints), and social assistance payments; and motorized transport (snowmobiles and power boats) in place of dog sledges and kayaks. An increase in alcohol and drug abuse, accidents, family violence, and other social problems began to emerge across the Arctic.

In the 1970s the conflict between the traditional land-based economy and modern large-scale industrial developments came to the fore when the rich potential of the Arctic seabed for oil and natural gas was discovered. A proposal to transport by pipeline natural gas from the Mackenzie Delta to markets in southern Canada sparked widespread opposition by indigenous and environmentalist groups and resulted in the Mackenzie Valley Pipeline Inquiry, which was chaired by Thomas

Berger, a noted Canadian jurist. The inquiry broke new grounds in giving credence to the voice of indigenous peoples. After extensive community hearings, it recommended delaying pipeline construction until after the settling of land claims. With the settlement of land claims, the pipeline project was resurrected in the early 2000s, proposed by a consortium of four oil and gas companies. An Aboriginal Pipeline Group was formed to represent the interests of Aboriginal communities and negotiate ownership shares in the project. Benefits and access agreements were entered into with various Aboriginal communities. The construction of the 1,220-kilometre long pipeline has been repeatedly delayed and its future remains uncertain.[3]

In southern Canada, the British colonial, and later Canadian, government entered into treaties with various First Nations as the country's territory expanded westward and northwards. Various Dene First Nations in what is now the western Northwest Territories participated in the signing of Treaty 8 (1899) and Treaty 11 (1921). With such treaties, the First Nations lost control of their lands in return for payments, various forms of assistance, and the setting up of Indian reserves. None of the territory occupied by the First Nations in the Yukon and by the Inuit had ever been ceded to Canada by treaty. For these groups, land claims became a core demand in their striving for political self-determination. Since the 1980s, a series of comprehensive land claims have been settled. The Inuvialuit Final Agreement (1984) was signed with the Inuit in the west and the Nunavut Land Settlement Agreement (1993) with Inuit in the eastern and central Arctic. Agreements were signed with Dene regional groups in the Northwest Territories: the Gwich'in (1992), the Sahtu/Métis (1993), and the Tlicho (Dogrib) (2005). In the Yukon, a series of agreements have been signed individually with Yukon First Nations since 1995, and the process continues. These land claim agreements generally involve the creation of regional corporations responsible for economic development, and the management and investment of the cash settlement. The indigenous peoples also gained legal title, surface and subsurface mining rights, and exclusive hunting and fishing rights to specific parts of the settlement area.[4]

Population Characteristics

The population of the three northern territories is characterized by its high proportion of indigenous or Aboriginal peoples, relative to the

Table 3.1   Selected demographic indicators of the three northern territories and
Canada, 2001

	Yukon		Northwest Territories		Nunavut		Canada
	Total	Aboriginal	Total	Aboriginal	Total	Aboriginal	Total
Population	28,670	6,980	37,360	18,965	26,750	22,855	30 million
% Aboriginal	24.3	–	50.8	–	85.5	–	4.4
% age <15 years	21.0	29.7	27.1	33.8	37.1	41.5	18.9
% age 65+ years	6.0	4.9	4.4	5.4	2.2	2.8	13.0

Source: Statistics Canada, 2001 Census of Canada
(www12.statcan.ca/english/census01/home/index.cfm).

whole of Canada (table 3.1). In Yukon, Dene First Nations constitute the
predominant Aboriginal group, while Nunavut is overwhelmingly Inuit.
Both Inuit and Dene are represented in the Northwest Territories. The
'settler' and indigenous populations tend to live in distinct communities.
Most non-indigenous people are found in the cities and in large towns
such as Whitehorse, Yellowknife, and Iqaluit, with populations of 20,500,
18,700, and 6,200, respectively, in 2006. Inuvik is Canada's largest town
north of the Arctic Circle, with a population of 3,500. (The proportion of
non-indigenous residents range from 40 per cent in Inuvik and Iqaluit to
over 80 per cent in Whitehorse and Yellowknife.)

Compared with the Canadian population, the population of the
northern territories is more fertile and more youthful (see also table 1.2
in chapter 1). The proportion of the population under fifteen years of
age is particularly large among the Aboriginal population, reaching 42
per cent in the predominantly Inuit Nunavut. The proportion of the
elderly (sixty-five years and over) is substantially lower in the North,
even among the non-Aboriginal population, reflecting the transient
nature of many residents who migrate to the North for occupational
reasons (table 3.1).

A variety of Aboriginal languages are spoken in the three territories.
The Northwest Territories in fact legislated nine Aboriginal languages
as official languages in addition to English and French (fig. 3.1). The
language of the Inuit is usually referred to as Inuktitut in Canada, particularly in the eastern and central Arctic. In the western Arctic, the
Inuit refer to their languages by the local names of Inuvialuktun and

Figure 3.1   Multiple official languages shown in a Northwest Territories public notice

CHIPEWYAN

JÁDIZI NÉNE XA DËNE YATI NEDHÉ XÉL
ʔEGHÁLADA KʼÉ TSʼɁ ʔASĺ KʼAUNETA-U/ ʔERIHTŁʼÍS
DËNE SÚŁINÉ YATI TʼA HUTSʼELKÉR XA BEYÁYATI
THEʔẠ ʔATʼE, NUWE TSʼÉN YÓŁTI.

CREE

Kispın kı nıtawıhtin ē nīhiyawıhk ōma
ācımōwın, tıpwāsınān - Masınahıkamıkos
ana ohcı Pikıskwēwına Ayısinēw Kıhcı
Okımānahk Ohcı ōti Kiwītınohk kıcı.

DOGRIB

TŁJCHQ YATI KʼĘ̀Ę̀, DI WEGODI NEWQ DÈ,
GOTSʼO GONEDE. EDZANÈ GOGHA YATI KAʔA XÈ
EGHÀLAHODA GINJHTŁʼÈKǪ̀.

ENGLISH

English: If you want this information in another Official
Language, call us - Office of the NWT Languages
Commissioner.

FRENCH

Si vous voulez ces renseignements en français,
contactez-nous - Bureau de la Commissaire aux langues
des T.N.-O.

GWICH'IN

JII GEENJIT GWICH'IN ZHIT GAVISHINDAI'
NIINDHAN JI'. NIKHWETS'ÀT GINÒHKHII NWT GINJIH
GUCOMMISSIONER GWITR'IT DEEK'IT DANH.

INUINNAQTUN

TAHAPKUAT TITIKAT PIYUMAGUVIGIT
INUINNAQTUN TITIGAGHIMAYUT
HIVAYAINAGIAQAQTUGUT - UQAUHILIRINIRMUT
KAMISINAUYUQ NUNATTIARMI.

INUKTITUT

ᐅᐧᑯᐊ ᐃᐅᑊᓇᒡᔪᓕᑦᒡ ᐱᐃᒍᒐᒡᓯ
ᐅᑊᓯ... - ᐅᐃᑊᐅᐱᕋᓇ...ᒡ ᐅᑉᑌᐱᐅᓴ
...ᕋᑯᕋᒡ ᒡᑊᓯᑊᕋᒡ.

INUVIALUKTUN

UVANITTUAQ ILITCHURISUKUPKU
INUVIALUKTUN, QUQUAQLUTA -
UQAUTCHITIGUN ANGALATCHIYIM SAVAKVIANI
NUNAPTINNI.

NORTH SLAVEY

Edırı kede ghǫ keorúzhá nahwhé nıdé, dúle
xáré nake kedé tʼá dene darahke

SOUTH SLAVEY

Edı gondı dehágh gotʼje zhatié kʼéé edatłʼéh
enahddhę nıdé, góhdlı ndéh gozhatié gha kʼaodhe tsʼę́
etsʼedehłí.

Source: Office of the Northwest Territories Languages Commissioner
(www.gov.nt.ca/langcom/offer.htm).

Figure 3.2   Selected socio-economic indicators of the three northern territories and Canada

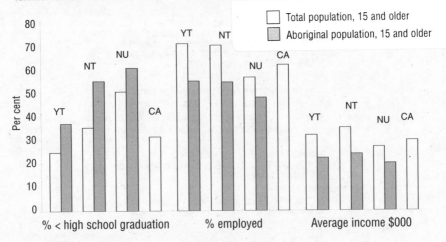

Source: Statistics Canada, 2001 Census of Canada
(www12.statcan.ca/english/census01/home/index.cfm).

Inuinnaqtun. While the languages of the colonizers were introduced and used in the administration of indigenous peoples' affairs, the Inuit by and large were able to maintain the viability and vitality of their language. Many of the Athabascan (Athapaskan) languages are seriously under threat. (Chapter 8 discusses further the distribution and current status of the Athabascan languages in Alaska and northern Canada.)

Socio-economic Conditions

Figure 3.2 compares three indicators of socio-economic status among the territories. In terms of education (measured by the proportion of the adult population who did not graduate from high school), Yukon fares better than Canada as a whole, while the Northwest Territories and Nunavut fare worse. However, within the territories, educational level is generally lower among the Aboriginal population than the total population of the territories.

In terms of the average income and employment rate, both Yukon and the Northwest Territories report higher levels than Canada as a whole; however, this is not the case for the Aboriginal population

Table 3.2   Selected health indicators of the three northern territories and Canada

	Yukon	NWT	Nunavut	Canada
General				
Life expectancy at birth (years)[a]				
Male	75.0	73.7	66.6	77.1
Female	80.5	78.1	70.0	82.1
Infant mortality rate (per 1000 live births)[a]	6.6	7.6	15.0	5.3
ASMR all causes (per 100,000)[b]	768.6	816.3	1183.3	605.2
Infectious Diseases				
Incidence of tuberculosis (per 100,000)[c]	5.2	21.1	108.0	5.2
Chronic Diseases				
Age-standardized prevalence of diabetes (%)[d]	3.8	4.0	1.3	4.8
ASMR ischemic heart disease (per 100,000)[b]	117.3	95.5	79.7	111.2
ASMR stroke (per 100,000)[b]	61.9	76.2	111.7	48.7
Age-standardized incidence of all primary cancers (per 100,000)[c]				
Male	324.1	339.4	359.6	456.2
Female	297.1	323.4	500.3	347.9
Injuries				
ASMR unintentional injury (per 100,000)[b]	59.3	53.6	62.4	25.6
ASMR suicide (per 100,000)[b]	18.5	20.8	80.2	11.3
Health Determinants				
Age-standardized prevalence of overweight and obesity (%)[e]	50.5	53.7	48.6	48.2
Prevalence of current smoking (%)[e]	27.5	36.6	64.7	22.9

[a]Life expectancy and infant mortality rates refer to mean of 2000–3 period.
[b]ASMR (age-standardized mortality rate, standardized to the 1991 Canadian population by the direct method) for all causes and selected causes refer to mean of 2000–2 period.
[c]Tuberculosis and cancer incidence refers to mean of 2000–4 period.
[d]Diabetes prevalence refers to 1999–2000 fiscal year, based on health care utilization administrative databases.
[e]Obesity and smoking prevalence refers to 2003.
Sources: Statistics Canada (Vital Statistics; Canadian Cancer Registry; Canadian Community Health Survey; available from the Health Indicators publication [Cat.No.82-221-XIE] available online at www.statcan.ca) and the Public Health Agency of Canada (Canadian Tuberculosis Reporting System, available in the document Tuberculosis in Canada, various years, available at www.phac-aspc.gc.ca/tbpc-latb/surv_e.html; and the National Diabetes Surveillance System, available at www.phac-aspc.gc.ca/ccdpc-cpcmc/ndss-snsd/english/index_e.html).

within these territories. This situation reflects the in-migration of non-Aboriginal people from other parts of Canada seeking employment; those who are no longer employed or who are retired tend to leave the North. The disparities with the rest of Canada are worst in Nunavut, which has only a small proportion of the non-Aboriginal population.

Planners in the Canadian Department of Indian and Northern Affairs developed a composite index of community well-being (CWB) obtained from the Census and based on aggregate income, education, housing, and labour force participation, with a maximum score of 1.0. In the North, the mean score for 31 Inuit communities was 0.70 (range 0.62–0.87), 33 Dene communities, 0.74 (range 0.63–0.89), and 13 predominantly non-Aboriginal communities, 0.88 (range 0.78–0.95). In the rest of Canada, the mean score was 0.81 (range 0.48–0.96), excluding Aboriginal communities. Counted in the category of non-Aboriginal communities are the cities of Yellowknife and Whitehorse and several mining towns.[5]

Health Status

Table 3.2 presents several health indicators and highlights the health needs of the population in the North. The disparities in health status relative to the Canadian population, exemplified by life expectancy at birth, infant mortality rate, and tuberculosis incidence, are least in Yukon and greatest in Nunavut, with the Northwest Territories occupying an intermediate position. This ranking generally reflects the proportion of Aboriginal people in each of the territories. Some chronic diseases (e.g., cancer, diabetes) are generally less prevalent than the national average, while others (e.g., stroke) exceeds it. Injury mortality rates, whether intentional or unintentional, are generally higher in the North. In terms of risk factors, northern populations are comparable to all Canadians with regard to obesity, while smoking prevalence is generally high, reaching 65 per cent in Nunavut, which does not bode well for the future.

While the gradation in risk of disease across the territories is influenced by the relative size of the Aboriginal population, such a generalization tends to overlook the fact that the Inuit and Dene populations differ in many significant ways in both disease burden (e.g., high stroke mortality and low diabetes prevalence among the Inuit) and risk factor prevalence (e.g., high smoking rates among the Inuit). In their statistical reports, the territorial governments have generally not distinguished between Aboriginal and non-Aboriginal residents and, when reporting on the Aboriginal population, have not always acknowledged differences between Inuit and First Nations, even though ethnic identifiers are available. However, Aboriginal data are presented in some reports, notably on cancer (see chapter 17) and injuries (chapter 18) in the Northwest Territories.

Health Services

Until the 1950s, health services in northern Canada were available sporadically from traders, missionaries, the police, and the military. As early as 1902, an Anglican hospital was opened in Cumberland Sound. The Canadian government, however, supplied medicines, paid the salaries of the medical staff of the mission facilities, and in times of hardship provided funds for relief administered by traders and missions. During an influenza epidemic in Coronation Gulf and the Mackenzie River in 1926–8, the Royal Canadian Mounted Police offered medical assistance to the Inuit.[6]

In Canada, an Indian Health Services has existed south of the 60th parallel for Indians living in reserves since the early twentieth century. It is operated by the Department of Indian Affairs. In the early 1920s Indian Affairs extended some medical services to the eastern Arctic. The first government physician among the Inuit initially made annual visits to Baffin communities by ship and took up residence in Pangnirtung in 1926. In the western Arctic, a physician was stationed in Aklavik in the 1930s. In 1945, the Department of National Health and Welfare assumed health care for Indians and Inuit and established a branch named Northern Health Services to serve all citizens, Native and non-Native, in the Northwest Territories and Yukon.

A unique aspect of health care in the Arctic has been the reliance on ships to service the widely scattered communities. Since the 1920s, ships of the Eastern Arctic Patrol usually had on board medical officers who treated patients in the villages along their route during a brief ice-free season. The ship most extensively equipped for medical work was the coastguard vessel the *C.D. Howe*, which was in service between 1950 and 1969. It undertook X-ray screening for tuberculosis, and patients thus diagnosed were evacuated with the ship.

The federal government's health services in the North expanded exponentially in the post-war years, with a vast network of health aid posts, nursing stations, and regional hospitals. There was also a refer-

Table 3.3   Health systems performance indicators for northern Canada

		Yukon	NWT	Nunavut	Canada
(A) Satisfaction with overall health care (%)					
quality rated as excellent/good	M	88.7	79.2	76.9	86.3
	F	80.8	79.5	60.5	86.2
very/somewhat satisfied	M	88.8	82.6	82.8	85.0
	F	82.1	80.4	70.9	84.8
(B) Use of preventive services (%)					
of women aged 18–69 with Pap					
smear within last 3 years		82.9	79.1	69.6	74.5
women aged 18–69 who never had					
Pap smear		8.7	9.5	23.4	12.1
women aged 50–69 with no mam-					
mography for at least 2 years		45.4	31.7	83.3	26.9
(C) Hospitalization for ambulatory					
care sensitive conditions					
(per 100,000)	M	556	1220	232	367
	F	472	1021	245	325

Note: All rates and proportions are age-standardized to the 1991 Canadian population, except mammography, which is a crude rate for a rather narrow age range.
Sources: (A) and (B) from the Canadian Community Health Survey 2003; (C) is from the Canadian Institute of Health Information hospital discharge database. Statistics Canada, *Comparable Health Indicators 2004* (Cat. No. 82-401-XIE), available online at www.statcan.ca.

ral hospital in Edmonton – the Charles Camsell Hospital, originally a National Defence hospital which was turned over to the Department of National Health and Welfare in 1946 – serving Inuit and Indians from the western Arctic. Beginning in the late 1960s and early 1970s, the federal government also contracted with southern universities to provide general physicians and visiting specialists to the northern regions; for example, McGill University serviced the Baffin region and the University of Manitoba, the Keewatin region.

In the 1980s the federal government initiated a process of transfer of control of health services to the territorial governments, which was completed in the Northwest Territories by 1988 and in Yukon by the early 1990s. In the first decade of the twenty-first century, the northern health care system is fundamentally different from that in the provinces. Salaried physicians are the rule rather than exception, and nurse practitioners, while supported by visiting physicians, by and

Table 3.4   Ethnic differences in health care use in northern Canada

| | Territories | | Canada |
	Aboriginal	Non-Aboriginal	Canada
Contact past 12 months			
General practitioner	58.8	75.9	78.7
Eye specialist	35.3	39.1	38.0
Other physician	15.1	24.1	28.9
Nurse	49.0	22.0	9.8
Dentist	45.0	53.5	59.4
Has regular doctor	31.1	67.0	83.9
Unmet health care needs	18.4	13.6	12.7

Source: Statistics Canada, Canadian Community Health Survey 2000/01,
from Tjepkema (2002).

large function quite independently of them in health centres (formerly
known as nursing stations) in the communities. Nurses are indeed the
backbone of the health service. There are regional hospitals in all the
territorial capitals, staffed by a limited number of medical specialists.
The referral pattern tends to run north-south, to teaching hospitals in
Vancouver, Edmonton, Winnipeg, Ottawa, and Montreal. The 'glue'
that keeps this geographically dispersed and tiered service delivery
system together is transportation and communication. Another critical
issue is cross-cultural interaction, as the majority of health care
providers are non-Aboriginal, recruited from outside the territories,
and generally for short duration.

How well is such a health care system working? The availability of,
and accessibility to, health services can be gauged by several indicators derived from surveys and also from institutional statistics on
health care utilization.

As table 3.3 shows, northerners are generally satisfied with the
overall health care they receive, compared to all Canadians, and
Yukoners tend to be more satisfied than residents in the other two territories. Nunavut women are particularly less likely to rate their health
care as excellent or be satisfied with it. In terms of the use of preventive services for women, Yukon and the Northwest Territories have
performed well in the coverage of Pap smears, but not so Nunavut,
where almost a quarter of the women have never had a Pap smear. All
three territories fare worse than Canada in mammography services,

and again there is a great unmet need in Nunavut. An indicator of the adequacy of ambulatory care is the rate of hospitalization for certain 'ambulatory care sensitive conditions,' which should be low if ambulatory care services are available and appropriately used. It can be seen that both the Yukon and Northwest Territories exceeded the Canadian national rate, while Nunavut reported a lower rate.

Within the North, there are some disparities between Aboriginal and non-Aboriginal people in their use of health services (table 3.4). These data also reflect the fact that in communities with a high proportion of Aboriginal people, the main source of primary care is nurses, while in towns and cities where most non-Aboriginals live, physicians are the primary source of care.

NOTES

1 For further details on the regional geography of the Canadian North, see Bone (1992, 2002).
2 A general history of the Canadian North is provided by Morrison (1998).
3 For an update on the pipeline project, visit www.mackenziegasproject.com.
4 Further information on Indian treaties and land claims in Canada can be found on the Indian and Northern Affairs Canada website: *Historic Treaty Information Site* (www.ainc-inac.gc.ca/pr/trts/hti/site/mpindex_e.html) and *Comprehensive Claims Policy and Status of Claims* (www.ainc-inac.gc .ca/ps/clm/brieft_e.html).
5 For a detailed description of the methodology of the Community Wellbeing Index, see O'Sullivan and McHardy (2004). Senécal and O'Sullivan (2005) performed an analysis of CWB in Inuit communities. These papers and also the database of all communities in Canada with their CWB score and individual components are available on the Indian and Northern Affairs Canada website: http://www.ainc-inac.gc.ca/pr/ra/pub4_e.html.
6 For an overview of the historical development of health services for Aboriginal people in Canada, see Waldram, Herring, and Young (2006). The biography of Otto Schaefer describes vividly the health care conditions during the 1950s (Hankins 2000).

4 Alaska

JAMES BERNER

Alaska is the only state in the United States containing lands that are considered arctic. As discussed in the introduction, the entire state falls within the purview of this book (map 6). Alaska is the largest but least populated state in the United States, with an area of 1.52 million square kilometres, about one-fifth the total area of all the forty-eight contiguous states combined (usually referred to as the 'lower-48'), and two and a half times the size of Texas.

Geographic Features

Successive portions of the earth's crustal plates that migrated to the north-western edge of the North American plate now form the land mass of Alaska. Because the formation of Alaska's land mass involved a great deal of tectonic plate movement, the active edge of the tectonic plate interface resulted in an arc of some seventy potentially active volcanoes extending from the Aleutian Islands into the south-central region. The result of this tectonic activity is seismic instability and frequent earthquakes, extending into the central part of Alaska. In 1964 North America's strongest earthquake, registering 9.2 on the Richter scale, and the ensuing tsunami devastated the city of Anchorage.[1]

Much of the state is mountainous, with over thirty-five mountain ranges, containing North America's highest peak, Mount McKinley (6,200 metres). Across the border in Yukon is Mount Logan, Canada's highest peak (6,000 metres). The Yukon River, the third-longest river in the United States, and its tributaries pass through much of Alaska.

Within the span of some 20 degrees of latitude (52°–72° N) can be found diverse environments, which can be broadly divided into several regions:

1 South-east Alaska, often referred to as the 'panhandle,' is a mountainous archipelago with deep, narrow fjord-like inlets, not unlike the coast of Scandinavia. Its temperate coastal rainforest is sustained by the wet maritime climate.
2 South-central Alaska is a mix of coastal rainforest, mountain ranges (such as the Chugach and Kenai Mountains), glacial lakes and hills, with mixed evergreen, birch, and alder forests.
3 The Aleutian Islands and the Alaska Peninsula are much less forested, with grassy, windswept mountains and a temperate northern maritime climate.
4 South-western Alaska has large areas of flat tundra, with small lakes and streams. The trees, mostly willow and alder, are short. Warming climate over the last fifty years has permitted the gradual northward movement of the treeline.
5 The interior and north-west Alaska, south of the Brooks Range and north of the Alaska Range, has a much colder winter and a short warm summer; it has mountains, rivers, small glacial lakes, and mixed birch and evergreen forests.
6 Northern Alaska, north of the Brooks Range Mountains, is treeless tundra, with small ponds and lakes and a typical Arctic winter, with a very short, cool summer, and very low annual precipitation.

There are also windswept, treeless islands out in the Bering Sea, such as the Pribilof, St Lawrence, and Diomede Islands. The Big and Little Diomedes are separated by the International Date Line and by the United States–Russian border.

Historical Development

The many archaeological sites that have been found on the eastern edge of the Beringia land bridge testify to the fact that Alaska was visited by migrants from north-eastern Asia who eventually peopled the Americas. The oldest confirmed archaeological site, dated as 12,000 years old, is located in Swan Point, near Fairbanks. When found, it contained artefacts associated with the microblade technology that originated in Asia (the Dyuktai culture, chapter 1). In this same period, humans were probably camping along the Nenana Tanana River valleys in central Alaska. Between 10,000 and 11,000 years ago, by which time the Beringia land bridge had been completely submerged, a coastal, marine-hunting-based culture known as the American Paleo-Arctic Tradition developed around Kotzebue Sound. At about the same time in the Alaska Range and Tanana Valley of the interior, the Denali culture arose, consisting of small, dispersed, and mobile populations that subsisted on freshwater resources and caribou hunting. Close to 4,500 years ago, the Arctic Small Tool Tradition emerged, which in Alaska was represented by the Denbigh complex near Norton Sound; this marked the beginning of the Paleo-Eskimo people who, within a few centuries, developed the pre-Dorset cultures throughout the Arctic. They, in turn, were replaced by the highly successful Thule culture, which eventually colonized the whole of Arctic North America all the way to Greenland.[2]

The recorded history of Alaska can be divided into three periods: Contact, the Russian period, and the American period.[3] Contact occurred at different times for different groups. The Aleuts were the first group to be contacted by Europeans in the mid-eighteenth century, when the Russians extended their influence across Bering Strait into Alaska. Vitus Bering, a Danish captain in Czar Peter the Great's navy, explored the sea and strait that now bear his name but was shipwrecked and perished in 1741. Subsequent explorations by Spanish, British, and American ships resulted in competing claims of sovereignty. In 1778 Captain James Cook sailed into the inlet that now bears his name. By the late eighteenth century, the southern Eskimos had been contacted, and by the end of the nineteenth century, all groups, including Eskimos in the far north, had been contacted. American whalers, even during the Russian period, were also active in the northern waters. In 1888 they rounded the North Cape and established a base on Herschel Island. Scientists also played an important role in the exploration of the Arctic. The Jesup North Pacific Expedition during the 1900s was an early example of Russian-American collaboration. It involved Franz Boas of the American Museum of Natural History and Waldemar Bogoras of the Imperial Academy of Sciences in St Petersburg and provided a rich source of ethnographical and geographical data.

The Russian period began in the late eighteenth century with the arrival of fur hunters, known as *promyshlenniki*, who swarmed into the Aleutian Islands and the Alaska mainland. They conscripted Aleut and Pacific Eskimo hunters, brutally exploited them and their kin, and almost exterminated the sea otter by the second decade of the nineteenth century. The first Russian settlement was established in 1784 on Kodiak Island, after a pitched battle with the indigenous inhabitants. With the shift to hunting terrestrial fur bearers, a monopoly in the fur trade was given by imperial decree to the Russian American Company in 1799 under the direction of Aleksandr Baranov.

The Russian influence in Alaska dwindled in the nineteenth century when the imperial government became disenchanted with the low profit. In 1867, Czar Alexander II sold Alaska to the United States for $7.2 million. Under the terms of the treaty of cession, 'uncivilized tribes' (i.e., those not yet under Russian control) were accorded protection by the United States. Almost immediately North-west Coast Indians objected to their land being sold by one country to another, neither of which legitimately owned it.

The U.S. government initially did not show much interest in Alaska either, and for years Alaska was referred to as Seward's Folly, after Secretary of State William Seward who negotiated its purchase. It became somewhat of an administrative orphan, and was variously under the control of the army, customs, and the navy. It finally was granted territorial status in 1912. Economically, fur was supplanted by the discovery of gold in the late 1800s, and Alaska's abundant salmon and crab fisheries became co-dominant with gold in the early 1900s.

The U.S. government pursued a policy of assimilation towards Alaska Natives through schools and missions, which was considerably more benevolent than its treatment of many American Indian nations in the West. The *Organic Act* of 1884 did recognize land rights of Alaska Natives but was unable to restrict non-Native encroachment. Alaska Native lands were never organized into reservations as in the lower-48, with the exception of the Metlakatla Indian community in southeastern Alaska. In the early decades of the twentieth century, the gold rush – the most famous one being the Klondike from 1897–8 – brought in miners and prospectors. Natives played a marginal role in the new wage economy, as they watched their traditional resources being depleted. Alaska Natives experienced an ever-increasing Americanization of their lives with the introduction of schools, Christianity, health care, and more extensive communication with the outside world.

With the advent of the Second World War, Alaska's strategic location became evident. A brief and bloody land campaign was fought in the Aleutian Islands in 1942 when the occupying Japanese forces were driven out of the western islands. Many Aleuts were relocated to temporary camps in south-east Alaska for the duration of the war and endured severe hardships. The construction of the Alaska Highway in the interior also accelerated the modernization of the Native population.

In the post-war years there was considerable population growth and the development of new economic activities related to oil and gas development and military defence. In 1959, the Territory of Alaska became the 49th state, beginning a new relationship between Natives and non-Natives. Statehood soon led to conflict over the selection of so-called vacant, unappropriated or unreserved lands by the state, lands also claimed by Alaska Natives, over and beyond those that were already legally held by them or held in trust for them by the federal government. After the discovery of oil in North Slope in the late 1960s, the economy was rapidly transformed, adding an element of urgency to the need to settle land disputes. In 1966 the Alaska Federation of Natives was formed, which took the lead in negotiations with the state, leading up to the *Alaska Native Claims Settlement Act* (ANCSA) of 1971. In return for agreeing to extinguish all claims of Aboriginal title, Alaska Natives were given direct ownership over some 10 per cent of the area of the state and $962.5 million in cash compensation. The land and cash would be channelled through regional Native (for-profit) corporations and smaller village corporations. The settlement had a substantial impact on the life of Alaska Natives.[4]

The Trans-Alaska Pipeline from Prudhoe Bay in the North Slope to Valdez was opened in 1977. Oil royalties benefited some Native regional corporations immensely and fuelled much of the state's economy during the 1970s and 1980s. In 1989 the oil tanker *Exxon Valdez* ran aground in Prince William Sound, resulting in an environmental disaster of unprecedented magnitude, negatively affecting the ecosystem, especially the fisheries of the region, on which residents were highly dependent. The economy of Alaska cooled as North Slope oil production declined in the 1990s.

Population Characteristics

The total population of the state was 626,900 in 2000, of which Anchorage alone accounted for 261,500. The state capital, Juneau, with a population of only 31,000, is located on a narrow coastal lowland on the panhandle, with no road access to the rest of the state. The only other large city is Fairbanks in the interior, with a population similar to that of Juneau.

Alaska Natives constitute 19 per cent of the state's population and number about 119,000 according to the 2000 Census. Alaska Natives form a larger percent of the state's population than the Native American population of any other state in the U.S. Among those who identified themselves further by tribal affiliation, 50 per cent were Eskimos, 39 per cent Indians, and 11 per cent Aleut.[5]

The 2005 American Community Survey provided a mid-decade population estimate of 641,700 for the state. Of these, about 122,140 reported their race as American Indian and Alaska Native either alone or in combination with another race.

The majority (58 per cent) of Alaska Natives live in small rural, remote communities, ranging in population from 50 to 5,000. Approximately 85 per cent of the non-Native population lives in larger centres. Very few of Alaska's small rural communities are connected by road to a major urban centre, and most depend on air or, less often, water transport.

Within Alaska there are some 47,000 Eskimos, and they belong to two major groups – the Inupiat who inhabit the northern and western coast as far south as Norton Sound, and the Yupik who inhabit the coast from Norton Sound to Prince William Sound in the south-east. The Yupik population is almost twice that of the Inupiat. Yupik can be further differentiated linguistically into Siberian Yupik, spoken on St Lawrence Island and also across the border in Chukotka, Russia; Central Yupik, spoken in west and central Alaska; and Alutiiq (or Sugpiag) on Kodiak Island, part of the Alaska Peninsula, Kenai Peninsula, and Prince William Sound (see map 3).

American Indians in Alaska number about 36,000 and they belong to the Athabascan language family and the linguistic isolates of Tlingit, Haida, Tsimshian, and Eyak. Some linguists lump Athabascan, Tlingit, Haida, and Eyak into a larger family of 'Na-Dene.' Athabascan Indians inhabit the interior and portions of the south-central coastal region, consisting of tribes such as Koyukon, Tanaina, and Ahtna (map 3). According to the Census, among those who identified with a specific tribal group, there were roughly equal proportions of Athabascans and North-west Coast Indians. (The Eskimos and Athabascans are discussed in greater detail in chapters 7 and 8 as examples of indigenous populations who are found in more than one circumpolar country.)

The Aleut people are the numerically smallest Alaska Native group, with an estimated population of 11,000. They inhabit the Aleutian Islands. The Aleut language is related to the Eskimo, and together they constitute the Eskimo-Aleut language family. Studies of mtDNA suggest that the Aleut are genetically closer to the Chukchi and Siberian Eskimos than North American Indians and Eskimos, and that they likely entered the Aleutian Islands from the east rather than 'island hop' from Kamchatka. Aleut are similar to Eskimos in the distribution of various mtDNA haplogroups in having predominantly haplogroups A and D, with the others (B, C and X) either very rare or absent all together. However, while haplogroup A predominates among Eskimos (60–90 per cent), D predominates among Aleuts (as much as 100 per cent in some groups).[6]

The Aleut culture thrived on highly successful maritime adaptation, using skinboats for hunting and fishing. It was estimated that at the time of Russian contact, there were between 15,000 and 18,000 Aleuts. Warfare, disease, and starvation resulted in drastic and rapid depopulation. Aleut resistance ended by the end of eighteenth century, and the people were either indentured to the Russian American Company or relocated to the Pribilof Islands where they remain today. The term Aleut today is also used to cover the Alutiiq-speaking Koniags on Kodiak Island and the Chugach of Prince William Sound, as well as some Yupik-speakers on the eastern Alaska Peninsula.

The Tlingit, Haida, and Tsimshian Indians inhabit the south-east Alaskan region popularly known as the 'panhandle,' which is completely outside the arctic/subarctic climatic and ecological zone. The majority of the population is to be found across the border in British Columbia. They are linguistically distinct but culturally very similar, belonging to the North-west Coast culture area, occupying its northernmost reaches. (Some linguists group the Tlingit, and sometimes the Haida, with the Athabascan languages into a Na-Dene family.) They are particularly known for their totem poles. Traditionally, they lived in permanent winter villages of plank houses and travelled by dugout cedar canoes. They subsisted on salmon from the rivers, but also on marine (herring, halibut, seaweeds) and intertidal resources (clams, cockles).[7]

The crude birth rate is consistently higher among Alaska Natives than the general population of Alaska or the United States nationally, although there has been a downward trend in all populations (fig. 4.1). Between 1960 and 1970, the growth rate of the non-Native population

Figure 4.1   Trend in crude birth rates: Alaska Natives, Alaska, and United States

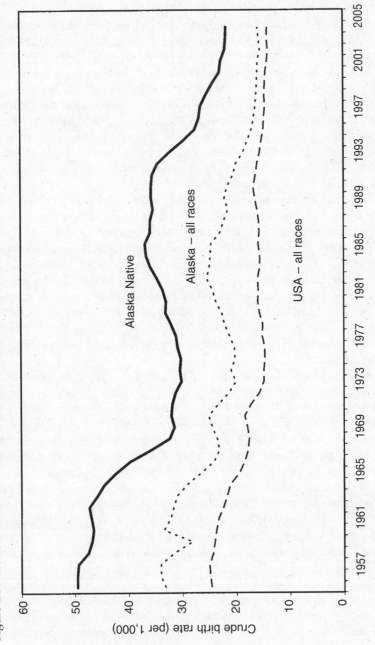

Sources: U.S. Indian Health Service; Alaska Area Native Health Service; Alaska Department of Health and Social Services.

was almost twice that of the Native population, due to the high immigration to the state. In the period 1990–2000, the situation was reversed, with the growth rate of the Native population more than twice that of the non-Native population. Similar to other indigenous populations, the Alaska Native population is also a young one. In 2000 its median age was twenty-four years, compared with the national age of thirty-five years. The population pyramid is shown in figure 4.2. The Alaska all-races population is also young, and it occupies a position intermediate between that of the Alaska Native and American all-races population in terms of proportion of children and elderly (see table 4.1). The Alaska Native population has aged, with the median age increasing from seventeen in 1960.

Socio-economic Conditions

The modern economy of Alaska is predominantly resource-based. Its development has been hampered by the geographic isolation – there is no international railroad connection and only one highway runs through Canada linking the state to the lower-48. In terms of air distance, it is closer to Japan than to the rest of the United States.

Since the Second World War, oil and gas have driven the development of Alaska and dominated the economy, now providing 85 per cent of Alaska's tax revenue; forestry, fishing, tourism, and mining provide the remaining 15 per cent.[8] Alaska's oil wealth allows the state to not levy a state income tax, and the Alaska Permanent Fund, established in the 1970s from oil royalties, makes periodic payouts to individual Alaskan residents. However, such dependence has dire consequences. In 2006, leakage in a pipeline led to the shutting down of the Prudhoe Bay refineries for months, costing the state millions of dollars per day in lost revenue.

A major issue in economic development is the control of land use. When the United States acquired Alaska, much of the territory was under federal control and private ownership had been severely restricted for over a century. Since statehood, there continues to be a politically complex struggle between the federal and state governments, settlers and Natives, and environmentalists and developers over the balance between environmental protection and the pace of economic development. One contentious issue, for example, is the drilling for oil in protected lands like the Arctic National Wildlife Refuge.

Figure 4.2   Age–sex distribution of Native and total population of Alaska

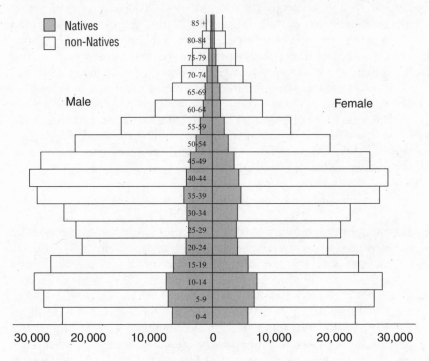

Source: U.S. Census Bureau, 2000 Census.

Table 4.1 compares several key socio-economic indicators between Alaska Natives and the total population of Alaska and the United States. It is evident that while the Alaska Native population fares poorly in terms of these indicators, Alaska enjoys a better socio-economic status than the United States nationally.[9]

Health Status

The health history of Alaska's peoples has been meticulously documented by medical historian Robert Fortuine. The Aleuts and Pacific Eskimos bore the brunt of the Russian onslaught in the eighteenth century that introduced syphilis, tuberculosis, and alcohol. The enslavement of hunters by the fur traders led to starvation among the families left behind. Warfare between Natives and Europeans was an

Table 4.1   Selected demographic and socio-economic indicators: Alaska Native, Alaska, and U.S. populations

	Alaska Native		Alaska		United States	
	2000	2005	2000	2005	2000	2005
Median age (years)						
% of population <5 years	24	27	32	34	35	36
% of population <18 years	10.4	10.0	7.6	7.7	6.8	7.0
% of population 65+	5.5	6.8	5.7	6.6	12.4	12.1
Education: % population aged 25+						
high school graduate or higher	72.4	78.7	88.3	91.0	80.4	84.2
with bachelor's degree or higher	5.9	5.5	24.7	27.3	24.4	27.2
Employment and income						
% adults aged 16 + employed	46.3	49.1	61.5	63.5	60.9	61.0
median household income	$33,769	$38,397	$51,571	$56,234	$41,999	$46,242
per capita income	$12,289	$14,287	$22,660	$26,310	$21,587	$25,035
% families below poverty level	17.7	21.4	6.7	8.3	9.2	10.2
% individuals below poverty level	19.9	25.3	9.4	11.2	12.4	13.3

Note: Data for Alaska Native from those reporting AIAN race alone.
Sources: U.S. Census Bureau, 2000 Census, and 2005 American Community Survey (www.census.gov).

uneven match, the latter possessing superior firearms that included cannons and that resulted in much loss of life. By comparison, the northern Inupiat survived the century relatively unscathed.

In the nineteenth century a number of great epidemics swept through most Native communities of Alaska. Most were caused by viruses that were highly contagious and spread rapidly through a population that had no prior immunity to them. Two of these epidemics – smallpox in 1835–40 and influenza and measles in 1900 – caused such devastation that they rank among the most significant single events in the history of the peoples they affected. Tuberculosis, syphilis, and gonorrhea were also prominent causes of illness during this period. Alcohol was widespread in the Native communities where it was the most sought-after of the Western goods that the traders offered in return for fur, ivory, and baleen.[10]

In common with the other circumpolar indigenous peoples of the Western hemisphere, the health status of Alaska Natives generally improved between the 1950s and the 1990s. Over this period, profound economic and technological changes, especially in transportation and communication, resulted in widespread lifestyle changes in terms of diet, physical activity, and other health-related behaviours. The inevitable result of the exposure to the pervasive Western culture in rural Alaska Native villages, however, has been the stress on traditional Native culture and values.

The section that follows provides trend data for several key health status indicators and highlights the disparities between the current health of Alaska Natives and the total population of Alaska and the United States.[11]

Life expectancy has dramatically improved since 1950, and the gap between the life expectancy of Alaska Natives and the all-races population in the U.S. has narrowed from twenty-two years in the 1950s to under seven years in the 1990s. As shown earlier in chapter 1 (table 1.2), there is little difference between the all-races population in Alaska and that in the United States as a whole.

Since 1945, infant mortality has improved for all U.S. populations, including Alaska Natives, as shown in figure 4.3. Age-adjusted mortality rates are considerably higher among Alaska Natives than among non-Natives for many causes of death, including cancer, respiratory diseases, and injuries. The risk of death from diabetes and cardiovascular diseases, for the moment, are lower.

Most of the mortality causes have known risk factors, and trend data is available for some of these, especially obesity and tobacco use. Obesity is a national problem throughout the U.S. as well as in Alaska, and, as figure 4.4 shows, the prevalence in Alaska is increasing. A survey among Alaska Natives demonstrated that the combined prevalence of obesity and overweight during 2001–3 among men was about the same between Alaska Natives and non-Natives, whereas among women, the prevalence was 62 per cent for Alaska Native compared with 51 per cent for non-Natives.[12] As the rate of obesity has increased, the rate of diabetes in Alaska Natives has increased from 15.7/1,000 population in 1985, to 31.4/1,000 in 1999. The U.S. all-races rate has increased by a smaller amount during the same interval, from 25.7/1,000 to 30.1/1,000.

Tobacco use is epidemic among Alaska Natives, although there was a slight decrease between 1991 and 2000, when the rate dropped from 45 per cent to 42 per cent. The rate of tobacco use is significantly greater than in the non-Native population, particularly among Alaska

Figure 4.3 Trends in infant mortality in Alaska and United States

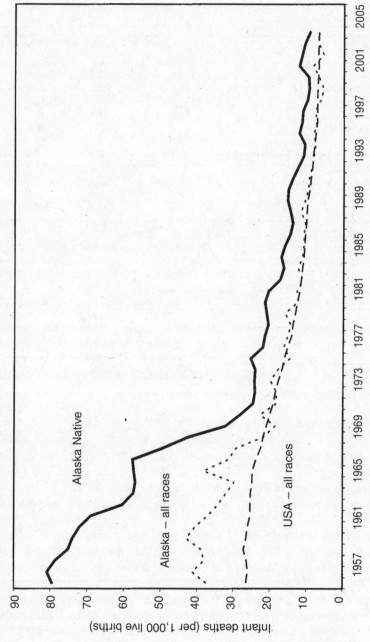

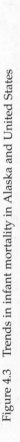

Sources: U.S. Indian Health Service; Alaska Department of Health and Social Services; and National Center for Health Statistics.

Table 4.2   Age-standardized mortality rates for selected causes: Alaska Native,
Alaska, and U.S. populations

Cause	Alaska Native	Alaska	United States
Cancer	247.4	186.0	185.8
Diabetes-related (underlying cause)	20.0	25.1	24.5
Heart disease	199.8	175.2	217.0
Stroke	76.7	56.1	50.0
Influenza and pneumonia	38.2	17.3	19.8
Chronic lower respiratory diseases	54.0	43.1	41.1
Chronic liver disease and cirrhosis	22.7	9.3	9.0
Unintentional injuries	84.6	55.1	37.7
Suicide	42.8	22.1	10.9
Homicide	12.3	6.6	5.9
All causes	1,079.6	790.7	800.8

Note: Age-standardized mortality rates (per 100,000) standardized to the 2000 U.S.
population. Alaska data are mean of 2003 and 2004; U.S. data are for 2003.
Sources: National Center for Health Statistics (various years), National Vital Statistics
Reports; Alaska Department of Health and Social Services (various years); Bureau of
Vital Statistics (various years).

Native women, 10 per cent of whom use it, compared with less than
0.5 per cent of non-Native women. Among Alaska Native teenagers,
the rate of tobacco use fell from 61.9 per cent in 1995 to 44.2 per cent in
2003, while among non-Native Alaska teenagers it decreased from 32.4
per cent to 12.3 per cent over the same period.

Health Services

For the non-Native population of Alaska, health care is a mix of private
and publicly funded systems. Public health is the responsibility of the
State Department of Public Health. Because of the sizable Native population, the federal government plays an important role in health care
in the state.

The Alaska Native population is provided publicly funded health
care by the U.S. Indian Health Service (IHS), an agency of the Public
Health Service, Department of Health and Human Services. The IHS
has been in existence since 1955, having been transferred from the
Bureau of Indian Affairs of the Department of the Interior. Since that
time, IHS has grown substantially, covering much of the United States
in a network of direct service and contract facilities and programs

Figure 4.4   Trend in prevalence of obesity and overweight in Alaska

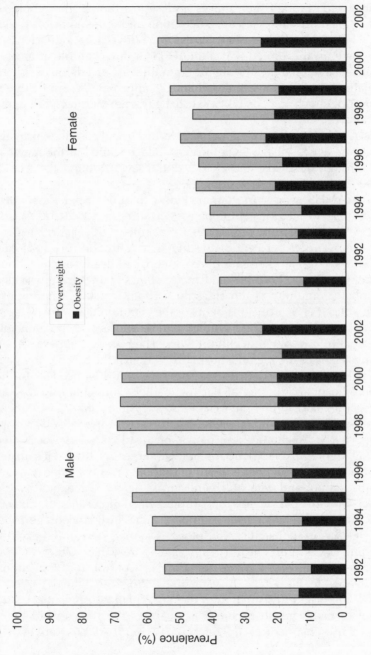

Note: Self-reported data; body mass index computed from height and weight; overweight – BMI 25.0–29.9; obese – BMI 30+

Source: Centers for Disease Control Behavioral Risk Factor Surveillance System (www.cdc.gov/brfss).

administered through area offices and service units. The whole of Alaska constitutes one such area, operating under the name of Alaska Area Native Health Services (AANHS), with its headquarters in Anchorage. In the United States the IHS is a rare example of a comprehensive, national health care program directed at a defined civilian population. In the 1990s, the policy of 'compacting' was instituted, transferring much responsibility to tribal governments and Native corporations.[13]

The AANHS and the regional Native health corporations provide health care at the village level through village clinics, at the regional level through hospitals, and at the central level through the Alaska Native Medical Center in Anchorage.

The AANHS works in conjunction with nine tribally operated service areas to provide comprehensive health care to 120,000 Alaska Natives. Under a variety of funding arrangements, Alaska tribal agencies administer 99 per cent of the Indian Health Service funds earmarked for Alaska. There are thirty-three tribal health organizations operating six rural hospitals and many clinics staffed by physicians and tribal community health aides throughout the state. Community health aides are, as a rule, residents of the communities who undergo a special training program, including twenty weeks of instruction and several months of practical clinical work. Their work is supervised by the physicians of the regional hospitals who visit the community on a regular basis and who provide telephone support as needed. In the regional hospitals (located at Barrow, Bethel, Dillingham, Kotzebue, Nome, and Sitka), family physicians and specialists provide in-patient and out-patient care while patients requiring more specialized care are transported to Anchorage, Fairbanks, or Seattle. The Alaska Native Medical Center (ANMC) in Anchorage serves as the area's major source of specialty services (including radiation therapy, bone marrow transplantation, and care of severe burns). It is co-managed by the Alaska Native Tribal Health Consortium, which represents all tribes in Alaska, and the Southcentral Foundation, the local Anchorage tribe. ANTHC has responsibility for other essential statewide services, including community health services and research. Other federal agencies such as the Centers for Disease Control and Prevention (CDC) operate the Arctic Investigations Program, which has conducted important research into the surveillance, prevention, and control of many health problems relevant to the state's residents.[14] Map 7 shows the medical care referral pattern for Alaska Natives.

Funding support for the Alaska Native tribal health care system in 2006 exceeded U.S.$328 million, of which less than 50 per cent represented resources transferred from the federal Indian Health Service. The majority of the remainder came from billing private and federal health insurance for medical care at ANMC.[15]

NOTES

1 Much of the general information about the State of Alaska is derived from a variety of sources. The Statewide Library Electronic Doorway (http://sled.alaska.edu), operated by the Alaska State Library and University of Alaska Fairbanks, serves as an excellent entry point to information resources. Visit also the state government website: www.state.ak.us.

2 The archaeology of Alaska is well discussed in the circumpolar review by Hoffecker (2005); for eastern Beringia, see Dixon (2006).

3 For a general popular history of Alaska, see Borneman (2003).

4 In 1983 the Canadian jurist Thomas Berger (see chapter 3) was asked by the Inuit Circumpolar Conference to consult the people and report on their views on the benefits and costs of ANCSA (Berger 1985). See McNabb (1992) for an appraisal twenty years later.

5 A variety of sources of census data on the Alaska Native population are available: special tabulations from the U.S. 2000 Census American Indian and Alaska Native Summary File (AIANSF) Sample Data, U.S. Census Bureau, American Fact Finder (http://factfinder.census.gov/servlet/DatasetMainPageServlet); U.S. Census Bureau (2003); Alaska Area Native Health Service (2001) provides a breakdown by Indian, Eskimo, and Aleut from 1970 to 2000, available online from www.ihs.gov/facilitiesservices/areaoffices/alaska/dpehs/population_reports/census.asp.

6 For details of the study on Aleut mitochondrial DNA, see Rubicz et al. (2003). Merriwether (2006) tabulated mtDNA distributions in indigenous Siberians and North Americans.

7 For a short succinct introduction to Alaska Natives culture and history, see Langdon (1987). The Smithsonian Institution's project Crossroads of Continents has produced lavishly illustrated volumes on the Native cultures of Alaska and Siberia, see Chaussonnet (1995) and Fitzhugh and Crowell (1988).

8 Additional economic data are available from the Alaska Office of Economic Development website; www.commerce.state.ak.us.

9 For a comprehensive review and compendium of the demographic,

health, and socio-economic data of Alaska Natives, see Goldsmith et al. (2004). The American Community Survey, conducted annually, provide updates on socio-economic and demographic data during the years between the decennial census.

10 See Fortuine (1989) for a comprehensive medical history of Alaska, and Fortuine (2005) on the impact of tuberculosis.

11 Data are obtained from the Alaska Bureau of Vital Statistics's *Annual Reports*; the Alaska Area Native Health Service's *Alaska Native Births and Infant Deaths 1980–1997*; 'Infant mortality 1993–2002,' *Alaska Vital Signs* 1 (1) (March 2005), 1–5; and the websites of the Indian Health Service (www.ihs.gov), the Alaska Native Tribal Health Consortium (www.anthc.org), and the National Center for Health Statistics (www.cdc.gov/nchs).

12 Data area available from the Behavioral Risk Factors Surveillance System (BRFSS), an annual telephone interview survey. Selected results from the 2001–3 surveys among Alaska Natives were compiled by the Alaska Native Health Board (2004).

13 For an overview of the Indian Health Services, see Rhoades, Reyes, and Buzzard (1987), and the IHS website: www.ihs.gov. Kunitz (1996) offers a critique of the system of 'compacting.' See Fortuine (2006) on the evolution of the various branches of the Public Health Service in Alaska and its commissioned officers.

14 The health care system for Alaska Natives is described in *Alaska Area Profile* available from the Indian Health Service website: www.ihs.gov/facilitiesservices/areaoffices/Alaska/dpehs/index.asp. Descriptions of the activities of the ANTHC and CDC can be found on www.anthc.org and www.cdc.gov/ncidod/aip.

15 Financial data are from ANTHC, *2006 Annual Report*, Financial Summary.

5 Arctic Russia

ANDREW KOZLOV AND DMITRY LISITSYN

The Russian North (*Sever*) stretches across the Eurasian landmass (see map 8). The Ural Mountains, which extend north-south for some 2,000 kilometres, are regarded as the dividing line between Asia and Europe. 'Siberia' (*Sibir*), as a geographical term, is generally used to refer to all of Russia east of the Urals and sometimes in a more restricted sense, excluding the Far East. In this chapter, the focus is on those parts of Russia located to the north of 60° N.[1]

Geographical Features

The European North of Russia extends from the Kola Peninsula and Kareliya in the west, across the Vychegda Lowland and Pechora Basin to the Urals in the east, with its northern shores washed by the White, Barents, and Kara Seas. Much of the land is low lying and swampy, with tundra in the north and taiga in the south.

Siberia can be subdivided into three large geographical regions: West, Mid, and North-east Siberia. These regions are very different in terms of their physical features. West Siberia is a low-lying flat plain, extending between the Ural Mountains and the Yenisey River, much of which is swampy. The north of Mid Siberia is occupied by the Central Siberian Plateau and the Putorana Plateau; further to the north is the Northern Siberian Lowland, and still further north, the Byrranga Mountains on the Taymyr Peninsula. North-east Siberia is a huge system of mountain ranges (such as the Verkhoyansk and Cherskiy) and highlands (such as the Kolyma and Chukotka). To the north, between the mountains and the Arctic Ocean, lies the Yana-Indigirka and the Kolyma Lowlands.

Several major rivers drain into the Arctic Ocean – the Northern Dvina, Mezen, Pinega, and Pechora in European Russia, and the Ob, Yenisey, and Lena in Siberia. Throughout history and even today they continue to be important transport arteries that traverse the huge northern expanses.

The climate, which is severe across the whole territory, can be characterized as continental, with typically long freezing winters and short cold summers. Winter temperatures decrease as one moves eastwards, and reach their lowest in the north-east (as low as –70° C). Permafrost occurs extensively throughout the region.

Vegetation varies from the Arctic deserts on the islands in the Arctic Ocean and the mountains of the Taymyr Peninsula to forest-tundra and northern taiga in the more southerly areas. The vegetation in the tundra consists of lichens and mosses, sedge, and low-growing dwarf birch, willows, and aspens. In the forest-tundra and taiga, firs, pines, and spruce prevail in Europe, while in Siberia the most widespread are larches and Siberian cedar.

The fauna of the Eurasian North is in many respects similar to the North American one. Among large mammals are reindeer, elk, mountain sheep, and brown bear. Fur bearers include sable, marten, fox, arctic fox, and ermine. The rivers and lakes are rich in fish, including such valuable food species as sturgeon and salmon.

Defining the North

The Russian Federation is composed of different types of administrative divisions, which is explained further in box 5.1. Defining 'North' in Russia can be problematic. Decision No. 1029 of the USSR Council of Ministers adopted in 1967, and a number of statutory acts that followed, defined the 'Far North districts and equivalents' in terms of awarding residents certain special privileges such as higher wages and longer duration of paid vacation. There are anomalies under this concept of 'The Far North.' For example, the whole Khanty-Mansi AO belongs to 'The Far North,' while only three districts of the Komi-Permyak AO have the same status, even though the whole AO lies almost on the same latitudes on other side of the Urals. (In 2005, the Komi-Permyak AO and Perm O merged to form the Perm K; and in 2007, the Taymyr AO and Evenki AO merged into the Krasnoyarsk K.) To add to the confusion, there are also 'territories of primary residence of indigenous, numerically small peoples,' with yet another set of boundaries. Thus, only part of the Khanty-Mansi AO is considered to be one such area, whereas in the Komi-Permyak AO no such entities are recognized.

Box 5.1   Administrative divisions in the Russian Federation

According to the constitution of 1993, the Russian Federation is divided into more than eighty territorial-administrative units called federal 'subjects' (*subyetkty*), with the designation of republic, *kray*, *oblast*, autonomous *okrug*, and federal city. These have varying degrees of autonomy, and they each send two representatives to the Federal Council (*Sovet Federatsii*), the upper house of the Russian parliament. The next level is the *rayon*, or district.

In this book, *kray*, *oblast*, and *okrug* are used as Anglicized terms (with 's' added to form the plural) rather than their translations as 'territory,' 'region,' and 'area,' which are not consistently used in the literature (for example, *oblast* is sometimes translated as 'province' and *okrug* as 'region'). The abbreviations R, K, O, and AO are used in referring to republic, *kray*, *oblast* and autonomous *okrug*, respectively. The shorter geographical names are used without the adjectival endings in the more formal Russian versions – for example, Murmansk Oblast instead of Murmanskaya Oblast; and Koryak AO instead of Koryakskiy AO.

Autonomous *okrugs* (with the exception of Chukotka) are generally part of some other federal subjects, and usually represent the traditional territories of some indigenous ethnic groups. In 2000, a presidential decree divided the country into seven 'federal districts' (*federalnyy okrug*): Central, North-West, South, Volga, Urals, Siberia, and Far East. The use of the term *okrug* at the supra-regional level thus adds further to the confusion.

Table 5.1 lists all the territories designated as 'northern' by the 1967 decree, those that lie predominantly north of 60° N and those that are recognized as territories of primary residence of indigenous peoples. In this chapter, when reporting demographic and health statistics, the type of regional aggregation being referred to depends on the data available.

Table 5.1 Territorial-administrative divisions designated as northern and areas of primary residence of indigenous peoples*

	North (1967 decree)	North (>60° N)	Indigenous area	
			(n=26)**	(n=40)**
Northwestern Federal District				
Kareliya R	all	all	–	yes
Komi R	all	all	yes	yes
Arkhangelsk O	all	all	yes	yes
Nenets AO	all	all	yes	yes
Leningrad O	–	part	–	yes
Vologda O	–	part	–	–
Murmansk O	all	all	yes	yes
Volga Federal District				
Perm O	part	part	–	–
Komi-Permyak AO	part	part	–	–
Urals Federal District				
Sverdlovsk O	part	part	yes	yes
Tyumen O	part	part	yes	yes
Khanty-Mansi AO	all	part	yes	yes
Yamalo-Nenets AO	all	all	yes	yes
Siberian Federal District				
Altay R	–	–	–	yes
Buryatiya R	part	–	yes	yes
Tyva R	–	–	–	yes
Khakasiya R	–	–	–	yes
Altay K	–	–	–	yes
Krasnoyarsk K	part	part	yes	yes
Taymyr AO	all	all	yes	yes
Evenki AO	all	part	yes	yes
Irkutsk O	part	part	yes	yes
Kemerovo O	–	–	yes	yes
Tomsk O	part	part	yes	yes
Chita O	part	–	yes	yes
Far East Federal District				
Sakha R	all	part	yes	yes
Primorskiy K	part	–	yes	yes
Khabarovsk K	part	part	yes	yes
Amur O	part	–	yes	yes
Kamchatka O	all	part	yes	yes
Koryak AO	all	All	yes	yes
Magadan O	all	All	yes	yes
Sakhalin O	all	–	yes	yes
Chukotka AO	all	All	yes	yes

*Areas enclosed by dotted lines constitute the Russian North for the purpose of this book; they are included in tables 1.1 and 1.2 and in map 8.
**n refers to number of officially recognized indigenous groups.

Ethnic and Linguistic Groups

According to the 1996 federal law *On the Bases of State Regulation of Social and Economic Development of the North of the Russian Federation*, the indigenous, numerically small peoples (*korennye malochislennye narody*) of the North, Siberia, and the Far East are those 'living on the territories of traditional residence of their ancestors, adhering to their original way of life, and believing themselves to be independent ethnic entities; their total number in Russia is less than 50 thousand people.' Between 1926 and 1993, this group included twenty-six peoples of various origins, languages, and cultures (table 5.2) who occupy an enormous territory, from the Kola Peninsula to Chukotka.[2]

Since 1993 the list has expanded considerably. By 2000, forty groups had been recognized and they were included in the 2002 Census. Many among the fourteen new groups are resident in the southern parts of Siberia. Some are previously grouped with other groups, for example the Alyutors and Kereks with the Koryaks, and Kamchadals with the Itelmens. The Veps are a Finnic-speaking European group resident in the north-west. In 2005, the forty-first such group – the Izhma-Komi in northern Komi Republic – was accorded the status. There are also four groups who are considered indigenous, but they are in the non-northern parts of European Russia. Few demographic and health statistics are available for the newly included peoples.

According to the 2002 Census, the total number of people in the original twenty-six ethnic groups mentioned above was 208,980, whereas the sum of all forty numerically small peoples of the North, the Far East, and Siberia totalled 252,222. There are also ethnic groups resident in the North who are considered neither indigenous nor numerically small (i.e., <50,000), but who are nevertheless ethnic minorities within Russia. Notable northern examples are the Komi (population 418,000) and the Yakuts (population 444,000).

Prehistory and Early History

The Russian North was first settled in the late Palaeolithic Age. The most ancient sites are found in the basin of the Pechora River: Byzo-vaya (28,000–29,000 years before present), Medvezhya (Bear) cave (16,000–18,000 years before present), and Pymva-Shor I (10,000–14,000 years before present). These are the northernmost Palaeolithic sites in Europe. In eastern Siberia, the best-known sites are of the Dyuktai culture (10,000–35,000 years before present). Since the 1990s, many

Table 5.2 Linguistic affiliation, territories of primary residence, and population of 26 indigenous, numerically small peoples of the North, Siberia, and the Far East

Language family/branch[a]	Ethnic group[b] (other names)	Territory of residence[c]	Population (2002)
Altaic			
Tungu	Evenks (Tungus)	Sakha R, Evenki AO, Krasnoyarsk K, Amur O, Khabarovsk K, Chita O, Buryatiya R, Irkutsk O, Sakhalin O, Tomsk O, Tyumen O	35,527
	Evens (Lamuts)	Sakha R, Magadan O, Chukotka AO, Khabarovsk K, Kamchatka O, Koryak AO	19,071
	Nanais (Golds)	Khabarovsk K, Primorskiy K, Sakhalin O	12,160
	Negidals	Khabarovsk K	567
	Oroki (Ulta)	Sakhalin O	346
	Orochi	Khabarovsk K	686
	Udege (Kekar)	Khabarovsk K, Primorskiy K	1,657
	Ulchi (Mangus)	Khabarovsk K	2,913
Turkic	Dolgans	Taymyr AO, Krasnoyarsk K	7,261
	Tofalars (Karagas)	Irkutsk O	837
Uralic			
Samoyed	Enets (Yenisey-Samoyeds)	Taymyr AO	237
	Nenets (Yurak-Samoyeds)	Yamalo-Nenets AO, Nenets AO, Arkhangelsk O, Taymyr AO, Khanty-Mansi AO, Komi R	41,302
	Nganasans (Tavgi-Samoyeds)	Taymyr AO, Krasnoyarsk K	834
	Selkups (Yenisey-Ostyaks)	Yamalo-Nenets AO, Tyumen O, Tomsk O, Krasnoyarsk K	4,249
Finnic	Sami (Lopars)	Murmansk O	1,991
Ugric	Khanty (Ostyaks)	Khanty-Mansi AO, Yamalo-Nenets AO, Tyumen O, Tomsk O, Komi R	28,678
	Mansi (Voguls)	Khanty-Mansi AO, Tyumen O, Sverdlovsk O, Komi R	11,432

Table 5.2 (continued)

Chukotko-Kamchatkan			
Northern	Chukchi (Lauravetlans)	Chukotka AO, Koryak AO	15,767
	Koryaks	Koryak AO, Kamchatka O, Magadan O, Chukotka AO	8,743
Southern	Itelmens	Koryak AO, Kamchatka O, Magadan O	3,180
Eskimo-Aleut	Eskimos (Siberian Yupik)	Chukotka AO	1,750
	Aleuts (Unangan)	Kamchatka O, Koryak AO	540
Language isolates			
	Kets	Krasnoyarsk K	1,494
	Yukagirs (Omoks)	Sakha R, Magadan O	1,509
	Chuvans	Chukotka AO, Magadan O	1,087
	Nivkhi (Gilyaks)	Khabarovsk K, Sakhalin O	5,162

[a]Linguistic terms and classification are based on *Ethnologue* (Gordon 2005). Some linguists group Yukagir with the Uralic in an Uralic-Yukagir family. Chukotko-Kamchatkan is also referred to as Palaeoasiatic. Chuvan was a Yukagir dialect that had become extinct and the people today speak Chukchi and Russian.

[b]English spelling of names of ethnic groups are based on ANSIPRA database.

[c]Population and territories of residence based on 2002 Census.

other Upper Palaeolithic sites have been discovered in eastern Siberia, including some to the north of the Arctic Circle.[3] According to archaeological data, the ancient population of the Siberian Arctic regions must have been the Yukagirs' ancestors who inhabited the territories from the Taymyr Peninsula to the Anadyr River in the first millennium AD.

The settlement of ancient Eskimos on the coast of the Bering Sea dates back to the second and first millennium AD. The ancestors of the Chukchi and the Koryaks lived in the interior areas of Chukotka, and later (first millennium BC) a branch left for the coast of the Sea of Okhotsk.

The Sami are considered the most ancient population of northern Europe. The majority of Uralic languages developed outside the Arctic regions, in taiga and even forest-steppe areas. In West Siberia their advance is well documented by archaeological records. Settlements of ancient Samoyeds (fifth century BC to the fifth century AD) have been found in the Mid Ob area. Similar artefacts in the north, in the lower reaches of the Ob, date back to the third and second centuries BC. The inhabitants of the Mid Ob area can be recognized as Selkups by the sixth to eighth centuries AD. The main Khanty groups were formed in the second half of the first millennium AD. The Mansi originated in the southern and mid Urals as a result of mixture of the ancient native hunters and fishers with the cattle herding population in the steppes. The advance of the Mansi, Khanty, and Selkups northwards was recorded in Russian documents of the seventeenth and eighteenth centuries.

The last to appear in the Arctic regions were the peoples speaking the languages of the Altaic family. The Evenks' ancestors originated in the Baykal area and Transbaikalia, and about the first millennium AD they appeared in mid and eastern Siberia, where they mixed with the local taiga population (probably related to the Yukagirs). Tungusic tribes settled in the huge expanses up to the Taymyr in the north, where they contributed to the formation the Nganasans and Dolgans. Further to the east, as far as the Sea of Okhotsk coast, Chukotka, and Kamchatka, they gave rise to the Evens.

In the first half of the second millennium AD, the Mid Lena basin was penetrated by Turkic groups from the Baikal area, which assimilated the local Tungus and Yukagir population. As a result of several migration waves, the Yakut tribes formed here about the fifteenth century. The Yakuts continued to settle farther to the north after the

Russian settlers started arriving in the seventeenth century. Now the northern Yakuts inhabit the lower reaches of the Lena River and the valleys of the Yana and Indigirka Rivers.

Traditional Lifestyles

The traditional economy of the northern peoples in Russia was almost exclusively based on animal resources. Several subsistence patterns in this economy have been identified.

Maritime hunters (Eskimos, Coastal Chukchi, Koryaks): These hunters lived in permanent settlements consisting of dugouts or ground dwellings with a frame made of whale bones. They engaged in seasonal seal and walrus hunting on ice and on rookeries and hunted whales from skin boats (*baydara*, akin to the Inuit's *umiak*). They preserved the animals' fat and meat (*kopalkhen*) in special holes dug in the ground outside the dwelling. Whale skin was also a part of their diet.

Seal and walrus skins were highly valued for their versatile uses, such as in the making of harness straps, lassos for catching reindeer, *baydara* covers, and footwear. Some Sami, Nenets, and Even groups also engaged in seasonal or periodic sea mammal hunting to provide themselves with skins for straps and footwear, although their basic occupation was reindeer herding and reindeer hunting.

Tundra reindeer hunters (Tundra Yukagirs, Evens, Nganasans, Tundra Enets, and some Sami groups): Reindeer hunting was widespread across northern Eurasia in ancient times. Initially, permanent settlements originated next to where migrating wild reindeer herds crossed rivers, thus making it easy to organize big seasonal hunting using boats and nets. Meat was processed so that it could be kept either dry or frozen. Later, various hunting schemes were developed, including those with domestic draught reindeer, decoy reindeer, mobile camouflage shields, and firearms. Tundra reindeer hunters lived in dugouts, semi-dugouts, and portable conical huts (called *chooms*) made of pole frames covered with reindeer skins.

Taiga hunters and fishers: The subsistence of these peoples relied on reindeer, elk, and mountain sheep hunting as well as fish from rivers and lakes. With the spread of reindeer herding, many groups became semi-nomadic or nomadic. They changed their seasonal camps or moved along a circle route (part of the Yukagirs, Evenks, Evens, Enets, certain Sami groups). However, reindeer herding provided a means of transportation, while the basic source of meat and skins was still wild ungulates. The Khanty, Mansi, and Kets settled on riverbanks and used artificial fences (*abatis*), crossbows, and hunting pits for hunting.

The dwellings of these nomadic groups were *chooms*, covered with deer skins in winter and birch bark in summer. The settled groups lived in dugouts and semi-dugouts of various design, and later, log huts (Khanty, Mansi, Okhotsk Evens).

Reindeer herders: These groups tended large reindeer herds that numbered in the hundreds and thousands. They constantly drove their herds to new, untrampled pastures. Some groups (Kola Sami, Nenets, Enets) made seasonal trips from the taiga zone to the tundra and back, while others (Chukchi, Koryaks) left the tundra for the sea coast in the summer.

Large-scale reindeer herding developed throughout northern Eurasia in the seventeenth and eighteenth centuries, primarily for transportation purposes (riding, packing, or sledding). Herding developed at different stages in different areas. This is evident from the various types of sleds and harnesses used for transportation, and by the distribution of reindeer herding. Population growth and migration of peoples in this period resulted in the reduction of the wild deer population. Social stratification helped concentrate reindeer herds in the hands of individual owners. These factors led to a reorientation of the economy from herding wild reindeer to raising them as domesticated animals. Not only were their pastures overtaken by domesticated herds, but wild reindeer also suffered further depletion as a result of intensive hunting.

Reindeer herders exerted strong cultural influence on hunters, especially tundra hunters. Almost all of them began to use reindeer relays, the outer clothing worn by reindeer herders (*malitsa, sokui, kukhlyanka*). They also began to cover their folding dwellings with reindeer skins. Even those groups that continued hunting as a way of life became much more mobile.

Historical Development

The first to contact the Russian state among all northern peoples were the Sami. Some Sami groups paid tribute to the Great Novgorod principality as far back as the twelfth century. The milestones in the history of Siberia were Yermak's penetration beyond the Urals (1581) and the later conquest of the Siberian Tatar Khanate (1598), one of the successor states of the Golden Horde. As a result, the peoples of West Siberia

(Siberian Tatars, Mansi, Khanty, Selkups) fell under the sphere of influence of the Moscovite state. Later, the established practice of governing the Siberian peoples and extracting tribute (*yasak*) from them was expanded to the whole territory of Siberia, which lasted till the nineteenth century. Originally *yasak* consisted of valuable furs, mainly sables. After sables became scarce, furs of other animals began to be accepted as well as cash payments. The amount of *yasak* and its compulsory nature varied considerably. In remote and poorly controlled areas, *yasak* was gathered sporadically. Sometimes *yasak* payment was purely symbolic or actually a form of trading. In the seventeenth century the *yasak* people were given the 'tsar's gifts' that included fabric, cauldrons, bread, vodka, and adornments.[4]

Once a new territory was annexed, Russian servicemen (*sluzhilye*) built a small fortress (*ostrog*) and tried to win local princes and elders to their side. The privileges of local heads were kept intact and they were charged with gathering *yasak*. The tsar's authorities did not interfere with the self-governing of Siberian peoples. The tsar's *voyevodas* (the chief military, fiscal, and judicial officials) adjudicated only commercial cases involving large sums, capital offences such as murder, revolt, or treason, and disputes between Russians and the *yasak* people. In the seventeenth century Russian control expanded rapidly to the east and northeast of Siberia. By the end of the century, Russian *ostrogs* were constructed in East Siberia and in Kamchatka.

Generally, the penetration of Russians into northern lands did not resemble military occupation. The authorities and traders aspired to make Siberian peoples supply them with furs and never tried to eliminate them or push them from their land. The economy of many indigenous peoples gradually changed because of the influence of trading connections with the Russians. Fur hunting, which used to be of secondary importance, became one of the major occupations. In the seventeenth and eighteenth centuries large-scale reindeer herding became wide spread, which led to significant reduction of the number of wild reindeer in many areas.

Russian *voyevodas* and cossacks actively involved conquered peoples in their campaigns. This often caused bloody wars between various tribes. In the seventeenth and eighteenth centuries the ethnic map of Siberia changed considerably as a result of such wars, as well as migration of a number of Siberian peoples to thinly populated territories, and mass fleeing of the population from *yasak* collectors (and in some places also from forced Christianization). The most prominent among such migrations was the expansion of reindeer-herding groups and the reduction of the territory occupied by settled hunters. The population of Yukagirs and maritime Koryaks dropped considerably, while the Yakuts settled farther and farther to the north, and the Chukchi moved southwards and westwards. As a result of mixing with the ancient Taymyr population, the Evenks, Enets, Nenets, and Yukagirs produced a new ethnic group, the Nganasans. The last to appear (in the late nineteenth and early twentieth centuries) were the Dolgans, who spoke the Dolgan dialect of the Yakut language. This group developed as a result of assimilation of the Evenks, the Yakuts, certain Enets families, and the Russian *old settlers* living in the lower reaches of land bordering the Yenisey, Pyasina, Khatanga, and Kheta Rivers.

In the nineteenth century special laws were passed in an attempt to preserve the Natives' economic well-being and way of life, and to protect them against the arbitrariness of Siberian authorities and fur traders. In 1822, the Charter or *Regulations on Governing Indigenous Peoples* was proclaimed, on which was based the *Statute of the Indigenous Peoples* (1892), which operated up until the 1917 Revolution. In practice, these laws were constantly broken, not only by traders and settlers but also by Siberian officials who were supposed to take care of indigenous peoples' rights on behalf of the government. Many groups of northern Natives preferred to leave and migrate deep into the tundra or taiga. They appeared in Russian settlements only if they needed to exchange furs for guns, ammunition, foodstuffs, and fabrics. On the whole, the policy of the imperial government towards the Natives of the northern frontiers can be regarded as one aimed at assimilation or acculturation.

Significant and drastic changes occurred in the North after the 1917 Revolution. In November 1917, *The Declaration of the Rights of Peoples of Russia* was adopted. It proclaimed the right 'of national minorities and ethnic groups occupying the territory of Russia to free development.' The constitution adopted in 1918 guaranteed 'equal rights for citizens, irrespective of their racial or national identity.'

During the Civil war of 1917–22, the Soviet government could not control the situation in the far-off margins of the country and, naturally, did not pay attention to the indigenous population of the North. Traditional trade connections were broken, northerners faced acute shortages of imported goods, hunters did not have enough ammunition, and the exchange of reindeer herders with the settled population stopped. In many places the new authorities confiscated furs, hunting weapons, and sled deer. In some areas, famine started as a result of unreasonable actions of the authorities and epidemics of deer murrain.

In 1924, mainly on the initiative of a distinguished ethnographer Vladimir G. Bogoraz, the Committee for Aid to Peoples of Far North Areas (commonly known as the Committee of the North) was formed, bringing together statesmen, scholars, and scientists. The goals of the committee were:

- to study the history, culture, everyday life, problems, and needs of Northern peoples,
- to plan and implement measures promoting economic development of the North,
- to protect peoples of the North from exploitation, and
- to develop the bases of administrative and judicial structures.

The activities of the committee brought about significant improvements in the life of indigenous northerners.

In the first decades of the twentieth century, all northern Natives were illiterate and there were no schools in their settlements. In 1930 the Committee of the North started to create the system of 'cultural bases' (*kultbaza*), a complex of institutions engaged in economic, educational, medical, veterinary, and research work. A network of schools offering education in the languages of the indigenous population was organized in the Far North. For the nine most widespread languages, a uniform northern alphabet was developed and textbooks were published. The Institute of Northern Peoples established in Leningrad became the centre for preparing educators to teach in the North. In 1931 there were already 123 schools in the Far North where about 3,000 children studied (approximately 20 per cent of all children of school age). The curriculum and the school year were designed in such a way that they would not affect the everyday life and traditional activities of the local population.

The system of public health services was also extended to the regions inhabited by indigenous northerners in the late 1920s. While their health status improved substantially, they still lagged behind the average rates for the country as a whole right up to the end of the twentieth century. Figure 5.1 compares the life expectancy of the northern Mansi with the Russian national average between 1930 and 1960.[5]

During the Soviet period, radical changes occurred in the economy

Figure 5.1   Trend in life expectancy among the northern Mansi compared with the Russian national average, 1930–60

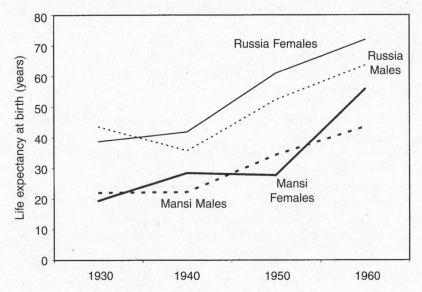

Sources: Kozlov and Vershubsky (1999); Prokhorov (2001).

of northern areas. In 1924 a law was promulgated on material support for the North; a year later all northerners were released from their tax payments. In 1929 private trade was forbidden everywhere and the state monopoly for industrial development of northern resources was established, including fishing, logging, and gold mining. The indigenous population was forced to join consumer cooperative societies or hunting and fishing cooperatives.

In 1929 the whole country became embroiled in the violent process of collectivization. It was accompanied by mass terror not only against prosperous peasants (*kulaks*) but also against those having just a few head of cattle. Government and party officials who carried out collectivization in northern areas came mostly from Central Russia. They did not understand the basics of Arctic reindeer herding which involved herds of several hundred heads, because in a Central Russian village having two or three cows and a pair of horses was considered a sign of 'prosperity.' This misunderstanding led to reprisals against

Figure 5.2   Placard promoting collectivization and denouncing shamans and *kulaks*, USSR, 1931

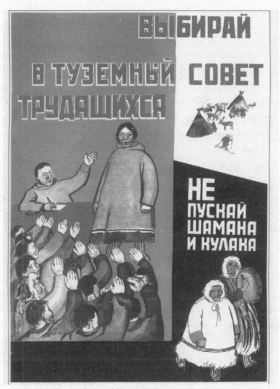

Source: Original by artist G. Khoroshevky. Slogan reads 'Elect a worker in the indigenous Soviet, do not let in a shaman or a *kulak*.'

many Native clans. Shamans were also the targets of ruthless campaigns in the North (fig. 5.2). Members of the Committee of the North tried to resist the collectivization of the northern Native economy or at least to soften the consequences of these measures, but it only brought about increased tension between the committee and the country's authorities.

Though the creation of collective farms in subarctic regions proceeded much more slowly than in the rest of the country, by the 1940s the overwhelming majority of reindeer herds already belonged to collective farms (*kolkhoz*). Just a few years of collectivization managed to push traditional social structures and the economy of reindeer herders to the brink of disappearance.

At the end of the 1920s the Committee of the North, trying to find a compromise between protection of indigenous peoples' interests and industrial development of northern regions, developed a model of national administrative-territorial entities – national areas (*okrug*) and national districts (*rayon*). Between 1929 and 1932, nine national areas and twenty national districts were formed. The Nenets national *okrug* was the first to be established. However, these regional and local authorities had no real influence on the central ministries that monopolized development of natural resources in the northern territories.

Owing to a mass inflow of population from the central regions to the so-called regions of new development, the northern Natives suddenly became ethnic minorities. In less than ten years, between 1926 and 1935, their share of the population in the national districts of the Russian North decreased from 56 per cent to 35 per cent. By 1970 it dropped to 15 per cent, and to 4.4 per cent by 1989.[6] Such drastic reductions occurred in the span of six decades, about two generations. In 1935 the Committee of the North was liquidated. Many scholars and scientists who had participated in its work were arrested in the course of political repressions.

The most radical transformations of the life of Natives in the Russian North happened after the Second World War. In the 1950s the system of boarding schools was developed. At first, children of nomadic reindeer herders and hunters studied in large settlements for several months a year. However, by the mid-1960s, boarding schools became the sole form of education in the North, obligatory for both the nomadic and settled population. Lessons in boarding schools were conducted in Russian (Native languages were taught as a separate subject only in the elementary grades). As a result, the number of Natives who could speak their mother tongue as their first language began to decrease quickly. In 1959, 76 per cent of Natives spoke their own languages, while in 1989 Native-language speakers accounted for only 52 per cent of northerners. Long stays in boarding schools and a growing language barrier among family members affected family cohesion and created a generation gap. By the mid-1970s, in many communities an entire generation had grown up who could not speak their mother tongue and used only Russian, which the older generation had mastered poorly.

It is incorrect to regard these processes as governmental actions aimed at the fastest possible assimilation of indigenous peoples of the North and the Far East. The Soviet cultural effort in the Arctic regions was a variant of *kulturtreger policy*, essentially no different from the practices of the European powers in their colonies. The only difference was the communist ideology, and also the idea of the USSR as an entity that required the cultural integration of peoples within the framework of a uniform society (*Soviet people*), and not just adaptation of colonized peoples to the needs of their metropolis. Aside from that, Soviet ethnic policy in the northern regions totally corresponded to the 'all-European outlook' of the epoch.[7]

Though language acculturation severely affected the traditional way of life and national cultures, it was not the acculturation itself that caused the catastrophe but a number of state campaigns that intended to enlarge settlements as a way of ending the nomadic way of life.[8] These campaigns were carried out under the slogan of 'improvement of the economy in northern areas.' In remote locations, medical aid stations, schools, and even shops were closed, and workplaces were liquidated. A number of territories could no longer practice traditional subsistence management under the pretext of hunting regulations or the need to protect state boundaries. As Soviet laws required all able-bodied citizens to work for either state or cooperative enterprises, Natives were forced to move to larger settlements where these enterprises were located. However, it was often impossible for them to maintain traditional occupations in those places, yet the state structures could not provide full employment for them. The policy of enlargement led to impoverishment, drunkenness, and loss of traditional livelihood all across the North.

What brought about the most radical change in the North was industrial development, which sharply increased in the mid-1950s. The state ministries and departments engaged in uncontrolled natural resources development, ignoring land rights of indigenous peoples or the ecological consequences of their activities. Employment of Natives in modern industrial production in northern regions has always been and remains minimal.

Changes in Russia as a result of the disintegration of the USSR had a significant impact on the indigenous northern population. Critiques began to appear in the press, and indigenous peoples began to form their own organizations. However, the economical chaos and collapse of a number of social structures led to a sharp deterioration of their economic well-being and indigenous northerners remain among the most vulnerable groups in the country.[9] What, then, is their situation at the beginning of the twenty-first century?

Economic Conditions

In 2003 in Russia, the GDP per capita was U.S.$3,018. However, the gross regional product (GRP) per capita varies tremendously among the constituent entities of the Russian Federation. The GRP in the richest region of the country is almost seventy times that of the poorest one (by comparison, the GDP per capita in the wealthiest country of Europe, Luxembourg, is only thirteen times that of the poorest, Moldova). In ten of the fifteen northern regions of the Russian Federation, GRP per capita is higher than the national average.[10] The overall statistics for both the Russian Federation and its regions do not reflect accurately the economic stratification of the population. Unfortunately, adequate data are lacking.

Local surveys in various localities suggest that the majority of Russian indigenous northerners live under conditions of severe economic hardship, and there is great disparity in income levels between Natives and migrants. As an example, we shall consider the situation in two regions of the Russian North: the relatively 'rich' Khanty-Mansi, and the 'poor' Chukotka AOs. According to the Federal State Statistical Service (*Rosstat*), in 1999 the per capita monetary income of the population of these regions exceeded the national average by three and two times, respectively. However, due to the high cost of living in the North and to uneven income distribution, the income of 16 per cent of the inhabitants of Khanty-Mansi AO and 71 per cent of Chukotka AO fell below the official definition of subsistence. (Across the whole of Russia, the income of 30 per cent of the population was below subsistence level.)

According to local surveys carried out among the Khanty-Mansi population in 1999, the per capita monetary income for rural Khanty and Mansi was 664 roubles a month (approximately U.S.$27). It amounted to only about 15 per cent of the regional average and 42 per cent of the average for the Russian Federation. All the surveyed Natives lived below the officially established monthly subsistence wage for this region (U.S.$51 in 1999), according to the *Russian Statistical Yearbook*. The per capita monthly income among the Chukchi was about the same (628.4 roubles, or U.S.$25.4).[11]

Table 5.3   Proportion of registered unemployed among total able-bodied adults in selected northern regions, 2002

Region	Indigenous peoples	Total population
Murmansk O	6.8	1.9
Kareliya R	–	8.1
Arkhangelsk O	4.0	1.2
Nenets AO	4.1	1.8
Komi R	–	5.3
Khanty-Mansi AO	6.0	1.0
Yamalo-Nenets AO	3.4	4.8
Taymyr AO	6.0	6.6
Evenki AO	9.7	5.6
Sakha R	3.9	4.8
Magadan O	12.0	7.4
Kamchatka O	12.8	6.6
Koryak AO	17.4	11.7
Chukotka AO	7.9	4.9

Source: Calculated from 2002 Census.

The income of the Natives living in villages in western Siberia is practically the same, irrespective of whether they are engaged in 'modern' trades or lead a traditional, or close to traditional, way of life. The monthly average monetary income among the 'westernized' and 'traditional' groups in 1999 was, respectively, U.S.$32 and U.S.$21. The difference of U.S.$10 could have no practical impact on the situation of a family oriented to the 'monetary' type of economy because of high prices of purchased products and essential commodities (clothes, hunting and fishing gear, gasoline, etc.). For example, 1 kg of bread, the most purchased product in Native villages, costs 8 roubles (about U.S.$0.32) at this time. The extremely low income of the Native rural population compels them to revert to a subsistence economy, which negatively affects their health and nutritional status.[12]

An important index of the well-being of a population is its labour employment status. It is important that we take special care while judging it on the basis of official Russian statistics, as official data are based on a very unreliable source, that is, the number of the unemployed who voluntarily register with the employment service. However, even if based on official statistics, it is possible to conclude that indigenous northerners face more acute problems in terms of labour employment than other groups (table 5.3) with the only exception of the Sakha Republic (Yakutia), the Taymyr AO, and the Yamalo-Nenets AO, where the proportion of unemployed in the economically active population is lower among indigenous northerners than the regional average. In the other northern regions, the proportion of the unemployed among indigenous peoples, compared with the average for the total population of the region ranged from 1.5 times higher to as much as 6 times higher in the Khanty-Mansi AO.

Long-term structural changes in employment of indigenous northerners are especially disturbing. The proportion of those who are engaged, either full-time or part-time, in unskilled manual labour and who occupy low-paid positions, such as janitors, loaders, and maintenance workers, is increasing.[13] Native workers in northern villages are excluded from management positions and lacks access to more prestigious occupations. The traditional occupations cannot provide full employment. For example, in the Khanty-Mansi AO, only 27 per cent of working Natives are engaged in traditional occupations, a proportion that is likely to be further decreased as the trend towards the reduction of fishing, hunting, and reindeer breeding continues.

Demographic Trends

The areas defined as the Russian North in this book (and listed in table 1.1 and shown in map 8) occupy some 53 per cent of the area of the Russian Federation. During the twentieth century, the Russian North was more heavily populated than other circumpolar regions of the world. The availability of cheap labour and neglect of human life resulting from massive deportation of people for political reasons created a unique situation. Even after the demise of the USSR and the outflow of a substantial number of people from the Arctic regions, some 5 per cent of the whole population of the Russian Federation (7.5 million people) continue to live in the North, compared with only 0.3 per cent of the Canadian population who live in the three northern territories.[14]

After 1989 the Russian Far North experienced a rapid population decline, primarily due to the outflow of non-indigenous settlers. During 1989–2000, the Chukotka AO and Magadan O lost 54 per cent and 40 per cent of their population (fig. 5.3), while other northern regions lost from 25 per cent to 15 per cent.[15] The general population decrease in the North has hardly touched the indigenous populations. As a result, the share of the indigenous population remaining in the

Figure 5.3   Population trends of Chukotka

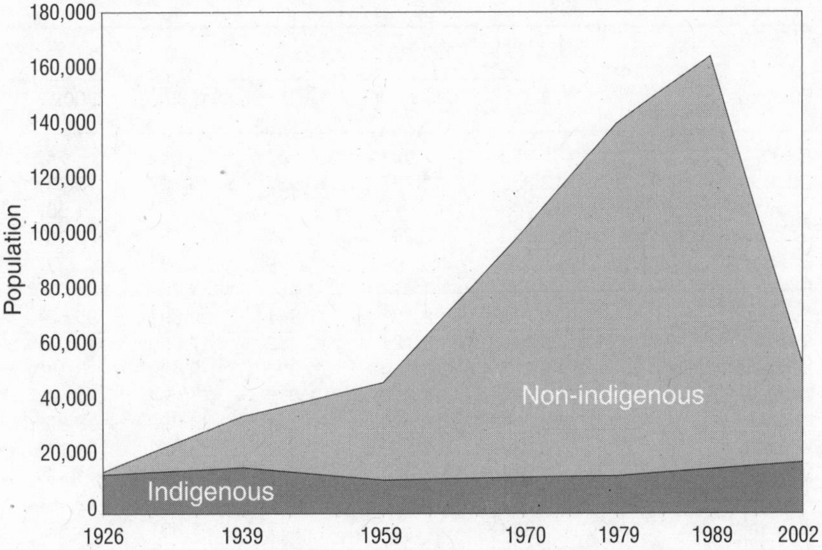

Source: Based on data in Bogoyavlensky and Siggner (2004).

regions of their historical residence has increased. According to the 2002 Census, the number of 'indigenous numerically small peoples of the North' is 252,222, of whom 165,923 live there, about 2 per cent of the northern population.

Since the 1920s, the population of 'indigenous numerically small peoples of the North' has steadily increased (table 5.4). Comparing 1959 with 1926, the decrease in some groups (for example, the Itelmens and Evenks) and sharp increases in others (such as a doubling of the Selkups and quadrupling of the Evens) are not the result of demographic processes such as fertility, mortality, and migration. The principal cause for these changes was the renaming of some ethnoterritorial groups, which in some cases happened because of forced administrative decisions. Many Itelmens, for example, were registered as Kamchadals, thus 'uniting' them with the Russian old settlers of Kamchatka. (Kamchadals were not considered indigenous until 2000.) The Enets were registered as Nenets before 1989. Another important reason was the growing ethnic consciousness of northerners. Thus, in

Table 5.4   Population trends for the 26 indigenous, numerically small peoples of the North, the Far East, and Siberia

Ethnic group	Population/date				
	1926	1959	1979	1989	2002
Aleuts	353	421	489	644	540
Chukchi	12,332	11,727	13,937	15,107	15,767
Chuvans	705	–	–	1,384	1,087
Dolgans	650	3,932	4,911	6,584	7,261
Enets	–	–	–	198	237
Eskimos	1,293	1,118	1,460	1,704	1,750
Evenks	38,746	24,151	27,941	29,901	35,527
Evens	2,044	9,121	12,452	17,055	19,071
Itelmens	4,217	1,109	1,335	2,429	3,180
Kets	1,428	1,019	1,072	1,084	1,494
Khanty	22,306	19,410	20,743	22,283	28,678
Koryaks	7,439	6,287	7,637	8,942	8,743
Mansi	5,754	6,449	7,434	8,279	11,432
Nanais	5,860	8,026	10357	11,883	12,160
Negidals	683	–	477	587	567
Nenets	17,566	23,007	29,487	34,190	41,302
Nganasans	–	748	842	1,262	834
Nivkhi	4,076	3,717	4,366	4,631	5,162
Orochis	647	782	1,040	883	686
Oroki (Ulta)	162	–	–	179	346
Sami	1,720	1,792	1,775	1,835	1,991
Selkups	1,630	3,768	3,518	3,564	4,249
Tofalars	415	586	576	722	837
Udege	1,357	1,444	1,431	1,902	1,657
Ulchi	723	2,055	2,494	3173	2,913
Yukagirs	443	442	801	1,112	1,509

Source: Compiled by authors and based on data from Russian censuses, 1926–2002.

the past, the self-designation 'Selkups' was used only by members of the northern branch of this ethnic group. When members of the southern branch (who used to call themselves Ostyaks and Ostyak-Samoyeds) accepted this ethnonym, there was a sharp non-demographic increase in the total number of the Selkups (for different reasons it occurred at the end of 1950s and the 1990s).

The natural increase in the population of northern peoples slowed considerably in the last two decades of the twentieth century because of a decrease by half in the birth rate and a small increase in the death

Table 5.5   Selected demographic indicators of the northern indigenous population

Period	Crude birth rate	Crude death rate	Natural increase	Infant mortality rate
1984–1988	30.2	10.5	19.7	41.1
1989–1993	25.7	10.8	14.8	30.4
1994–1998	19.8	12.6	7.2	32.5
1999–2002	17.6	11.7	5.9	27.6

Note: Crude birth rate, crude death rate, and rate of natural increase are per 1,000; infant mortality rate is per 1,000 live births.
Source: Estimated by Bogoyavlensky (2004).

rate. Infant mortality rates remained extremely high and declined very slowly (table 5.5). In 2003–4 the infant mortality rate was 20 per 1,000 live births among indigenous northerners, compared with 13.3 per 1,000 for the whole of Russia.[16] However, unlike the population of Russia on the whole, the rate of natural increase among the indigenous population remains positive. In the whole of the Russian Federation, the population has been negative since 1995; in 2005 it was –6 per 1,000.

In comparison with the population of the Russian Federation, the indigenous population is also considerably younger. The proportion of children under fifteen is almost twice that in the country, while the proportion of those aged forty-five and over is only half that observed in all of Russia. The population structure of indigenous peoples of the Russian North is shown in figure 5.4. There is, however, substantial regional variation in the pattern. The situation among the Sami in the Kola Peninsula during 1969–2005 is described in box 9. 2 in chapter 9.

Traditionally, many ethnic groups in the Russian North practise late marriages, resulting in comparatively low fertility rates. Thus, in the 1950–67 period, the age-specific fertility rate for women between 15 and 44 was 112/1,000 among Mansi women, and the median age of parents giving birth to their first child was 23.7 for mothers and 24.5 for fathers. Modern methods of family planning have spread slowly throughout Russia, particularly in the North. The typical methods used are intrauterine devices and induced abortions. In Russia, every 63 pregnancies per 100 women end in legal abortions – among the highest in the world. The frequency of abortions among northern indigenous women is about one-quarter to one-third the national

Figure 5.4   Age–sex structure of 26 indigenous populations of the Russian North

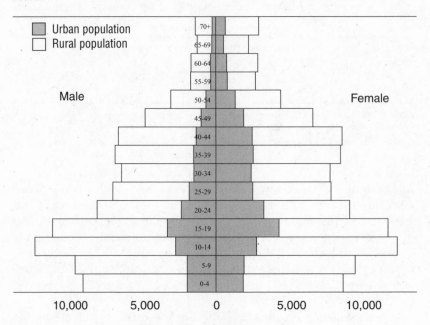

Source: 2002 Census of Russia (www.gks.ru).

average, similar to the other ethnic groups living in rural areas. During the 1970s and 1980s, among the Kola Sami, there were 25 abortions per 100 pregnancies, and among the Chukchi, there were 29 abortions per 100 pregnancies in 2000–3.[17]

There is pronounced gender imbalance in the northern indigenous population, which is manifested quite early among young adults because of the high death rate of men. From age thirty and over, the excess of women over men is pronounced (fig. 5.4).

The increase in population among some indigenous populations as registered by successive censuses may be the result of increased ethnic identity and pride. Among the Kola Sami, this is mostly connected with the increased possibilities of establishing contacts with Sami communities in Finland and Scandinavia after the fall of the Iron Curtain. In the north of western Siberia the major factor was an economic one. For example, on the crest of the oil boom, the administration of the

Khanty-Mansi AO undertook a number of measures for material support of indigenous peoples. As a result, the total non-demographic gain for the Khanty, Mansi, and Selkups turned out to be 3.8 times more than that for all indigenous northerners of Russia taken together. At the same time, in those regions of the Russian North where the economic situation remains adverse, populations of indigenous northerners suffer non-demographic losses.

The indigenous population of the Russian North is predominantly rural. In the 2002 Census, only 28 per cent of indigenous peoples within the territories of their primary residence was classified as urban, a proportion similar to that of the total USSR population in the late 1930s, compared with 73 per cent in the Russian Federation in 2002.

Among indigenous northerners living in cities, the proportion of women is more than half (58 per cent). One of the reasons for this is that young women are more eager than men to move from villages to cities to attend colleges and universities, and they tend to remain in the cities after finishing their education. The second important factor is interethnic marriages, primarily involving indigenous women and non-indigenous men. Families from such unions are more likely to move to the cities. Since the late 1980s, there has been a strong tendency among some northern indigenous groups towards interethnic marriages.[18] As shown in the population pyramid in figure 5.4, urban indigenous women tend to outnumber men, especially in the fertile cohort between ages fifteen and forty-four. Accordingly, the proportion of children from mixed marriages in the cities is especially high. Natives living in cities tend to be more satisfied with their ethnic origin than those living in rural areas.[19] It would appear that the urbanization process does not affect the rate of ethnic assimilation of indigenous northerners.

Health Status

In 1988–9, life expectancy for indigenous northerners was sixty years, some ten years less than the overall average in Russia. In the 1990s the situation became considerably worse. For example, in the Berezovo *rayon* of the Khanty-Mansi AO, in 1996–9 the average age at death was forty-eight for men and sixty for women. Both are approximately twelve years less than the corresponding all-Russian figures. Moreover, within the same region, the indigenous Khanty and Mansi died five to eleven years earlier than the Russian residents. Reduction of life expectancy among northerners is strongly influenced by external causes: traumas, accidents, poisonings, murders, and suicides. Thus, in 1990–3, 69 per cent of all deaths among the northern Mansi occurred among men between ages fifteen and fifty-nine, and 21 per cent of them were in their twenties.[20]

In 2003 there were 90 cases of injuries per 1,000 for the whole of Russia, but in the areas where indigenous northerners reside a lower rate was registered, 61 per 1,000, irrespective of the ethnic origin. As in the north, the death rate from injury is very high. We are inclined to explain these rather favourable morbidity figures by the fact that Natives are less likely to use the health services and that statistical reporting in northern hospitals is more likely to be poor. In 1998–2001, almost 37 per cent of all deaths among the Khanty, Mansi, and Nenets in the north of western Siberia were due to injuries, while across Russia the proportion was only 14 per cent.[21]

It is difficult to track the number of suicides among the indigenous population in the North. Some experts estimated that it likely exceeds the national average three- or even fourfold. The suicide rate in Russia is one of the highest in the world (36 per 100,000), with the highest rates reported in the northern regions of the country – the Komi R (110.3), the Koryak AO (133.5), and Nenets AO (95.7). Between 24 per cent and 55 per cent of all suicides among indigenous northerners happen while in the state of alcoholic intoxication.[22] The impact of alcohol on mortality is examined in further detail in box 5. 2.

In terms of morbidity, Russian statistical reports routinely provide the number of registered patients with a particular diagnosis established for the first time, thus offering an estimate of disease incidence. Table 5.6 compares the regions of primary residence by the twenty-six northern indigenous groups with Russia as a whole with regard to first diagnosis. Table 5.6 indicates that between 1999 and 2001, overall morbidity rates in the northern indigenous areas declined by almost 8 per cent. This contrasts with the worsening situation in the rest of the country, which has experienced consistent annual increases since the 1990s. This apparent 'improvement' is unlikely the result of fewer episodes of illness, but rather the result of under-reporting due to the shrinking of the health care system in the North, lack of access to and underutilization of health services by indigenous people, and the poor state of statistical services.

Table 5.6   Crude rates of first diagnosis by cause: Northern indigenous areas and
Russia

Diagnosis [ICD-10 codes]	Northern indigenous areas		Russia 2001
	1999	2001	2001
Total	744.6	687.5	725.6
Diseases of respiratory system [J00-J99]	347.6	296.4	300.0
Injury / poisoning / other external causes [S00-T98]	65.3	62.5	89.8
Diseases of digestive system [K00-K93]	44.9	48.4	35.9
Certain infectious / parasitic diseases [A00-B99]	47.6	42.3	41.4
Diseases of skin / subcutaneous tissue [L00-L99]	42.8	41.0	47.2
Diseases of genitourinary system [N00-N99]	34.5	35.5	41.0
Diseases of musculoskeletal system / connecting tissue [M00-M99]	33.6	34.5	35.3
Diseases of eye / adnexa [H00-H59]	30.3	31.1	33.7
Diseases of ear / mastoid process [H60-H95]	16.4	17.7	23.1
Diseases of circulatory system [I00-I99]	16.9	16.7	19.6
Diseases of nervous system [G00-G99]	18.1	12.1	15.7
Endocrine / nutritional / metabolic diseases [E00-E90]	8.1	7.6	10.8
Mental / behavioral disorders [F00-F99]	9.1	7.5	7.6
Neoplasms [C00-D48]	6.4	6.1	9.0
Diseases of blood / blood-forming organs / immune disorders [D50-D89]	5.2	4.5	5.1
Congenital malformations / chromosomal abnormalities [Q00-Q99]	1.4	1.1	1.7

Note: Rates are per 1,000; 'northern indigenous areas' refers to 'territories of primary
residence of indigenous, numerically small people of the North.' Since 2002, no information has been published on the Tyumen O, the Khanty-Mansi AO, and the Yamalo-
Nenets AO.
Source: Federal State Statistics Service (2005).

Among infectious and parasitic diseases, helminthiases appear to be
endemic in the North.[23] Since the demise of the Soviet Union, there has
been a resurgence of tuberculosis in Russia. Among the reasons are the
emergence of resistant strains, an overall decline in the quality of life,
and, a uniquely Russian factor, a reduction in preventive services
because of insufficient funding for the public health system. This has
resulted in delayed detection: up to 40 per cent of those initially diagnosed have disseminated the disease, and thus are highly contagious.

In 2004 the tuberculosis sickness rate in the areas inhabited by northern indigenous people was 78.5 per 100,000, which exceeded the all-Russian rate of 71.7 per 100,000 by 9.5 per cent.

One of the few categories of diseases which show an excess in the North, despite likely under-reporting, is digestive diseases. Of particular importance is gastritis, and less commonly, stomach and duodenal ulcers. The epidemiology of *Helicobacter pylori*, the main pathogenic organism causing a peptic ulcer, is poorly researched in the Russian North. Available data suggest that the carrier rate of *H. pylori* among Arctic Natives is very high, however the risk of development of peptic ulcers appears to be much lower than among the population of the temperate zone.

Box 5.2 Impact of alcohol on mortality among indigenous populations of the Russian North

Alcohol abuse has had a major impact on the mortality pattern of northern regions in general, and on indigenous communities in particular. In the mid-1970s, from 31 per cent to 57 per cent of violent deaths in various Chukchi groups were associated with alcoholic abuse. By the beginning of the 1990s the situation had become even more depressing: 73 per cent of murders, 55 per cent of suicides, 64 per cent of accidental injuries among indigenous northerners occurred in a condition of medium or strong alcoholic intoxication.[24]

Alcoholic death rates among inhabitants of the Berezovo *rayon* in the Khanty-Mansi AO in 1996–9 can serve as an example of a situation that was quite typical for the last decade of the twentieth century. Of 362 deaths among the natives (excluding infants under one year of age), 29 per cent were associated with alcohol, compared with only 15 per cent in the non-indigenous population. For women, the death rate from alcohol was five times higher among the indigenous population than among Russians living in the North (15.2 per cent and 3.5 per cent, respectively).

These results are similar to those obtained in Chukotka in 1994. Among both the Chukchi and Eskimos, deaths caused by alcohol were considerably more frequent than among the non-indigenous population. For Chukchi women, the death rate from alcohol in 1980, 1988, and 1994 exceeded the corresponding rates for all women in the AO by 2.3 times. As of 1994, alcohol caused 19 per cent of women's deaths in the AO and 42 per cent of indigenous women's deaths.

Health Care

According to the federal law *On Guarantees of Rights for Indigenous Numerically Small Peoples of the Russian Federation*, indigenous peoples have the right to receive free medical care in state and municipal health care facilities, including annual prophylactic medical examinations. The structure of health care services in the northern regions corresponds to the all-Russia structure. Small villages have qualified medical help stations equipped with a number of beds, where people are cared for by medical assistants (*feldshers*) and midwives. These stations are subordinate to local hospitals, which are staffed by one or more general physicians, a surgeon, and a gynaecologist, and equipped with clinical laboratory and radiology units. There is a tiered system from *rayon* to *oblast*, with increasingly specialized personnel and facilities. There are usually specialized medical dispensaries or clinics for cancer care, skin diseases, sexually transmitted diseases, tuberculosis, and psychiatry, and so on.

The distinctive feature of northern health care is the use of mobile teams. These are not obligatory and are most often created by *okrug*-level health authorities. There are no uniform standards: some teams may consist of only one or two medical assistants and nurses, while better-equipped teams may contain entire polyclinics with medical specialists. Their functions also vary, and may include distribution of medications, lung examinations by fluoroscopy, and more complex diagnostic and treatment services.

The mobile teams are not responsible for evacuation of emergency patients from far-off villages to hospitals. These functions are assigned to 'flights of sanitary aircraft,' carried out, as a rule, by crews of regular light planes and helicopters at the request of hospitals. There is no specialized medical aircraft service in the Russian North.

The majority of medical assistants and nurses working in medical stations and local hospitals in predominantly indigenous areas are themselves also indigenous. However, the proportion of the Natives among doctors is very low. Since the overwhelming majority of the Natives are Russian-speaking or bilingual, they do not experience language problems in their communication with doctors. Nevertheless, there is a serious problem with the conflict of cultures, because doctors coming from other regions have insufficient knowledge of local customs and of the psychology of northerners. There is no evidence that Natives of the Russian North feel antagonistic towards 'Western'

Table 5.7 Selected health services indicators

Indicator (per 10,000 population)	Russia 2001	Indigenous areas*		
		1996	2001	2004
Doctors of all specialties	47.1	33.8	32.1	40.1
Paramedical personnel	107.3	116.6	105.8	123.5
Hospital beds	114.8	153.2	130.8	132.4

*Data refer to 'territories of primary residence of indigenous, numerically small populations of the North.'
Source: Federal State Statistics Service (2005).

medicine. Problems and misunderstandings occur most frequently on the part of the doctors. Physicians training at medical universities in Russia are not exposed to any courses on 'northern medicine' nor are they trained to work with indigenous peoples. Much empirical learning occurs on the job.

Table 5.7 summarizes several health services indicators in the areas inhabited by 'indigenous, numerically small peoples of the North.' The disintegration of the USSR has caused a mass outflow of professionals (including doctors) from the Arctic regions of Russia. In Soviet times, a significant proportion of these specialists came from Ukraine and other republics who had suddenly turned into citizens of newly independent foreign countries. Also, in the first half of the 1990s, the Russian government pursued a policy aimed at reducing the 'superfluous' population in the high-latitude regions of the country, negatively affecting the infrastructure in health care as well as other sectors. All this occurred against the background of the general economic decline of the country – total public expenditures on health care accounted for only 3 per cent of GDP in the Russian Federation. Between 1996 and 2001 there was an overall decrease in the number of doctors and paramedical personnel and the closing of some hospitals, although the number of hospital beds was still 12 per cent higher than the national average. By 2004 the number of health workers showed an increase, after almost fifteen years of continuing decline.

NOTES

1 This chapter uses mainly Russian-language sources. A wide variety of statistical data are available from the website of the Federal State Statistical Service (www.gks.ru), which has an abbreviated English version. The Russian version has an interactive site to allow region-specific data retrieval. There are fourteen volumes of data (both print and electronic) from the 2002 Census. Particularly useful for this chapter are volumes 4 (*Nationalities*), 13 (*Indigenous Peoples*), and 14 (*Summary*).

2 The Arctic Network for the Support of the Indigenous Peoples of the Russian Arctic (ANSIPRA) website at the Norwegian Polar Institute (www.npolar.no/ansipra) provides a comprehensive listing and description of all Russian indigenous peoples in English, including population, distribution, history, and lifestyle. The spelling in this table is based on this listing. See also the website of RAIPON (www.rapion.ru), the Russian Association of Indigenous Peoples of the North. English-language publications on Russian indigenous peoples are limited. An English translation of the standard Soviet-era ethnography, *Narody Sibiri* by Levin and Potapov (1956; translation 1964), is available. The joint Soviet–US exhibition 'Crossroads of Continents' produced a lavishly illustrated handbook (Fitzhugh and Crowell, 1988), containing chapters written by leading Soviet ethnographers.

3 See Pavlov and Indrelid (2000), Mangerud, Svendsen, and Astakhov (1999), and Molchanov (1977). For a succinct introduction to the field in English, see Hoffecker (2005). Note that dating of Dyuktai sites earlier than 25,000 years ago is disputed (see Dixon 2006).

4 For a general history of Siberia in English, see Forsyth (1992). A short report prepared for the Minority Rights Group International by Vahktin (1992) offers a critique of Soviet policies from the Bolshevik Revolution to Glasnost.

5 Kozlov and Vershubsky (1999); Prokhorov (2001).

6 Vakhtin (1993); Vojnova, Zacharova, and Rybakovsky (1993).

7 See Cheshko (2000) for an analysis of Soviet ethnic policy.

8 Kozlov, Vershubsky, and Kozlova (2003).

9 Kozlov (2004).

10 Gadjiev and Akopov (2005).

11 *Russian Statistical Yearbook 2000* (Federal State Statistics Service 2003); Chukotka data are from Litovka (2001).

12 Kozlov and Zdor (2003); Kozlov (2004).

13 Pika and Prokhorov (1994).

14 Trevitch (2002).
15 Vishnevsky (2001); see also Bogoyavlensky and Siggner (2004).
16 Calculation based on *Economic and Social Indicators ... 2004* (Federal State Statistics Service 2005).
17 Davydova (1989); Maksimova (2005).
18 Kozlov and Vershubsky (1999).
19 Kharamzin and Khairullina (2002).
20 Pivneva (1995).
21 *Economic and Social Indicators ... 2004* (Federal State Statistics Service 2005); Bogoyavlensky (2004).
22 Pika and Prokhorov (1994); Kozlov (2006); Kozlov and Vershubsky (1999).
23 Feschbach (1995); Kozlov and Vershubsky (1999).
24 Data in box 5.2 are based on the review by Kozlov and Vershubsky (1999). The study in Khanty-Mansi AO was reported by Kozlov (2006) and Chukotka AO by Demina et al. (1998) and Lensky et al. (1998).

6 Northern Fennoscandia

SVEN HASSLER, PER SJÖLANDER, AND URBAN JANLERT

As a geographic term, 'Scandinavia' has different meanings and usages. In its broadest sense, it encompasses all the Nordic countries and their dependent territories. More narrowly, it refers to only Denmark, Norway, Sweden, and Finland, or only the three contiguous countries of Norway, Sweden, and Finland. Sometimes Finland is excluded; when Finland is included, the term 'Fennoscandia' is often used. For the purpose of this book, Scandinavia will be used interchangeably with Fennoscandia to refer to Norway, Sweden, and Finland collectively (map 9).

Geographic Features

We define northern Scandinavia, which does not exist as a single political-administrative unit, as comprising the six counties of Nordland, Troms, and Finnmark in Norway; Norrbotten and Västerbotten in Sweden; and Lappi in Finland (Lapin *lääni*; Lapland in English), with a total of more than 1 million inhabitants.[1] This region is located on the northern tip of mainland Europe. It is demarcated to the north by the Barents Sea and the Arctic Ocean, to the east by the Russian border, to the west by the Atlantic Ocean, and to the south more or less by 65° N latitude.[2]

The land area of the region is approximately 380,000 square kilometres in total, which is about the size of Poland or one-third the total area of the three countries of Norway, Sweden, and Finland. The region exhibits a variety of landscapes – islands and fjords along the Norwegian Atlantic coast, alpine mountain regions separating Norway and Sweden, low-lying mountains in Finnmark, vast coniferous forests in northern Finland and Norrbotten, as well as archipelagos in the Gulf of Bothnia.

The Scandinavian mountain range, Skanderna (also known as the

Kjolen), is part of the Caledonian mountain range that stretches all the way to the British Isles. It was formed 400 million years ago and has eroded down to mostly smoothly formed shapes with peaks not exceeding 2,000 metres. To the east of the mountains the climate is more continental, with less rainfall, colder winters, and warmer summers than in the coastal regions west of the mountains. Thanks to the Gulf Stream that sweeps up along the Norwegian coast, the climate in northern Scandinavia is generally warmer than other regions located at the same latitude. The average twenty-four-hour temperature on the coast (Tromsø) is about 12°C in the summer and about –4°C in the winter, while inland (Jokkmokk), the average twenty-four-hour temperature reaches 14°C in the summer and –15°C in the winter. However, the coldest winter temperatures in Europe are recorded in northern Scandinavia at latitude 68° N.

Historical Development

The history of human activity in northern Scandinavia can be traced back to the end of the last Ice Age, around 10,000 years ago. Old rock carvings found, for example, in the town of Alta show people living in settlements along the fjords of northern Norway, making their livelihood out of hunting and gathering. The history of the region is also strongly characterized by the indigenous people of the region, the Sami (see chapter 9). Their land, Sápmi, stretches over most of the region and also into the northwestern tip of Russia, the Kola Peninsula.[3]

Nowhere else on earth are agriculture and forests found as far north as in northern Scandinavia. The waterways in the north of Norway are ice-free all year round, which is not seen anywhere else at those latitudes. This unique climate has probably contributed to the long process of moving the cultural border between indigenous arctic and European civilizations northward that has been going on for close to 6,000 years. The culture of northern Scandinavia is partly arctic and partly on the fringe of a European centre. It is part of a circumpolar community but at the same time identifies with southern nations. As soon as the coastal areas were exposed from the inland ice, reindeer hunters from the northern parts of present-day Germany moved in and followed the melting ice northward. The areas along the Norwegian coast and the Gulf of Bothnia were inhabited first, followed by settlement in the interior of Scandinavia, reaching the northern tip of Scandinavia by the Barents Sea around 2500 BC.

While southern Scandinavia during the Neolithic period experienced agriculture and domestication of animals, people in the north still survived as hunters and fishers. It seems as if there were a climate border dividing Scandinavia into two parts, which kept away the encroachment of agricultural society. During the first centuries AD, farming, domestication, and the establishment of small ironworks reached the northern regions. It was also during this time that the first signs of a Sami community could be observed with reindeer herding being one of its characteristics. By the tenth century, Sami settlements were generally located in the highlands while other groups occupied the coasts and river valleys. Sami households generally lived off a combination of fishing, farming, and nomadic reindeer herding, a pattern that is familiar even today.

During late medieval times and until the fifteenth century, the region attracted increasing interest from traders and merchants from the south and Russia in search of furs and fish. The long arm of the state was not far behind, and the king began taxing the Sami. Like the Norsemen in Norway and the Karelians in Finland, the Swedish Birkarlar were a group of traders that travelled the region extensively to trade and to gather tax for the Swedish king. The introduction of a trading economy in the region had a major impact on the living conditions as well as on the social structures of the people. At this time Christianity was also spreading. This period, which marks the beginning of the process often referred to as the colonization of the north, saw rising ethnical conflicts over land between the Sami on the one side and Norsemen, Swedes, and Finns on the other.

During the fifteenth century northern Scandinavia, especially Finnmark, was drawn into the arena of international politics. Through conquests, Sweden had left Russia with no sea exits other than the northern shores. At this time, it was thought that there was a sea passage to China and India north of Finnmark. As the base for taxation of the Sami and trading declined, the state shifted its interest towards the region's strategic geopolitical position and its wealth in minerals, fish, and timber.

The borders between the neighbouring countries in the 1400s were somewhat fluid. Norway belonged to Denmark, and Finland to Sweden, and land was either jointly controlled by two or three countries or exclusively controlled by one nation. Through the treaty of 1751 between Denmark-Norway and Sweden-Finland, more fixed borders were established, of which the one between Norway and Sweden is the longest and one of the oldest in Europe. Through this treaty an agreement named the Lapp Codicil was signed, giving the Sami the right to move freely across the border with their herds while being taxed in only one of the countries, and securing for them civil rights in both countries. When the border between Russia and Norway was fixed in 1826 and that between Russia and Finland in 1944, the division of the region was finalized, setting the scene for a stable and peaceful region. However, national borders were generally ignored by the Sami. When Finland came under Russian rule in 1809, the Codicil that allowed the nomadic Sami to move freely across the borders was disputed. First, Russia decreed that the Finnmark Sami were not allowed to use the winter grazing grounds in Finnish Lapland, and, in 1889, Russia closed the border between Finland and Sweden for the moving of herds.

The colonization of the region was supported by policies of new settlements in the north by the national governments, motivated by a lack of resources in the south. In the fifteenth and sixteenth centuries, Finnish farming settlements were established in Tornedalen in the north-western part of Sweden as well as in Finnmark in the very north of Norway. The expansion of settlers into traditional Sami areas also created conflicts and partly pushed the Sami away from the inland to the fjord areas along the coast. Such conflicts have persisted in many communities in the region up to the present day.[4]

Christianity was introduced as early as the fifteenth century and spread among the Sami in the region. In the late nineteenth century, a priest named Lars Levi Laestadius founded a conservative movement oriented towards revival of the Lutheran belief with strong scepticism of modernism. This Laestadian movement attracted Sami and Finnish settlers and had a major influence on the lifestyle of the people in the region.

Since medieval times the region has attracted exploration of the rich resources of the sea and the minerals in the ground such as iron, copper, silver, and gold. With industrialization came the development of sawmills, mines, and ironworks, mostly along the Gulf of Bothnia. These developments drew in labourers and caused great demographic changes as people moved from inland to the towns along the coast to work in the new industries. In the twentieth century, hydroelectric power was explored and today only a handful of rivers have been spared from being regulated by dams and power plants. Major rivers that are still unharnessed include the Kalix (Sweden), Torne (Sweden and Finland), Ounasjoki (Finland), and Tana (Norway).

Population Characteristics

The population density of Norway, Sweden, and Finland is low in comparison to other European countries, and the northern regions of these countries are even more sparsely populated (see table 1.1 in chapter 1).

For instance, Finnish Lapland covers about 30 per cent of Finland's land area but contains only 3.5 per cent of its population. The relative population density is similar in the northern counties of Norway and Sweden. Moreover, within counties there are considerable regional differences in population density. In most counties there are one or two more urbanized regions where half or more of the population of the county resides; for example, Tromsø in Troms, Umeå in Västerbotten, and the Luleå-Boden-Piteå region in Norrbotten. This implies that the rural parts often hold less than one inhabitant per square kilometre.

While the northern region in Norway shows a very similar age distribution and birth rate as Norway in general, the northern counties in Sweden and Finland are characterized by a somewhat older population and a lower birth rate compared with national statistics (see table 1.2 in chapter 1).

The number of indigenous peoples (the Sami) in the Nordic countries is not well known since ethnicity is not recorded in national population registers in these countries. Various estimates give the total Sami population to be between 80,000 and 110,000. A high estimate would locate about 60,000 in Norway, 36,000 in Sweden, and 10,000 in Finland (see table 1.1 in chapter 1, and further discussion in chapter 9). The majority of the Sami live in the northern areas of the countries, totalling approximately 89,000 or 85 per cent of the population. The highest density of Sami can be found in the region of the Tana River, where they are the ethnic majority in two Norwegian municipalities (Karasjok and Kautokeino) and in Utojoki, Finland. The density of Sami gradually decreases with the distance from this core region, particularly towards the eastern and southern parts of the northern region.

Northern Sami is the most widespread of the Sami languages (see chapter 9), and is spoken by most Sami-speaking people in Norway, Sweden, and Finland. The number of Sami who regularly speak Sami is not known, but they are probably less than half of the Sami population. Although the number of Sami speaking Sami has decreased over the last decades, there is optimism that the language will survive since it is protected by national legislations in all three countries. In practice, this means that the local authorities are obliged to provide interpreting services, if necessary, when Sami are using municipal and public services in their home districts.

Socio-economic Conditions

Figure 6.1 compares three indicators of socio-economic status among Norway, Sweden, Finland, and their main counties. The level of edu-

Figure 6.1   Selected socio-economic indicators in Norway, Sweden, and Finland and their northern regions

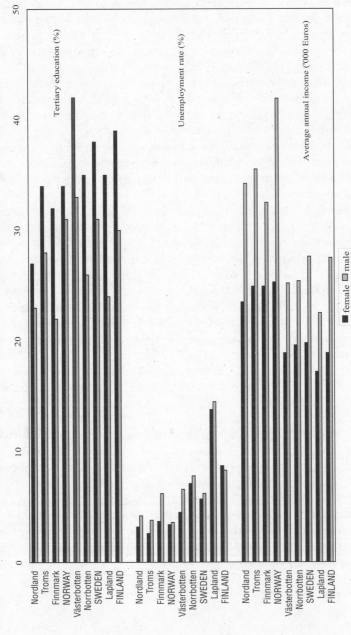

Notes: Data on education (25–64 years) and unemployment (16–64 years) are for 2005, and on income (≥ 20 years) for 2004.
Sources: Statistics Norway (www.ssb.no); Statistics Sweden (www.scb.se); and Statistics Finland (www.stat.fi).

cation is generally high in these countries, and it is higher for women than for men. A large majority of the adult population has graduated from high school and, at a national level, more than 30 per cent have studied in university. The proportion of people with university education is lower in northern Scandinavia, particularly for men, than in the countries as a whole.

The unemployment rate shows a west-east gradient with the lowest rates in Norway and the highest in Finland. There is also a somewhat larger unemployment rate in the more rural parts of these countries, which is demonstrated by the relatively high rates in Lappi, Norrbotten, and Finnmark.

The average annual income is highest in Norway; the figures for Sweden and Finland as a whole are very similar to each other. Although there are on average smaller incomes in the northern regions in all three countries, the disparities are modest. In contrast to what would be expected from the gender differences in the level of education, men report significantly higher incomes than women. This might appear surprising in countries that are known as being among the most 'gender neutral' in the world.

Socio-economic data for the Sami people of the three countries are not readily available. Box 6.1 presents data obtained from an epidemiological study on the association between socio-economic factors and cardiovascular diseases in the Swedish Sami population.[5]

Box 6.1 Ethnic differences in socio-economic conditions in Sweden

The annual net income for Sami men and women (reindeer herders and non-herders) between 1970 and 2000 was compared with that of a demographically matched non-Sami population and of Sweden as a whole. Among men, there were small differences in the median net income among non-herding Sami and non-Sami, whereas the income for the reindeer-herding Sami men was considerably lower throughout this period. Among women, reindeer-herding Sami did not fare much worse than the other groups, and they experienced a much steeper rate of increase between 1990 and 2000. More importantly, since the late 1980s the net income of reindeer-herding Sami women has exceeded that of their men, and in 2000 the difference was considerable. Within reindeer-herding Sami households, the largest proportion of the family's net income is derived from regular work done by women.

Figure 6.2   Trend in net median income among reindeer-herding Sami, non-herding Sami, non-Sami, and Sweden as a whole

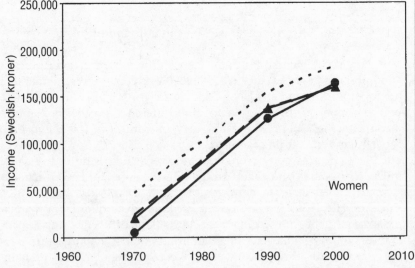

In terms of education, there were very little differences in the distribution of educational levels among women belonging to the four comparison groups. Moreover, the proportion of reindeer-herding Sami women with tertiary education was the largest, and the proportion of those with only primary education the smallest. Reindeer-herding Sami men reported the lowest proportion of tertiary education and had the highest proportion of those with only primary education.

Figure 6.3   Relative frequency of tertiary, secondary, and primary education among reindeer-herding Sami, non-herding Sami, non-Sami, and Sweden as a whole

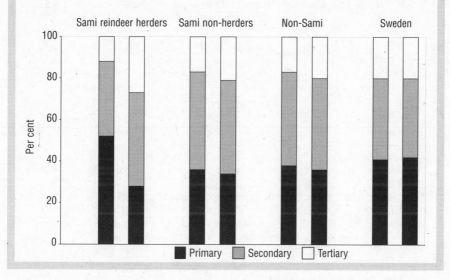

Health Status

The regional differences in health are relatively small. Mortality rates show a general tendency to be highest in Finland while the differences between Norway and Sweden in most cases are smaller (table 6.1). The northern regions have slightly higher rates than the national figures. The suicide rate is considerably higher in Finland, especially in Lapland, than in the other two countries.

The trend for IHD mortality is favourable in all three countries with Norway being the most positive example. The trend for cancer is similar for most forms of cancer. In general, the frequency has increased with time, with a few exceptions of decreasing incidence

Table 6.1   Age-standardized mortality for selected causes in Norway, Sweden, and Finland and their northern regions .

	Finland		Norway		Sweden	
	National	North	National	North	National	North
All causes	671.0	693.0	633.3	666.2	593.4	626.6
Infectious diseases						
Tuberculosis	1.2	1.9	0.6	0.9	0.5	0.9
Pneumonia	28.8	22.1	26.0	26.9	14.2	12.9
Chronic diseases						
Ischemic heart disease	162.2	172.4	105.5	125.5	117.2	129.7
Stroke	62.2	59.8	53.3	58.0	54.9	60.6
Cancer						
All sites	147.3	155.3	174.0	174.6	156.1	147.2
Breast	12.2	10.3	12.8	9.1	11.8	11.0
Prostate	10.2	11.7	14.6	14.2	14.9	15.3
Lung	27.9	33.1	34.8	38.5	25.2	19.3
Injuries						
Unintentional	43.1	50.2	28.7	30.3	22.2	29.6
Suicide	20.4	25.2	11.2	11.4	11.9	9.9

Note: Mean annual age-standardized mortality rates (per 100,000) for the period 2001–3, standardized by the direct method to the European Standard Population of EUROSTAT.

Sources: National data for Finland, Norway, and Sweden from EUROSTAT; regional data for Norway (Troms, Nordland, and Finnmark) and Sweden (Norrbotten and Västerbotten) from EUROSTAT (http://epp.eurostat.ec.europa.eu); regional data for Finland (Lappi) are special tabulation requested from Statistics Finland.

such as cancer of the stomach. The incidence of breast cancer, prostate cancer, and colorectal cancer is increasing in almost all countries. Dietary factors are probably significant for this development, but for breast and prostate cancers, hormonal factors also play an important role. As well, the incidence of testes cancer are increasing and tobacco-related cancers, such as lung cancer, is high in all three countries. However, the incidence of lung cancer among men is decreasing corresponding to an earlier decrease of smoking among men.

With regard to alcohol consumption, the statistics are unreliable, as the available data are based on sales figures. These figures indicate that the largest consumption/sales are to be found in Finland, followed by Sweden and Norway. Accordingly, the number of treatment

Table 6.2   Selected health indicators in Norway, Sweden, and Finland

Indicator	Norway	Sweden	Finland
Life expectancy at birth[a]			
Male	77.5	78.4	75.3
Female	82.3	82.7	82.3
Infant mortality rate (per 1000 live births)	3.3	3.1	3.3
Sales of alcoholic beverages (litres per capita per year)[b]	6.2	6.5	9.9
Prevalence of current smoking (%)[c]			
Male	27	15	27
Female	25	18	20

[a]Life expectancy data are for 2004.
[b]Alcohol consumption converted to equivalent of litres of 100 per cent pure alcohol per capita aged 15 years during 1995–2004.
[c]Percentage of daily smokers in 2004, age 15–64 (Finland), age 16–74 (Norway), age 16–84 (Sweden).
Source: NOMESCO (2006).

periods/discharges from hospital for alcoholic liver diseases are higher in Finland (see table 6.2).

Although the number of smokers in the Nordic countries has been decreasing during recent years, there are still large differences in the number of smokers. Norway has the highest prevalence of smokers and Sweden the lowest, among both men and women. Finland shows the most significant sex gap (see table 6.2).

The population structure varies somewhat between the Scandinavian countries, Sweden having the oldest population and the lowest fertility rates. Sweden accordingly also has the lowest natural increase while net migration contributed to population growth in Sweden as well as in Norway and Finland. Life expectancy has increased significantly during the last decades and during the last 100 years life expectancy has increased by almost thirty years.

Life expectancy is highest in Sweden for both females and males. The female advantage (i.e., how many years longer females will live compared with men) is about five years for Sweden and Norway and seven years for Finland. Fertility rates and infant mortality rates are quite similar in all three countries (see table 6.2).

In all the Scandinavian countries, it is possible to obtain treatment for infertility, which is paid for by the public health services. More

Table 6.3   Available health care resources in Norway, Sweden, and Finland and their northern regions

	Finland		Norway		Sweden	
	National	North	National	North	National	North
Physicians per 1000 inhabitants	3.2	1.8	3.3	3.5	3.1	2.9
Nurses per inhabitant	8.1	7.9	13.3	13.8	10.4	11.8
Dentists per inhabitant	0.8	0.7	0.8	0.8	0.8	0.8

Sources: Data for Finland are for 2004, from Statistics Finland (www.stat.fi); data for Norway are for 2003, from EUROSTAT (http://epp.eurostat.ec.europa.eu); data for Sweden are for 2003, from the National Board of Health and Welfare (www.social styrelsen.se).

and more people are receiving such treatment, and a significant proportion of live births are the result of in vitro fertilization (IVF). A large number of births resulting from IVF are still multiple births. Internationally, the Nordic countries are characterized by having very low perinatal mortality.

Since the middle of the 1970s, induced abortion has been available in most of the Nordic countries. In Sweden, it is a requirement that the abortion take place before the end of the eighteenth week of gestation, while it must be performed before the end of the twelfth week of gestation in the other Scandinavian countries. Abortion can also be carried out after the twelfth and eighteenth week of gestation, but only following special evaluation and permission.

In Norway and Sweden, it is solely up to the pregnant woman herself to decide whether an abortion is to be performed, while in Finland permission is required. Such permission is given on the basis of social and/or medical criteria. Abortion rates vary somewhat in the Nordic countries.[6]

Health Services

In the Scandinavian countries, health services are a public matter, although a private sector does exist, more so in Finland (about 23 per cent of health expenditures) than in Norway or Sweden (about 15 per cent) (see table 2.1 and fig. 21.2 in chapters 2 and 21, respectively). All countries have well-established systems of primary health care. In addition to general medical practitioner services, preventive services are provided for mothers and infants and school health care and dental care are provided for children and young people. Preventive occupational health services and general measures for the protection of the environment exist in all the countries. Table 6.3 compares several health care indicators in the three countries and their northern regions.

The countries generally have well-developed hospital services with advanced specialist treatment. Specialist medical treatment is also offered outside hospitals. The health services are provided in accordance with legislation, and they are largely financed by public spending or through compulsory health insurance schemes. In all countries, however, there are some patient charges for pharmaceutical products. Between 75 and 85 per cent of health care expenditure is publicly financed. In 2003, the level of public financing was lowest in Finland with 75 per cent, while the proportion in the other Scandinavian countries was over 80 per cent.

For many years, there has been a trend towards fewer hospital beds. Resources have been concentrated in fewer units, often involving a division of work in the most specialized areas. Units have often been merged administratively, not necessarily leading to fewer physical units. Another trend is that psychiatric hospitals have been closed down to varying degrees.

The municipalities have responsibility for primary health care, including both preventive and curative treatment such as children's health, health education, advice concerning contraceptive measures, health surveys and screening, medical treatment (including examination and care), medical rehabilitation, and first aid. General medical treatment is provided in health centres, in inpatient departments, or as home nursing services.

NOTES

1 The European Commission and its agencies (e.g., EUROSTAT) have also defined various levels of regions within Europe. At the NUTS-2 level, the three Norwegian counties of Nordland, Troms, and Finnmark constitute region NO-07 Norge-Nord; and the two Swedish counties of Norrbotten and Västerbotten constitute region SE-08 Övre Norrland. For Finland, there is FI-15, called Pohjois-Suomi. It includes three lower-level divisions: A1 Keski-Pohjanmaa (Central Bothnia), A2 Pohjois-Pohnjanmaa

(northern Bothnia), and A3 Lappi (Lapland). It thus includes also parts of Oulu county.

2　Our grouping of the six counties (*fylke* in Norwegian, *län* in Swedish, and *lääni* in Finnish) differs from the informal notion of North Calotte ('cap'), originally proposed by a Finnish parliamentarian in 1957 for cooperation among the five northernmost counties (excluding Västerbotten) of the three countries. The Barents Euro-Arctic Council (established 1993) is currently represented by the three northernmost Norwegian and two northernmost Swedish counties, as well as by both the Lapland and Oulu counties in Finland.

3　Much of the historical information in this chapter is based on Salvesen (1995) and Simonsen (1976). Vahtola (1992) focused specifically on northern Finland.

4　The historical evolution of interethnic relations in northern Scandinavia are discussed in detail in Tägil (1995), Lantto (2000), and Lange (1998).

5　Details on the construction of the Sami population, health, and living conditions database can be found in Hassler, Sjölander, and Ericsson (2004), and discussed in box 9.1 in chapter 9.

6　NOMESCO (2006).

PART TWO

Peoples

7 Inuit

PETER BJERREGAARD AND KUE YOUNG

The word *Inuit* is the plural of *inuk*, which means a person. The term is today used to denote a number of closely related population groups inhabiting the circumpolar region. These groups are known under a variety of self-designated names, including Kalaallit (in Greenland), Inuit and Inuvialuit (in Canada), Inupiat and Yupik (in Alaska), and Yuit (in Siberia). The older term 'Eskimo' is generally perceived to be derogatory in Canada, while in Greenland it refers to historical populations, and in Alaska it continues to be acceptable. In this book, we will use the term Inuit, which is also the term used by the international organization, the Inuit Circumpolar Council (formerly Conference).[1]

The traditional homeland of the Inuit comprises the coast of the Chukotka peninsula in eastern Siberia, the western and northern coasts of Alaska, the Arctic coast and Arctic Archipelago in northern Canada, and the narrow coastal strip of Greenland (map 3). The majority of the Inuit live in coastal villages while some in Canada and Alaska also live in more inland communities along rivers and lakes. In addition, a significant number of Inuit have emigrated to large cities such as Anchorage, Ottawa, and Copenhagen.

Origins and History

Chapter 1 outlined the Asian origins of the indigenous populations of the Americas. The details of the migration – its date, the number of 'waves,' the point(s) of entry, the routes of dispersion, and the time required to populate the length and breadth of the Americas – have been the subject of much debate. The issue is complex and requires a synthesis of geological, archaeological, anthropometric, genetic, linguistic, and ethnographic evidence.

How closely the Inuit are related to other populations in the Old and New World has long fascinated and preoccupied scientists. An older generation of physical anthropologists measured physical traits in living populations and skeletal remains – for example, craniofacial dimensions and dental morphology. Earlier studies on single genetic markers identified some unique patterns in the Inuit – for example, the blood group gene *ABO*B* is present in Inuit and Aleuts but very rare among North and South American Indians, whereas the *DI*A* gene of the Diego system that is present among Amerindians is very rare among Inuit and Aleuts. There is also a vitamin-D-binding protein gene ('group-specific component') called *GC*IGL* (first identified in Igloolik), which is unique to the Inuit, though in low frequency (<1%) but is not found in non-Inuit. Genetic distance analyses of multiple genetic markers in the pre-genomics era suggest that Chukchi, Inuit, and Dene are closely related, forming a continuum that extends across the Bering Strait. In Cavalli-Sforza's reconstruction of human evolution globally (figure 1.1), the Inuit and Chukchi are closely related, and they belong to a larger grouping of Arctic, northeastern Asiatic peoples, separate from the Amerindians of the western hemisphere.[2]

In the 1980s, the 'three-wave' theory of migration proposed by Greenberg and colleagues ignited much debate. It suggested that the Eskimo-Aleuts were the last group to come over from Asia via the Beringia land bridge, following two earlier waves of Palaeo-Indians and Na-Dene. Since the 1990s, a new generation of analytical techniques involving mitochondrial DNA (mtDNA) and the non-recombinant region of the Y chromosome (NRY) added substantial new data but did not resolve the issue. Multiple waves, as many as four, were invoked by some researchers, while another school indicated that a single migration most likely between 10,000 and 17,000 years ago and subsequent geographical isolation and genetic drift (a random process that, in small populations, can substantially increase the frequency of certain markers over successive generations) could account for the observed pattern.[3]

Studies on mtDNA and NRY rely on the identification of mutations on segments of DNA called haplotypes that are transmitted together. Such haplotypes can be assigned into haplogroups, which correspond to genetic lineages of people who can trace their common origin to the time those mutations occurred and were perpetuated in subsequent generations. Haplogroups A, B, C, D, and X in the mtDNA system occur in different frequencies among indigenous North Americans.

However, among the Inuit, Dene, and Chukchi, haplogroup A predominates, while B is absent or very rare. Within haplogroup A, there are certain sublineages that are specific to certain groups, for example the 16265G in A2 that is found in all Inuit groups. In the NRY system, haplogroup Q and C are present in indigenous peoples in North America, with Q in particularly high frequencies (more than 50%) in all groups, while C is extremely rare among Inuit.[4]

Regardless of when and where the Inuit's ancestors separated from their Asiatic kin, it was only relatively recently that the Inuit arose as a culturally and biologically distinct population in North America. Archaeologists generally divide Inuit pre-contact history into two major traditions, the Palaeo-Eskimo and Neo-Eskimo. About 4,500 years ago, the Palaeo-Eskimos emerged from the Bering Sea region and began to migrate across and occupy the rest of the Arctic. They underwent a series of gradual cultural changes and adaptations, recognized as the Independence I, Saqqaq, Pre-Dorset, and Dorset cultures.

About AD 1000, the Neo-Eskimo tradition entered the western Arctic, again from Alaska, and proceeded eastwards relatively rapidly in the following centuries. The precipitating cause was likely climatic change (the so-called Medieval Warm Period) that resulted in an eastward shift of the range of the bowhead whale and those who hunt them. Known as Thule, these people replaced the Dorset culture and were the direct ancestors of the present-day Inuit. While there is broad consensus on the cultural sequence and major timelines, there are still some unresolved issues around the transition from the Late Dorset to the Thule. The Dorset culture likely survived into the second millennium AD (as late as AD 1500 in northern Quebec and Labrador), to be met and displaced by the new Thule arrivals. There are indications of material exchanges and even social interactions between the two groups, and indeed some Inuit oral histories described contact with people very different from themselves who were known as 'Tuniit.' Some archaeologists, however, dispute the radiocarbon dating and propose that there was a 150-year hiatus between the two groups, with the Late Dorset people dying out by AD 800.[5]

The Thule people were technologically more advanced than the Dorset, especially with regards to hunting at sea. They lived in permanent villages throughout the winter in houses made of stone, whalebones, and sod. They used tools made of metal (meteoritic iron from northwest Greenland and implements obtained from the Norse settlers through trade or warfare). Their social organization involved some degree of status differentiation and formal leadership, with a developed sense of territoriality and intergroup competition.

There is some contemporary relevance to the issue of the timing of the Dorset culture's termination. If it did not persist past the first millennium AD, it would suggest a failure to adapt to the climate-induced environmental changes. However, had they been successful in overcoming nature, they would have survived a few centuries more, only to be supplanted by the socially better organized, technologically more advanced, and demographically more prolific Thule people.

The transformation of the Thule into the Inuit was a complex process which began probably in the fifteenth century and involved population movements and changes in subsistence strategies and settlement patterns that varied in timing and speed in different regions. The trigger for these changes may again be climate-related, as they occurred at the same time as the 'Little Ice Age' (ca. 1450–1850). There was, for example, abandonment of the northernmost Thule territories. The decline of the whale population led some groups to leave the coast and move inland to live off the caribou. Others stayed on the coast and hunted smaller mammals such as seals and walruses. Also occurring at the same time was the beginning of European explorations and increasing interactions between the Inuit and these newcomers with their new materials, techniques, ideas, and diseases. (The history of the Inuit after European contact and under European colonization in each region is discussed in greater details in chapters 2 to 4.)

The Smithsonian Institution's *Handbook of North American Indians* estimated that at contact the Inuit population of the Arctic culture area from Alaska to Greenland numbered approximately 72,000. It was more than halved by the beginning of the twentieth century, when the population reached its nadir of some 34,000.[6]

Contact and colonization were accompanied by culture change, which proceeded at a different pace across the circumpolar region. The Inuit adopted some items of European material culture, especially iron tools, firearms, and fabrics. These were superimposed on the traditional way of life and made it more efficient. The hunting life remained largely intact well into the twentieth century in most regions. Christianity in its various forms (Russian Orthodox, Moravian, Lutheran, Catholic, and Anglican, among others) began to displace traditional beliefs and shamans. Missionaries also built schools, introduced written scripts for the language of the Inuit, compiled dictionaries and grammar books, and provided medical aid and welfare relief in times of hardship. A Western concept of law and justice was imposed and enforced by non-Inuit police and military personnel. While the languages of the colonizers, whether Danish, English, French, or Russian, were introduced and used in the administration of Inuit affairs, the Inuit by and large were able to maintain the viability and vitality of their language.

Despite their vastly different experiences, some more benign than others, all Inuit groups struggled for political changes which allowed them to regain much of the autonomy that had been lost to the modern state, be it Danish, Canadian, American, or Russian. The process of self-determination has gone the furthest in Greenland, which achieved Home Rule in 1979. The process only began in the last decade of the twentieth century in Chukotka, where the Inuit, among other northern Natives, emerged from decades of Soviet rule, only to be plunged into the social, political, and economic chaos of the post-communist era.

In Alaska, the Inuit witnessed statehood in 1959 and participated in the subsequent land claims negotiations that resulted in the *Alaska Native Claims Settlement Act* (ANCSA) of 1971 and the establishment of regional Native corporations. In Canada, Inuit in both the western (Inuvialuit) and eastern Arctic settled major land claims in 1984 and 1993, respectively. In 1999, the new Nunavut Territory was inaugurated with an overwhelming Inuit majority population. In 2005, the Inuit in Labrador also signed a comprehensive land claims agreement with the federal and provincial governments and established the regional government of Nunatsiavut.

The political development of the Inuit, given its distribution in four countries, has a strong international dimension. In 1977 the Inuit Circumpolar Conference (ICC) was formed to address common issues affecting Inuit and to present a unifying voice. Not until the end of the Soviet era were the Inuit in Chukotka able to join and meet freely their cousins elsewhere. The Inuit are also actively involved in international forums advocating and safeguarding the rights of indigenous peoples everywhere. In the 1990s, they actively participated in efforts to monitor and mitigate threats to the fragile Arctic environment. In 1996, the Arctic Council was formed and the ICC was one of several 'permanent participants' along with other cross-national indigenous peoples' organizations.

Table 7.1   Subdivisions of the circumpolar Inuit population

Cultural group	Language	Political division
East Greenland	Inupiat-Inuit	Greenland
West Greenland	Inupiat-Inuit	
Polar	Inupiat-Inuit	
Labrador Coast	Inupiat-Inuit	Canada
Northern Quebec	Inupiat-Inuit	
Baffinland	Inupiat-Inuit	
Iglulik	Inupiat-Inuit	
Netsilik	Inupiat-Inuit	
Caribou	Inupiat-Inuit	
Copper	Inupiat-Inuit	
Mackenzie Delta	Inupiat-Inuit	
North Alaska Coast	Inupiat-Inuit	Alaska
Interior North Alaska	Inupiat-Inuit	
Kotzebue Sound	Inupiat-Inuit	
Bering Strait	Inupiat-Inuit	
Nunivak	Central Alaskan Yupik	
Mainland Southwest Alaska	Central Alaskan Yupik	
Pacific	Alutiiq	
St Lawrence Island	Siberian Yupik	
Siberian	Siberian Yupik	Russia

Note: Categories under 'cultural group' refer to 20 'tribe-like' groups defined by the Smithsonian Institution (Damas 1984).

Cultural and Linguistic Groups

Ethnologists generally recognize some twenty tribe-like groupings of Inuit across the Arctic, who differ in terms of language/dialect, technological repertoire, pattern of subsistence, and social organization. In pre-contact times, such groups were nomadic and generally did not exceed 1,000 members each. Table 7.1, using the terminology of the Smithsonian *Handbook*, lists the subdivisions of these groups.

The languages of the Inuit belong to the Eskimo-Aleut or Eskaleut family (see map 3), which has three main branches: Aleut, Yupik, and Inuit-Inupiaq. Aleut is spoken by the inhabitants of the Aleutian Islands in Alaska and Commander Islands in Russia. Linguists ascertained that Aleut and Eskimo split about 4,000 years ago. Siberian

Yupik is spoken by Siberian Eskimos in Chukotka and on the St Lawrence Island in the Bering Sea. Central Alaskan Yupik is spoken in west-central Alaska between Norton Sound and Bristol Bay. Pacific Yupik, or Alutiiq, is also known as Sugpiaq. Its speakers are often considered to be Aleuts. There are two dialects – Koniaq, spoken on Kodiak Island and the Alaska Peninsula, and Chugach, spoken on the Kenai Peninsula and in Prince William Sound. Inupiat-Inuit is a largely mutually intelligible continuum of dialects across northern Alaska, Canada and Greenland. In Canada the term Inuktitut is generally used to refer to the language spoken by the Inuit, although strictly speaking, it should only refer to those dialects spoken in the central and eastern Arctic. Two other major dialects are used in the western Canadian Arctic: in the Mackenzie delta (Inuvialuktun) and the Kitikmeot region of Nunavut (Inuinnaqtun). The national language of Greenland is called Kalaallisut, and it has three main dialects spoken in North, East, and West Greenland.[7]

In Canada, Inuktitut is one of the few Aboriginal languages which is relatively secure. According to the 2001 Census, among Inuit nationally, 51 per cent declared it as their mother tongue (first language learned in childhood and still understood), 26 per cent used it most often or on a regular basis at home, and 10 per cent had sufficient knowledge to conduct a conversation. These percentages were even higher in Nunavut – 82, 33, and 15 respectively.

Today, most Inuit of the younger generations have English, Danish, or Russian as their second – or even first – language, while the older generations predominantly still speak their indigenous languages. In Alaska, many young Inuit have only limited knowledge of Inupiat or Yupik, while in Greenland it is only young Inuit in some mixed families and those who grew up outside Greenland who do not have Greenlandic as their mother tongue. A thorough knowledge of one of the European languages is important since higher education is usually offered in those languages.

Population Distribution

The world Inuit population numbered around 165,000 at the beginning of the twenty-first century, comprising those with self-identified full or partial Inuit heritage (table 7.2). The Inuit are a fairly young population compared with western European and North American populations. Figure 7.1 compares the relatively broad-based popula-

Table 7.2 World distribution of Inuit population

Country/region	Population		
Russian Federation[a]	1,750		
Chukotka Autonomous Okrug		1,590	
United States[b]	54,760		
State of Alaska		46,730	
Canada[c]	51,390		
Northwest Territories		3,500	
Inuvialuit region			2,670
Nunavut		22,450	
Kitikmeot region			4,290
Kivalliq region			6,740
Qikiqtani region			11,420
Quebec		10,170	
Nunavik region			8,620
Newfoundland and Labrador		6,170	
Nunatsiavut region			4,165
Greenland[d]	50,400		
Denmark[e]	7,000		
Global total	165,300		

[a]Russian Census, 2002 (Federal State Statistical Service www.gks.ru).
[b]U.S. Census, 2000 (U.S. Census Bureau http://factfinder.census.gov): Race recorded as 'Eskimo alone or in any combination.' Note that not all Alaska Native respondents provided additional information about tribal affiliation.
[c]Census of Canada, 2001 (Statistics Canada www.statcan.ca): including 'Inuit single origin' and 'Inuit and non-aboriginal origins'; Kivalliq is formerly known as Keewatin, Qikiqtani (also known as Qikiqtaaluk) as Baffin, and Nunavik as Ungava. Nunatsiavut is the Inuit region of Labrador.
[d]Greenland population as on 1 January 2006 (Statistics Greenland www.statgreen.gl): Inuit identified as 'persons born in Greenland.'
[e]Inuit population in Denmark based on estimates in Togeby (2002) and Bjerregaard, Young, and Hegele (2003).

tion pyramid of Canadian Inuit with the more cylinder-shaped population pyramid of Canada. In the 2001 Canadian Census, 41 per cent of the Inuit population was under 15 years of age, compared with 19 per cent among all Canadians, whereas only 3 per cent of the Inuit population was 65 years and over, compared to 13 per cent in Canada.

Figure 7.1   Age–sex structure of Canadian Inuit population compared with
all Canadians

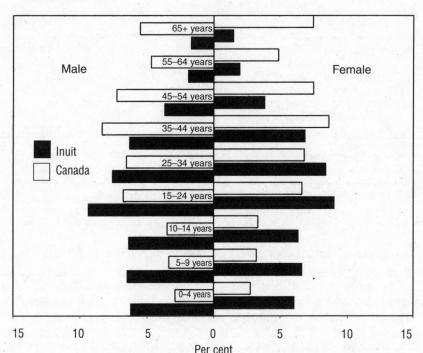

Source: Census of Canada 2001 (Statistics Canada www.statcan.ca,
Cat. No. 97F0011XCB2001004).

Socio-economic Conditions

Until fairly recently, the economy of the Inuit was based on subsistence
hunting and hunting for furs, whale blubber, and other commodities
sought for by the European and North American markets. In the 1920s,
large shoals of cod were discovered in the coastal waters of West
Greenland and the economy was transformed into a cash economy.
After the cod had all but disappeared, shrimp became the major export
item. In other regions, fossil oil and minerals form the basis of the
modern cash economy. Although there are few full-time hunters,

Table 7.3   Selected demographic and socio-economic indicators of Inuit population in Alaska, compared with all-race populations of Alaska and the United States

	Alaskan Inuit	Alaska	United States
Median age (years)	22	32	35
% of population <5 years	10.6	7.6	6.8
% of population <18 years	43.4	30.4	25.7
% of population 65+	5.2	5.7	12.4
Education: % population aged 25+			
with high school graduate or higher	69.6	88.3	80.4
with bachelor's degree or higher	5.0	24.7	24.4
Income			
Median household income	$33,398	$51,571	$41,994
Per capita income	$10,838	$22,660	$21,587

Source: 2000 Census (U.S. Census Bureau http://factfinder.census.gov).

leisure time hunting is widespread both as a pastime and to provide an important supplement to the diet.

The Inuit living in their traditional regions are generally less well educated and less affluent than their fellow citizens in the southern parts of their respective countries and than the southerners living in the North (see table 7.3). Nevertheless, the socio-economic development since the 1950s has been significant. Modern, well-insulated houses with piped water and sewage as well as electricity have almost entirely replaced the small stone-and-turf or wooden houses of poorer quality.

Inuit communities do vary in terms of their economic well-being across regions. In Canada, the mean community well-being (CWB) index – a composite index of education, housing, and employment (see chapter 3) – was 0.67 for Nunavik, 0.70 for Nunavut, 0.72 for Labrador, and 0.73 for the Inuvialuit region. All Inuit regions had scores lower than the 0.80 for non-Aboriginal communities in Canada. However, the gap had closed between 1991 and 2001.[8] Within the Canadian North, the distribution of CWB scores among Inuit communities was very similar to that of Dene communities (see fig. 8.2 in chapter 8).

Health Patterns

Many health problems are common to Inuit in the circumpolar North. There are, however, significant differences, not only among the Inuit in

Table 7.4   Estimates of Inuit mortality by cause in Alaska

Census area	Cancer	Heart disease	Unintentional injuries	Suicide
North Slope (66%)	221.9	136.9	107.1	36.1
Ratio area/state	1.2	0.7	1.8	1.8
Northwest Arctic (81%)	196.5	187.1	101.3	75.8
Ratio area/state	1.0	1.0	1.7	3.7
Nome (75%)	227.0	166.4	125.6	77.5
Ratio area/state	1.2	0.9	2.1	3.8
Wade Hampton (87%)	260.8	211.3	81.8	70.7
Ratio area/state	1.4	1.1	1.4	3.4
Bethel (80%)	199.1	179.9	97.2	37.2
Ratio area/state	1.0	1.0	1.7	1.8
Alaska state all-races	192.6	188.7	58.8	20.5

Note: Mean of 2000–4, age-adjusted to U.S. 2000 population. Percentage in parentheses refers to Inuit population as proportion of total all-races population in the census area, according to 2000 Census. The Inuit population as a proportion of the Alaska Native population ranged from 93% to 98% in these areas.
Source: Alaska Department of Health and Social Services, Bureau of Vital Statistics (www.hss.state.ak.us/dph/infocenter).

Greenland, northern Canada, Alaska, and Chukotka, but also within individual regions. Living standards, and with them health and disease patterns, are subject to local conditions as well as to the economic and political framework of the four states in which the Inuit live. There is no readily available compendium of 'pan-Inuit' health indicators. Information about the health of the Inuit comes from official statistics and scientific studies. The routinely collected health statistics, however, differ among countries and over time as to how the Inuit are defined as an ethnic group. Indeed, in most jurisdictions, statistics are not generally available for ethnospecific groups.

In Alaska, all indigenous peoples are combined into one group as Alaska Natives. Except for a few disease registries (namely, cancer and diabetes), mortality and morbidity data are not available for Inuit separately. However, the Inuit make up the vast majority of Alaska Natives in certain jurisdictions and such regional data can be used as surrogate Inuit data. Data can be aggregated by service areas of the federal Indian Health Service (IHS), Alaska boroughs, and Census

Figure 7.2   Trend in life expectancy at birth of Canadian Inuit compared
with all Canadians

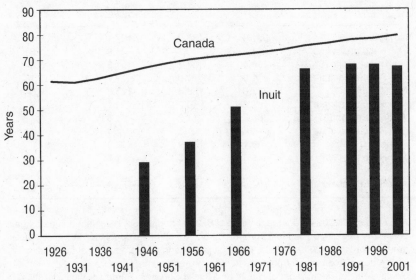

Source: Based on unpublished data by R. Wilkins, Statistics Canada.

areas (used by the state health department), or Native regional corporations. Such boundaries do not coincide and most serve a mixed
Native population. For example, the Barrow Service Unit of IHS, the
North Slope Borough, and the Arctic Slope Regional Corporation serve
a predominantly Inupiat population in the north of the state. The
Yukon-Kuskokwim Service Unit of IHS, the Wade-Hampton Census
Area, and the Calista Corporation serve a predominantly Yupik population in communities in the Yukon-Kuskokwim basin. Table 7.4 presents mortality data from five Alaskan census areas with large Inuit
populations.

   In Canada, health statistics on Inuit are available for the Northwest
Territories and Nunavut, although in routine publications of the territorial health departments, ethnospecific data are generally not provided. In Nunavut, which is 85 per cent Inuit, and in Nunavik in
northern Quebec, which is 90 per cent Inuit, regional data can essentially be interpreted as Inuit data. In the rest of the country, no health
data for Inuit are available.

Figure 7.3   Health expectancy for Greenland Inuit

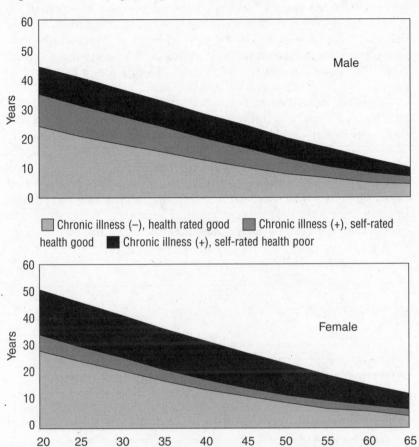

Source: Based on data in Iburg, Brønnum-Hansen, and Bjerregaard (2001).

Based on health expectancy as an overall measure of health status, the Inuit have experienced considerable progress, although substantial disparities still exist. The trend for the Canadian Inuit is shown in figure 7.2. The most impressive improvement occurred between the 1940s and 1980s, when life expectancy at birth among the Inuit more than doubled. At the end of the twentieth century, life expectancy was still some twelve years shorter than Canadians nationally, comparable to that of Canada in the 1950s.[9] In Greenland, almost 90 per cent of the population is Inuit and some routine statistics, including mortality statistics, are available separately by place of birth, with persons born in Greenland being a reasonably valid indicator of Inuit ethnicity, at least among the older generations. With time, this provides a less and less accurate approximation of Inuit-specific data.

Traditional measures of health such as life expectancy are based entirely on mortality and therefore do not reflect the full spectrum of health. In a study of the Greenland Inuit's combined life expectancy with survey-derived measures of self-rated health and the presence of chronic illness to produce a 'health expectancy' (fig. 7.3), it can be seen that, especially in the older population, as much as 60 per cent of their life could be spent in poor health or suffering from a long-term illness or disability.[10] Inuit health issues are more prominent and discussed in greater detail in most of the chapters that follow. Health care delivery for Inuit is discussed in the regionally focused chapters on Greenland, northern Canada, and Alaska.

NOTES

1 For simplicity, we use the spelling 'Inupiat' and 'Yupik' rather than the linguistically more correct 'Iñupiat' (singular 'Iñupiaq') and 'Yup'ik.' Within Alaska, the term Eskimo is often used by Alaska Natives themselves, and it appears in official publications. One hardly ever hears the term Inuit being used in Alaska. In Russia, *Eskimosy* is the official term used. The common belief that 'Eskimo' is an Algonkian Indian term meaning 'eater of raw meat' has no linguistic basis (see Damas 1984:7).

2 Historically important anthropometric data series, such as those collected by Franz Boas and Aleš Hrdlička in the nineteenth and early twentieth centuries, were reanalysed by Ousley (1995). Szathmary and Ossenberg (1978) analysed twenty-four discrete cranial traits collected from eighteen indigenous populations in Siberia and North America. Cavalli-Sforza, Menozzi, and Piazza (1994:99) constructed several genetic trees in the mammoth *History and Geography of Human Genes*. For a review of blood groups, immunoglobulins, and other classical markers among Native Americans, see O'Rourke (2006).

3 The three-wave theory of Greenberg, Turner, and Zegura (1986) was highly influential and also highly criticised. Szathmary (1993) provided a

comprehensive re-examination of the anthropological genetics of Aboriginal North Americans. For the multiple-migration view, see Torroni et al. (1992) and Schurr (2004); Mulligan et al. (2004), Zegura et al. (2004), and Merriwether (2006) argued in favour of a single migration.

4 Tables of mtDNA haplogroup frequency data on indigenous North Americans and Siberians can be found in Starikovskaya et al. (1998), Lorenz and Smith (1996), and Merriwether, Rothhammer, and Ferrell (1995). For NRY data, see Zegura et al. (2004) and Bosch et al. (2003).

5 For a discussion of the contemporaneity of Dorset and Thule cultures, see Friesen (2004). McGhee (1996) offered an overview of the archaeology and prehistory of the Palaeo-Eskimos.

6 These estimates, based on ethnohistorical research and the archaeological record, were aggregated by Ubelaker (2006) from various archival sources.

7 See Campbell (1997) for detailed description of Eskimo-Aleut languages. Note that there are actually two more branches of Yupik once spoken in Siberia – Naukanski and Sirenikski, after the villages of Naukan and Sireniki in Chukotka. These are now extinct. Siberian Yupik is more properly called Central Siberian Yupik, or Chaplinski, after the village of Chaplino.

8 See the report by Senécal and O'Sullivan (2005). The report and the statistical database are available from the Department of Indian and Northern Affairs website: www.ainc-inac.gc.ca/pr/ra/pub4_e.html.

9 Inuit data are for 1941–50, 1951–60, 1963–6, 1978–82, 1989–93, 1994–8, and 1999–2002. Data for 1941–82 are from Robitaille and Choinière (1985) and refer to Inuit in the then Northwest Territories; 1989–2002 data are from unpublished data by R.Wilkins of Statistics Canada, which refer to 'Inuit-inhabited areas' in the Northwest Territories, Nunavut, Nunavik, and Labrador.

10 Based on Iburg, Brønnum-Hansen, and Bjerregaard (2001). Life expectancy computed from 1991–5 life table, self-rated health and chronic illness data obtained from the 1993–4 Greenland Health Interview Survey. Five categories of self-rated health were collapsed into two: 'very good' and 'good' into 'good,' and 'fair,' 'poor,' and 'very poor' into 'poor.' Chronic illness refers to long-standing illness, sequelae from injury, disability or complaint that lasted six months or more.

8 Dene

KUE YOUNG

Dene (or Den'a or Dine, depending on the language) is a self-designation term, meaning 'the people.' This group is usually referred to by anthropologists as Athabascan (or Athapaskan or Athabaskan) Indians, a linguistic classification. Dene is now the term preferred by some indigenous organizations, especially in Canada – for example, the Dene Nation, which represents various First Nations in the Northwest Territories. The homeland of the Dene is referred to as Denendeh. For the purpose of this book, Dene will be used to refer to all Athabascan-speaking people in northern Canada and Alaska.[1]

Geographical Distribution

The Dene have a wide distribution throughout North America. There are three main branches: the first are the Northern Athabascans, speaking some twenty-three languages. Their homelands range from the Alaska Pacific coast, across the interior of Alaska, Yukon, the Northwest Territories, the northern parts of the Canadian provinces of British Columbia, Alberta, Saskatchewan, and Manitoba, to the western shores of Hudson Bay. Included in this group are the Tsuut'ina (formerly Sarcee), who are found today in southern Alberta, just outside the city of Calgary. The second branch are the Pacific Coast Athabascans, who include riverine tribes between Washington State and northern California and who speak some eight languages. Finally, the Southern Athabascans are found in the American south-west. They speak seven languages and include such well-known tribes as the Navajo and Apache, believed to have migrated to their present location only within the past 500 to 1,000 years or so.[2]

This chapter focuses solely on the Northern Athabascans within Alaska, Yukon, and the Northwest Territories. They occupy a variety of terrains – mountains, plateaus, and valleys. The dominant ecological feature is the boreal forest or taiga, punctuated by swamps, lakes, and rivers. Towards the east, it is mostly barren grounds, which merge into the tundra. Two major river systems traverse the Dene territory – the Yukon River, which drains into the Bering Sea, and the Mackenzie River, which drains into the Arctic Ocean. The Northern Athabascan habitats can be grouped as follows:

1 The lowlands of the Mackenzie River basin, where groups such as the Gwich'in (formerly Kutchin or Loucheux), Slavey, Tlicho (formerly Dogrib), and Dene Soun'liné (formerly Chipewyan) reside today in the Northwest Territories.
2 The Cordilleras, the south–north mountain chain that extends from British Columbia through the Yukon into Alaska, occupied by the Northern and Southern Tutchone, Kaska, Gwich'in, Han, Upper Tanana, and Tanacross.
3 The Yukon-Kuskokwim basins, inhabited by the Koyukon, Dene Hit'an (formerly Ingalik), and Tanana.
4 The Cook Inlet–Susitna River basin, where the Dena'ina (Tanaina) – as the only maritime-based Athabascan culture – can be found.
5 The Cooper River basin in south central Alaska, the homeland of the Ahtna.

Historically, the Dene existed as small bands of 25 to 100 people. Such bands might split up or coalesce, depending on game availability and the need for larger cooperative efforts. Named groupings are often taxonomic devices used by anthropologists and ethnolinguists, and are not 'tribes' with any implied degree of political organization and integration. Until recently there has not been any regional identity beyond the community. This changed with land claims negotiations and settlements in both Alaska and Canada. There are now state and territorial-level organizations (e.g., the Tanana Chiefs Conference in Alaska, the Sahtu Dene Council in the Northwest Territories), as well as cross-border ones, such as the Arctic Athabaskan Council and the Gwich'in Council International, both permanent participants of the Arctic Council, an intergovernmental organization of Arctic states.[3]

Traditional Subsistence

The traditional Dene livelihood is based on hunting and fishing, supplemented by gathering berries. The species harvested depends on the locality. A wide range of animals and fish are found in most regions: large game such as caribou, moose, and bears; smaller mammals such as rabbits, beavers, and muskrats; waterfowl such as ducks and geese; and aquatic species such as whitefish, pike, and trout. Muskoxen roam the barren grounds to the east, while mountain sheep can be found in the mountainous parts of Alaska and the Yukon. Riverine and coastal groups have access to salmon, and sea mammals (seals, sea otters, and sea lions) are hunted by the Tanaina. Subsistence activities revolve around seasonal cycles, which are dependent on fish and game migration (e.g., salmon, caribou), and families move among different camps at different seasons, which vary in size and composition.

The Dene adapted technologies from others in the same environment – for example, the Ingalik borrowed from the Yupik; the Ahtna constructed plank dwellings similar to those of the Tlingit; and the Tanaina used sea kayaks similar to the Yupik and Aleuts.

Genetic Affinities

The distinctiveness of the Dene as a people compared with other North American Indians and the Inuit is implicit in the three-migration model of the peopling of the Americas, purportedly based on linguistic, dental morphological, and genetic evidence. Under this scenario, present-day Dene (as part of a larger grouping called Na-Dene) are descendants of the second wave of Asian migrants, which took place perhaps some 5,000 to 10,000 years ago. Classical physical anthropological measurements of cranial and skeletal specimens have placed the Dene closer to the Aleut than to the Inuit. One mutation of the serum albumin gene *AL*Naskapi*, originally found in an eastern Algongkian Indian sample, is unique in being present only among members of the Algonkian- and Athabaskan-language families, albeit in relatively low frequency (<5 per cent). It has been suggested that the mutation probably originated in the north-western coast of North America in some ancestral group of these two language families.[4]

Of the four mtDNA haplogroups found among indigenous peoples in the Americas, haplogroup A was the most prevalent group among the Dene, at least in the few groups such as the Dogrib for whom data are available and among whom the frequency exceeded 90 per cent, with the remainder being group C, while the others are absent altogether. Even among their southern kins, the Navajos and Apaches, haplogroup A is still present in some 50 to 60 per cent of individuals. There are mtDNA variants which are specific to the Dene: 16129 A, which is shared with all other New World populations; 16129 T, which is shared with the Chukchi and Inuit; and 16331 G and 16233 G, which are specific to the Dene and Tlingit. Such data have been used to support multiple migrations, although the counter-argument was that the separation of ancestral groups sharing these mutations could have occurred prior to, or after, a single migration. Within the multiple-migration camp, mtDNA data have been used to support the Dene-as-second-wave model, while others proposed that the Dene and Eskimo-Aleuts entered together as part of a third wave. All dated the Dene's entry as after the Last Glacial Maximum when the ice-free corridor was already open.[5]

Interestingly, in 1999 an 'ice man' was found in a glacier in the area bordering Alaska, the Yukon, and northern British Columbia. It was dubbed *Kwäday Dän Ts'ìnchi* by the local Champagne-Aishinhik First Nation (meaning 'Long Ago Person Found'). Molecular analyses of bone and muscle tissues revealed that the DNA from the frozen human remains belonged to haplogroup A. His clothing was radiocarbon-dated to about 500 years ago.[6]

History and Politics

European explorers came to Dene regions in the eighteenth and nineteenth centuries. The fur trader Alexander Mackenzie travelled down the river that now bears his name (but is called Dehcho by the Dene) and reached the Arctic Ocean in 1789. In Alaska, the first European explorers who came into contact with the Dene were Russians. In 1833, the Russian-American Company established a post at the mouth of the Yukon River and began penetrating the interior. In the 1840s, the explorations of Lavrentiy Zagoskin resulted in the compilation of valuable ethnographic and linguistic information. Russian traders soon followed.

Life among the Dene underwent slow but significant changes after contact, with new material goods and technologies brought by traders and new religions introduced by missionaries. Most groups remained relatively isolated and had limited interactions with the external world until the 1950s. The anthropologist June Helm, writing primarily about the Mackenzie region, identified a general pattern in the changes effected by external influences:

1 first direct contact with an entering European into Dene territory often had little immediate impact;
2 trade activities, either through other indigenous groups acting as middlemen or directly with European traders;
3 hostilities, usually between indigenous groups, exacerbated by the European presence; these are rarely directed at the Europeans. European-initiated hostilities towards the Dene were generally limited to the Russian occupation of Alaska;
4 introduction of epidemic diseases;
5 arrival of missionaries and subsequent Christianization;
6 shock intrusion of non-indigenous settlers and others – examples include the various gold rushes, influx of homesteaders, and the growth of towns and cities;
7 initiation, and later, proliferation of government services in the areas of education, social welfare, health care, economic development, and so on;
8 advances in transportation – in the nineteenth century the two great river systems of the Mackenzie and Yukon greatly facilitated trade, travel, and settlement; in the twentieth century, it was the highways and, most importantly, air travel, that sustained the North.[7]

The Dene experienced colonization by the Russians (later Americans) and British (later Canadians) in their traditional homelands in Alaska and northern Canada. Formal treaty agreements ceding their lands were never signed in this vast territory, with the exception of Treaty No. 8 (1899) and Treaty No. 11 (1921). Treaty No. 8 involved only a small portion of the present Northwest Territories, south of the Hay River and Great Slave Lake. Treaty No. 11 covered much of the Mackenzie basin in the western part of Northwest Territories. The land in the area was deemed unsuitable for agriculture, and the Canadian government had shown little interest in concluding treaties there until 1920, when oil was discovered at Norman Wells.[8]

Land claims became a major political issue in both Alaska and northern Canada in the 1950s and 1960s. In Alaska, the landmark

Alaska Native Claims Settlement Act of 1971 settled land-ownership disputes between the federal and state governments and the indigenous inhabitants (see further discussion in chapter 4). In a departure from the Indian reservation system in the rest of the United States, for-profit, land-owning Native regional corporations were created to manage the resources of the land and promote the economic and social well-being of their 'shareholders,' the indigenous peoples. Two of these corporations (Ahtna and Doyon) covered exclusively Athabascan territory. Others (Cook Inlet, Chugach, Calista, and Bristol Bay) have varying mixture of Athabascan, Eskimo, Aleut, and Tlingit populations.

In Canada, the federal government entered into land claims and self-government negotiations with First Nations. This long drawn-out process has, since the 1990s, resulted in a series of final agreements with regional Dene groups in the Northwest Territories – with the Gwich'in in the lower Mackenzie and delta area in 1992; the Sahtu Dene and Metis in the central Mackenzie basin and around Great Bear Lake in 1993; and the Tlicho (Dogrib) in 2003. In the Yukon, the approach involves negotiations between the federal and territorial governments with individual First Nations, under a territory-wide umbrella final agreement signed in 1993.

These various land claims and self-government agreements have ushered in a new era in Dene history and have provided a framework that allows them to control to a large extent their own affairs and the resources on their lands. The implementation of these agreements remains fraught with uncertainties, and considerable obstacles still exist for the Dene to achieve full social and economic development.

Population and Languages

It is not an easy task to estimate the size of the Dene population in Alaska, Yukon, and the Northwest Territories. While the United States Census can identify an individual as 'American Indian and Alaska Native' (AIAN) under race, ethnic, or ancestry group, with further distinctions as to tribal affiliation, many AIAN individuals choose not to provide the latter information.

The 2000 U.S. Census identified 119,241 AIAN in Alaska: 36,301 Indians, 46,733 Eskimos, and 10,695 Aleuts. Among 'Indians,' 14,546 reported to be Athabascan either alone or in combination with some other group. However, this is likely an underestimate. An alternative

Figure 8.1   Age–sex structure of Dene population compared with all
Canadians

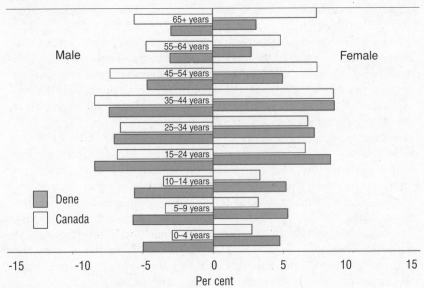

Source: Census of Canada 2001 (Statistics Canada www.statcan.ca,
Cat. No. 97F0011XCB2001004).

approach is one based on residence, where Indians residing in census
areas that fall within traditionally Athabascan territory are counted as
Athabascans. In practice, this amounts to considering all Indians living in
the Alaskan panhandle as Tlingit and Haida, and those in the rest of the
state as Athabascans. Using this method, the total count is 16,353, excluding the Indian population of Anchorage. As Anchorage is a melting pot
of Alaska Natives from all over the state, only a portion, although likely
a majority, of its Indian population (8,449) can justifiably be considered
Athabascans. Thus, as a rough estimate, the Athabascan population in
Alaska in 2000 could be somewhere between 14,500 and 24,000.

The Canadian Census of 2001 counted 6,175 people in the Yukon
and 11,950 in the Northwest Territories who reported North American
Indian origins. As all Yukon First Nations and all but one indigenous
community in the Northwest Territories are Dene, the combined population of Dene in northern Canada is about 18,000.[9]

Table 8.1   Estimated number of speakers of Northern Athabascan languages in
Alaska, Yukon, and the Northwest Territories (NWT) in the late 1970s*

Language	State/ Territory/Province	Estimated speakers
Koyukon	Alaska	700
Holikachuk	Alaska	25
Ingalik	Alaska	100
Tanaina (Dena'ina)	Alaska	250
Ahtna	Alaska	200
Upper Kuskokwim (Kolchan)	Alaska	130
Lower Tanana	Alaska	100
Tanacross	Alaska	120
Upper Tanana	Alaska	250
Han	Alaska, Yukon	30
Gwich'in (Kutchin, Loucheux)	Alaska, Yukon, NWT	1,200
Tutchone	Yukon	450
Tahltan-Kaska-Tagish	Yukon, British Columbia	350
Chipewyan	NWT, Alberta, Saskatchewan, Manitoba	5,000
Slavey**	NWT, Alberta, British Columbia	5,000
Dogrib	NWT	2,000

*Other Northern Athabascan languages found outside the northern territories include
Tsetsaut, Babine, Dalkelh (Carrier); Tsilhqot'in (Chilcotin); Sekani and Dunneza
(Beaver) in British Columbia; and Dunneza and Tsuut'ina (Sarcee) in Alberta.
**Slavey (or Slave) can be divided into South Slavey and North Slavey, which also
includes Bearlake and Hare. Tutchone can be divided into Northern and Southern
Tutchone. Yellowknife is considered a dialect of Chipewyan.
Source: 1979 data from the subarctic volume, Handbook of North American Indians
(Krauss and Golla 1981).

As with most other indigenous populations, the Dene population is a
young one (see fig. 8.1). In the Canadian North, 33 per cent of the Dene
population in 2001 were children under the age of fifteen (compared
with 19 per cent for all Canadians), and 6 per cent were aged sixty-five
and over (compared with 13 per cent of the national population). In
Alaska, the Athabascan Indians in 2000 had a median age of twenty-five
years, compared with the Alaska-all races median of thirty-two years.

As stated earlier in this chapter, Athabascan is primarily a linguistic
label. Athabascan belongs to the larger group called Athabascan-Eyak.
Eyak is a single language that used to be spoken near the mouth of the
Copper River in southern coastal Alaska – only one speaker is believed
to have been alive at the end of the twentieth century. Eyak and

Table 8.2   Selected socio-economic indicators of Dene in Yukon and the Northwest
Territories compared with Canada

Proportion (%) of adults aged 15 and above	Dene	Canada
With less than high school graduation	50.5	31.3
Employed	52.8	61.5
Income under $10,000	37.8	27.6
Income $40,000+	19.0	24.1

Source: 2001 Canada Census (Statistics Canada www.statcan.ca,
Cat. No. 97F001XCB1051, 97F001XCB1053, 97F001XCB1048).

Athabascan probably split around 3,500 years ago. Some linguists
group Athapaskan, Eyak, Tlingit, and Haida into a 'superfamily' of
Na-Dene. However, the practice is not universally accepted.[10] The
Smithsonian Institution's subarctic volume of the Handbook of North
American Indians recognizes twenty-three distinct Northern Athabascan languages. Of these, sixteen are found within Alaska, the Yukon,
and the Northwest Territories (see map 3).

The number of speakers of Athabascan languages has suffered a
relentless decline. Table 8.1 provides an estimate from 1979. Most of
the languages with fewer than 500 speakers were considered precari-
ous or even moribund then, and those with less than 100 clearly on the
verge of extinction. Two decades later, an assessment by the Alaska
Native Languages Center documented a continuing decline, with no
group within Alaska having more than 500 speakers.[11]

In Canada, during the 2001 Census, some 17,000 individuals
declared an Athabascan language as their mother tongue, of these
about 5,000 resided in the Yukon and Northwest Territories. Excluding individuals who reported 'Dene' or did not specify the language,
the languages with the most individuals reporting to be their mother
tongue were Dogrib (1,835), South Slavey (1,030), North Slavey
or more specifically Hare (830), Gwich'in (310), and Chipewyan
(300).

Socio-economic Conditions

The socio-economic disadvantage of Dene in terms of education,
employment, and income is evident in table 8.2, which compares all
Canadians with the combined First Nations population of the Yukon
and Northwest Territories. The mean community well-being index

Figure 8.2   Distribution of Aboriginal communities in the Canadian North
with non-Aboriginal communities in Canada by community well-being score

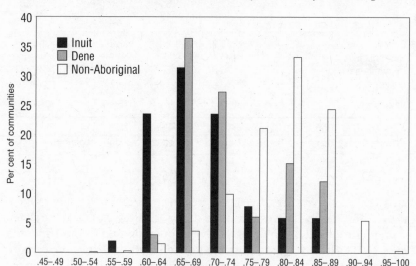

Source: Community well-being index database (Indian and Northern Affairs
Canada www.ainc-inac.gc.ca/pr/ra/cwb/db_e.csv).

(combining education, income, housing, and employment – first discussed in chapter 3) for Dene communities in the Canadian North was
0.74 (0.79 in the Yukon and 0.74 in the Northwest Territories), lower
than the 0.80 for all communities in Canada. The disparities are more
evident in terms of the distribution of communities (fig. 8.2). The Inuit
and Dene distributions generally overlap.

   In Alaska, among individuals who self-identified as Athabascans in
the 2000 U.S. Census, 73.8 per cent have high school graduation or
higher, compared with the state-wide proportion of 88.3 per cent. The
median household income was $29,196, considerably less than the
$51,571 for Alaska as a whole.

Health Patterns

It is difficult to construct a pattern of the major health conditions
among the Dene, even within a single jurisdiction, let alone one that

Table 8.3 Estimates of Athabascan Indian mortality, by cause, in Alaska

	Yukon-Koyukuk Census Area	Alaska State – all races	Ratio
Cancer	203.7	192.6	1.1
Heart disease	165.6	188.7	0.9
Unintentional injuries	173.2	58.8	2.9
Suicide	70.4	20.5	3.4
All causes	988.3	818.4	1.2

Note: Mean of 2000–4, age-adjusted to U.S. 2000 population.
Source: Alaska Bureau of Vital Statistics (www.hss.state.ak.us/dph/infocenter).

crosses national borders. In Alaska, health statistics are usually broken down into Alaska Natives versus all others, or all residents in the state, with no further division of the Native population into Eskimo, Indian, and Aleut. However, it is possible to use health statistics for certain service units of the Alaska Area Native Health Service, which serves primarily Athabascan communities (e.g., the Interior Service Unit). The state health department's vital statistics bureau also reports causes of death statistics by census area. There is one census area, the Yukon-Koyukuk area in the interior, whose population was about 70 per cent Native, of whom 95 per cent were Athabascans. Table 8.3 provides some mortality data for this census area.

In Canada, prior to the transfer of health care responsibilities from the federal to the territorial governments (see chapter 3), health statistics from Yukon and the Northwest Territories were reported separately for Inuit, Indians, and others. Since the 1990s, such reports are no longer publicly available. At best, some tables within reports provide data separately for Aboriginal and non-Aboriginal. Ethnic-specific health data are available for a few diseases, namely, cancer and diabetes, for which registries exist. The low rates of diabetes among Dene relative to other Native Americans in southern Canada and the lower-48 are discussed in chapter 16. Within Alaska, the Indian rate tends to be higher than the Eskimo one.

As for cancer, Alaska Indians (further breakdown into Athabascans, Haida, and Tlingit is not possible) are at an elevated risk. With all cancer sites combined, Alaska Indian men had 2.4 times the incidence of New Mexico Indians, and 1.2 times that of whites in the United

Figure 8.3   Standardized incidence ratios of selected cancer sites comparing Dene in the Northwest Territories and all Canadians

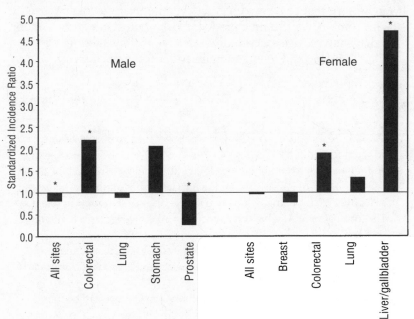

Note: Bars marked with an asterisk are statistically significantly different from 1.0 (p<0.05), indicating higher or lower risk among Dene compared with all Canadians.
Source: *Cancer in the Northwest Territories 1990-2000* (Northwest Territories Health and Social Services 2003).

States. For women, the ratios were 2.8 and 1.5. The largest differences were primarily in cancers associated with tobacco use.[12]

In the Northwest Territories, the cancer burden among Dene differs from that of Inuit and non-Aboriginal people. Among Dene men, colorectal cancers were commonest (35 per cent), followed by lung (19 per cent) and prostate and stomach (7 per cent). Among Inuit, lung cancer accounted for 25 per cent, followed by stomach (16 per cent). Among women, the distribution by sites is quite similar between Dene and Inuit, with breast and colorectal cancer equally common (22–24 per cent each), followed by lung (16–19 per cent). Figure 8.3 shows the risk of selected cancer sites relative to the Canadian population nationally. It can be seen that Dene men had an overall lower risk of cancer with all sites combined and a much reduced risk of prostate cancer. Among sites that showed an excess among Dene was colorectal cancer in both men and women, and liver and gallbladder for women.[13]

NOTES

1 In 1997, the Tanana Chiefs Conference based at Fairbanks, Alaska, adopted Resolution 97-35 designating *Athabascan* as the correct spelling and requesting that other entities follow that policy. In respect for that resolution, the Alaska Native Language Center has adopted Athabascan as its preferred spelling, which will also be the spelling used in this book. The international Athabaskan Arctic Council, however, uses a different spelling.

2 For further discussion of the archeology, history, languages, and culture of Athabascans, see the subarctic volume of the *Handbook of North American Indians* (Helm 1981).

3 More information about the Arctic Athabaskan Council can be found online at www.arcticathabaskancouncil.com and the Gwich'in Council International at www.gwichin.org. A chronology of Dene historical highlights is provided in the Dene Nation website, www.denenation.com.

4 Greenberg, Turner, and Zegura (1986) are the originator of the three-migration model in the pre-genomics era. Ousley (1995) reviewed the historical literature on the relationships between Amerindians, Eskimos, and Aleut. Szathmary and Ossenberg (1978) created dendrograms based on craniometric data and classical genetic markers. Smith et al. (2000) studied the Naskapi mutation. The genetic distance between Dene and other Amerindians has also been demonstrated in the distribution of HLA class II alleles and haplotypes (Monsalve, Eden, and Devine 1998).

5 See Merriwether, Rothhammer, and Ferrell (1995) for mtDNA haplogroup frequency data in the Dogrib, and Zegura et al. (2004) for NRY data from the Tanana. Schurr and Sherry (2004) and Torroni et al. (1992) offered different versions of the multiple-migration model. Starikovskaya et al. (1998) identified those mtDNA sequence variants specific to the Dene and other populations.

6 DNA analyses were reported by Monsalve et al. (2002). The 'ice man' was turned over to the Champagne-Aishihik First Nation for reburial.

7 Helm (2000) assembled and updated her lifelong studies on the Dene in the Northwest Territories.

8 Fumoleau (1975) provided a detailed historical account of Treaties 8 and 11.

9 Canadian and U.S. census statistical data can be accessed from the website of Statistics Canada (www.statcan.ca) and the U.S. Census Bureau (www.census.gov).

10 The concept of Na-Dene originated with the noted anthropologist Edward Sapir in 1915. Over time, the meaning of the term varied. A stricter grouping includes only Athabascan-Eyak and Tlingit. Adding Haida to the family is more controversial. See Campbell (1997) for a more mainstream view. Some 'lumpers' even attempted to link Na-Dene with Asian languages, for example, into something called 'Dene-Caucasian' – see, for example, Ruhlen (1994). The use of Na-Dene is particularly prevalent in discussions on the origins of North American Indians, influenced by the three-wave migration theory.

11 The 1997 estimates are from the Alaska Native Languages Center, based on Krauss (1997), available from www.uaf.edu/anlc/stats.html.

12 Kelly et al. (2006) is one of the few papers among the many on Alaska Native cancer epidemiology that provided data specific to Indians. New Mexico Indians are unusual in the country in having a very low prevalence of smoking.

13 See Northwest Territories Department of Health and Social Services (2003).

9 Sami

SVEN HASSLER, SIV KVERNMO, AND ANDREW KOZLOV

The Sami are the indigenous people of Scandinavia. 'Sami' is the name used in self-designation, by and large replacing the term 'Lapp,' which is of Finnish origin and now regarded as derogatory. In older studies and in official documents until the 1980s, 'Lapp' was most often used.[1]

Geographical Distribution and Population

The Sami homeland, Sápmi, today stretches over the northern regions of four countries – Norway, Sweden, Finland, and Russia (fig. 9.1). It extends from the fjords along the North Atlantic coast of Norway in the west to the Kola Peninsula of Russia in the east. It encompasses a wide variety of terrains, including coastal flats, mountain ridges and plateaus, dotted by lakes and criss-crossed by rivers and streams. From the treeless tundra in the north, the vegetation cover thickens and grows into the boreal forest to the south. The territory had contracted considerably in historic times – during the first millennium AD it covered much of central and southern Scandinavia and extended as far southeast as Lake Ladoga in present-day Russia.[2]

It is extremely difficult to estimate the population of the Sami in the Nordic countries, as ethnicity has not been identified in censuses or population registries since the 1970s. Various estimates give a range of 60,000 to 110,000 in the four countries. Table 1.1 uses the estimates of 60,000 for Norway, 36,000 for Sweden, and 10,000 for Finland. Of the total 106,000 in Scandinavia, 89,000 reside in the northern regions as defined in this book. We do know that in Russia there were exactly 1,991 self-identified Sami in the 2002 Census.[3]

Figure 9.1   Map of Sápmi, the Sami homeland in northern Norway, Sweden, Finland, and Russia

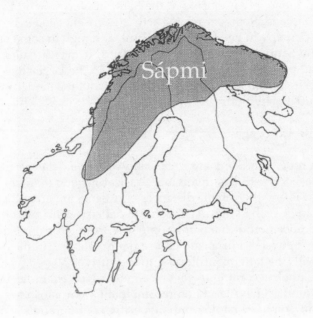

In Norway, about one-third of the Sami population live in Finnmark (Finnmárku) county, particularly in Kautokeino, Karasjok, Tana, Nesseby, and Porsanger municipalities. In Sweden, Sami are concentrated in various municipalities in Norbotten and Västerbotten, especially Jokkmokk, Arjeplog, Gällivare, and Kiruna. In Finland, the Sami region consists of the municipalities of Enontekiö, Inari, Utsjoki, and the northern part of Sodankylä, all within Lapland county (Lappi). In addition, the Skolt Sami, originally from Petsamo, were resettled in several villages in Inari after the Second World War when their territory was ceded to the USSR. Overall the Sami constitutes about one-third of the population of these municipalities, but it is only in Utsjoki that they constitute the majority.

Sami are engaged in a variety of livelihoods, depending on their locality, including farming, fishing, trapping, sheep and reindeer breeding and herding. Although considered as 'traditional' and a cultural marker of the Sami, reindeer herding was of relatively recent vintage, developing during the sixteenth century. It is a state-sanctioned monopoly exclusive to the Sami in Norway and Sweden, but not in Finland. Reindeer-related activities are engaged in by only a minority (perhaps 10 per cent) of the Sami, although in some regions, such as the Sami region in northern Finland, it may account for as much as 40 per cent. Today, many Sami live in the large cities, especially Stockholm and Oslo, and are involved in all the modern professions, occupations, and trades.

Origins and Languages

Within Europe, the Sami are genetically isolated relative to other groups. Based on studies involving classical genetic markers in the pre-genomics era, the genetic distances between Sami and other populations can be seen in figure 1.1. Some geneticists concluded that the genetic composition of the Sami population resulted from extensive admixture between European and Asiatic groups (from western Siberia), with the latter contributing to as much as 50 per cent of the Sami gene pool, according to some estimates. Newer studies involving mitochondrial DNA and non-recombinant Y-chromosomes found that certain common haplogroups (specific configurations of DNA variants) among the Sami are absent or very rare in Siberian Natives, but do occur in low frequencies in other European populations. Conversely, some common haplogroups among Siberians are not found at all among Sami. Yet another haplogroup, highly prevalent among Sami, is found widely distributed across Arctic Europe and Asia. A phylogenetic reconstruction based on such data suggested that the Sami are descendants of a narrow distinctive subset of Europeans with little evidence of gene flow from indigenous Siberian populations. A plausible route of migration into Fennoscandia was from western Europe via a detour through eastern Europe, which corresponded with archaeological evidence of the recolonization of the European north after the Last Glacial Maximum (end of the Ice Age).[4]

Sami belongs to the Finno-Ugric branch of the Uralic language family (see chapter 1). The closest linguistic neighbours of the Sami are Finnish, Karelian, and Estonian speakers. There are nine Sami dialects which are regarded as distinct languages by many linguists. These could be grouped into three main groups: South and Ume Sami in the

Southern Sami group; Pite, Lule, and North Sami in the Central Sami group; and Inari, Skolt, Kildin, and Ter Sami in the Eastern Sami group. The differences between them are profound, and other than neighbouring dialects, they are not mutually intelligible. It is estimated that half of the total Sami population speak at least one of the languages. The proportion of fluent speakers, however, has declined steadily during the twentieth century. North Sami is in the strongest position with the largest number of speakers, estimated at 15,000, followed by Lule Sami at around 3,000, while Ter, Pite, and Ume Sami are on the verge of extinction; the remaining Sami languages each have about 500 speakers. Depending on their location, the various languages have slightly different orthographies based on the Latin alphabet, except Kildin, which uses the Cyrillic alphabet.[5]

Much effort has been expended in sustaining the viability of the Sami languages. Today they are used in television, radio, and newspapers. There is an active literature and theatre. Education in Sami is available in all four countries, including a Sami college (*Sámi Allaskuvla*) in Kautokeino, Norway. Public services are available in Sami in certain municipalities in Finland and Norway where they are the majority.

History and Political Developments

Archaeologists identified the Komsa culture, which probably thrived in coastal Finnmark some 10,000 to 7,000 years ago, taking advantage of the receding and melting Fennoscandia icesheet. From 7,000 to 2,000 years ago, Arctic Norway was in its Late Stone Age, which was firmly based on the exploitation of marine resources (fish and sea mammals) although there was some reindeer hunting in the inland areas. The people lived in semi-subterranean houses, probably for extended periods and with some degree of social complexity. They also left behind rock engravings (e.g., in Alta Fjord) that document hunting, fishing, and various rituals. Major changes occurred about 2,000 years ago, which marked the beginning of the Iron Age in the region. The Kjelmøy culture of this era (in the vicinity of Varanger Fjord) is regarded by archaeologists as the direct antecedent of the Sami in historic times.[6]

There were early contacts with explorers and adventurers, and the Sami were known to the Romans in the first century AD. During the Middle Ages, the Sami were engaged in trading furs, but soon attracted the attention of the growing states of Norway, Sweden, and Russia (Novgorod). In the sixteenth and seventeenth centuries, Norwegian settlement began to spread northwards along the coast, establishing fishing villages. Russian influences (and the Orthodox Church) came from the east, while Swedish authority held sway inland to the south. These influences converged in the northern tip of Fennoscandia, where the Sami were subjected to taxation by two or even three jurisdictions at various times.

King Gustav Vasa of Sweden declared in 1542 that all unsettled land in the north belonged to the Swedish crown and no one else. His son, King Carl IX, worked hard to extend his power northwards in the early seventeenth century and titled himself 'King of the Lapps in the northern land' (*Lapparnas i Nordanlandens konung*). Christianization of the Sami was intensified in the sixteenth and seventeenth centuries, resulting in the majority of the Sami abandoning their old shamanistic religion. During the seventeenth and eighteenth centuries the Sami in Sweden and Swedish-ruled Finland were referred to as the 'tax-Lapp' (*skattelappar*) and they were obliged to pay tax for their use of land (*lappskatteland*) and mountains (*lappskattefjäll*).[7]

In 1751, a peace treaty between Norway (then part of Denmark) and Sweden (then ruling Finland) was signed, settling long-standing border disputes between the kingdoms. Appended to the treaty was the so-called Lapp Codicil, which guaranteed Sami cross-border movements for the purposes of reindeer herding and hunting, as well as other rights, while prohibiting them from being owner of taxable land in more than one country.

During the eighteenth century, the number of settlers started to grow and the need for more land and resources increased. The Sami became an obstacle for the expansion of 'civilization' and they were expected to assimilate. By the end of the nineteenth century, the Sami were outnumbered in many of the municipalities in Sápmi and conflicts over land, fishing, and hunting rights emerged between settlers and the Sami. Conflicts also appeared over issues such as language, religion, and other cultural matters.

During the latter part of the nineteenth century, the Sami were still considered a nomadic people who made their living from reindeer herding and, accordingly, were unsuitable for making a livelihood in other areas such as farming. The dominant Swedish view was reflected in a statement in a parliamentary session in 1907, 'The reindeer is made for the Sami and the Sami for the reindeer.' The connection between the two was considered to be so strong that herding was necessary for the survival of the Sami. The view that the Sami were to be kept as reindeer herders and as nomads resulted in a policy of segregation. Too much intercultural admixture was seen as a threat against the distinct Sami culture. These segregationist ideas were also expressed in school policies and the introduction of nomad schools with curricula suited for the nomadic lifestyle.[8]

The 'Sami should be Sami' policy of the Swedish government was clearly dualistic. It strived for segregation and assimilation at the same time. On the one hand, Sami were to be maintained as reindeer herders, while on the other, non-herding Sami were looked upon as a troublesome middle category between the Sami and the Swedes who should simply be absorbed into mainstream Swedish society. The most important instruments for implementing this Sami policy were laws regulating the right to breed reindeers in the late nineteenth century. It was also the first step towards giving reindeer herding the central position in the Sami policy while other aspects of Sami culture were marginalized. In 1928 this was stressed even more, when Sami other than reindeer herders were excluded from the Sami context and political demands outside the reindeer herding sphere were ignored. While earlier it was necessary to be a Sami in order to herd reindeers, it now became necessary to be a reindeer herder in order to be a Sami.

During the nineteenth century, across the border in Norway, 'Norwegianization' of the Sami was in full swing. From 1850 on, Norwegian was installed as the language of instruction (the banning of Sami in many schools persisted well into the 1950s). The *Land Act* of 1902 stipulated that property could only be transferred to Norwegian citizens, defined as those who could read, speak, and write Norwegian. Until the 1940s, proficiency in the Norwegian language was required to buy or lease state land for agriculture in Finnmark.

Early in the twentieth century, the beaver and wild reindeer population in northern Finland was depleted, and Sami used their land less and less. As a result taxes were decreased, and these were eventually repealed in 1924. However, the now non-tax-paying Sami were removed from land registers and their rights simply 'forgotten.' Some Sami founded homesteads like the Finnish settlers, but the state considered all land not owned privately as 'public.' In Finland, this land issue has been a major bone of contention, as Finnish law and the Finnish state do not recognize the Sami as having any special rights to public lands, which are open to all. Thus today, some 90 per cent of land in the Sami region remains 'public,' which can be used for reindeer herding.

Despite its remoteness, Sápmi was not spared the devastations of the Second World War. In 1944, the retreating Germans burned down much of Sápmi, and almost the entire Sami population in Finnish Lapland was evacuated to the south, creating considerable hardship. The scorched earth policy was also implemented in Finnmark, although some inhabitants managed to escape forced evacuation by hiding in the mountains.

In the post-war era of reconstruction, industrialization, and economic prosperity, the Nordic countries became the envy of the world, with their generous welfare state, advanced economy, and vibrant democracy. The nineteenth-century concept of the nation-state did not seem to have a place for the Sami as a distinct, indigenous people with special rights. Yet a monocultural and homogeneous 'homeland' (*Folkhemmet* in Swedish) no longer existed because of increased immigration and the influx of refugees, especially in Sweden. From successfully having avoided making politics out of the Sami issue, the Nordic governments now had to face more intricate questions of their responsibility towards the oldest ethnic minority in their midst.

The 1960s and 1970s witnessed the awakening of Sami activism and struggle for political rights. In 1979 the hydroelectric power project in Alta, Norway, which dammed and flooded traditional Sami lands and built roads that threatened reindeer grazing and calving, ignited Sami protests. On the political front, progress has been made. The Sami were granted some political influence through the establishment of Sami parliaments (*Sámediggi*) in all three countries: Finland in 1973, Norway in 1989, and Sweden in 1993. These assemblies are primarily consultative and advisory and are supposed to look after the interests of the Sami in a number of different matters, such as protecting the Sami languages and the usage of land and water for reindeer herding. There were symbolic milestones in the proclamation of the Sami anthem and flag in 1986 and Sami National Day (February 6) in 1993. The interest in old traditions, Sami languages, and cultural heritage has increased, not least among many young Sami and among Sami living in more assimilated areas. In Norway, the constitution was amended in 1988. Article 110a states: 'It is the responsibility of the authorities of the State to create conditions enabling the Sami people to preserve and develop its language, culture, and way of life.'[9]

Internationally, the Sami have also come to identify themselves with other indigenous populations around the world that have experienced colonialism. Among the Nordic countries, increasing contacts and collaboration between Sami movements across national boundaries culminated in the formation of the Nordic Sami Council in 1964. With the Kola Sami from Russia joining in 1992, the name was changed to the Sami Council. It has been active internationally in promoting indigenous peoples' rights and was a founding member of the World Council of Indigenous Peoples in 1975. It has sat as a permanent participant of the Arctic Council since its formation in 1996.

Health and Acculturation

The concept of acculturation offers a framework for explaining the health of the Sami population. Defined as culture change that results from continuous, first-hand contact between two or more distinct cultural groups, acculturation brings about social and psychological changes that in many circumpolar regions such as Sàpmi have been manifested in a variety of psychological and physical health problems. New diseases, changes of diet, accidents due to new technology, and new substances such as alcohol, tobacco, and drugs are all examples of possible health consequences related to acculturation. On a psychosocial level, changes in attitudes, culture, and identity may result in acculturative stress when original political, linguistic, religious, and social institutions become altered or new ones take their place. As health status linked to acculturation experiences in a culturally pluralistic society is expected to be better than in a culturally monistic one, which often pursues an assimilationist ideology, the outcome of the acculturative process is obviously dependent on the ideology of the dominant culture.[10]

One aspect of acculturation that the Sami shared with indigenous peoples in North America and other parts of the world is the removal of children from their families and communities and placing them in boarding schools located far away for extended periods of time. Such schools acted strongly as assimilation agencies by alienating children from their languages and traditional knowledge and skills, with long-term detrimental health consequences. The relationship between the boarding school experience and mental health is further explored in chapter 19.

Paucity of Health Data

An adequate description and understanding of the health of Sami is hampered by the lack of Sami-specific demographic and health data. Sami status is not identified in any of the health statistical reporting systems of the Nordic countries. Box 9.1 describes a research database that attempted to reconstruct the Sami population of Sweden from which epidemiological studies could be generated.

In a country such as Sweden, where its National Board of Health and Welfare (*Socialstyrelsen*) has identified the need to recognize and overcome health disparities between ethnic groups, the Sami are in fact not mentioned separately in any of its policy documents, nor in reports from the Institute of Public Health (*Folkhälsoinstitutet*).[11]

A national policy document titled *Health on Equal Terms* presented the future of public health in Sweden. Under the heading 'Ethnic Differences in Health,' the health situation of different immigrant groups was discussed but nothing was said about the Sami. In the Public Health Report of Sweden for 2005 (*Folkhälsorapport*), the distribution of health in the population was discussed under labels such as regional differences or foreign descent, while the health conditions of the Sami were only indirectly referred to in statements such as 'behind the regional differences, differences in culture and traditions could also be found influencing, for instance, the diet.'[12]

Knowledge of the health and living conditions of Sami is still very poor. Except for the government plan of action for health and social services for the Sami population in Norway, the establishment of the Center for Sami Health Research at the University of Tromsø, and the Sami-specific health service in Finnmark, there is a lack of other national initiatives with the purpose of studying and monitoring the health situation of the Sami. In the absence of long-term strategic initiatives, the available knowledge is anecdotal, which makes the overall picture defective and hard to capture. The poor interest in research on the health conditions of the Sami stands in stark contrast to the large number of scientific articles that have been published about the health issues of the indigenous populations in the U.S., Canada, and Greenland (see other chapters in this book).

Belatedly, there has been recognition that Sami-specific data are critically needed, and collaborative projects between government agencies and Sami organizations have been launched. For example, the Nordic Sami Institute (*Sámi Instituhtta*) is engaged in a joint project with Statistics Norway (*Statistisk sentralbyrå*) to develop a Sami Social Science Database with the capacity to collect Sami-specific social statistics. An extensive health survey of approximately 6,000 Sami in Norway has created possibilities of future knowledge of the health status and living conditions among Norwegian Sami.

Box 9.1 Creating a Swedish Sami population database

In order to facilitate health research on the Sami population of Sweden, Hassler and colleagues have created a Sami population database from several data sources, adopting a strategy that uses broad inclusion criteria to minimize the risk of excluding Sami who might satisfy one definition or another.[13]

As a starting point, they identified a group of 'index Sami' from:

1 the electoral register of the Sami parliament (*Sametinget*) – Swedish law stipulates that individuals who consider themselves to be Sami and speak a Sami language, or have lived in a Sami-speaking household, or have a parent or grandparent who spoke a Sami language, are entitled to vote,
2 the register of reindeer breeding companies, administered by the Department of Agriculture (*Jordbruksverket*) – the right to breed reindeer in Sweden is restricted to Sami who are listed in a previous official register of entitled breeders, or have forefathers who had this right, or are married to someone who has, and
3 the population censuses, conducted every five years by Statistics Sweden (*Statistika Centralbyrån*), identifies individuals who reported their occupation/source of income as reindeer herding or breeding.

Relatives (forefathers, siblings, and children) of non-duplicated individuals from these sources were then identified from the Swedish Kinship Register, a unique Scandinavian invention that is the envy of epidemiologists and geneticists worldwide.

This process resulted in a cohort of 41,721 Sami individuals who were alive at any time after 1941. For a given year, for example, 1998, the number of individuals alive totalled 36,000, which is twice as many as the official estimate of the Swedish Sami population.

Through electronic data linkage of this Sami population register with well-established national health databases (causes of death, hospital discharge, cancer registry), it was possible to investigate a variety of health events among the Sami and correlate them with various demographic, geographic, and socio-economic factors. The Sami can be further subdivided into reindeer herders and non-herders, not only as occupational categories but also as markers of 'acculturation.' For comparison, a non-Sami cohort was also assembled at a 4:1 ratio, matched on age, sex, and residence to the individuals in the Sami register.

Major Health Conditions

Life expectancy at birth was 74.9 years for Swedish Sami men and 80.0 years for Sami women, virtually identical to those of non-Sami men (74.6) and non-Sami women (80.3). When mortality rates for specific causes were examined, those of the Sami and their non-Sami neighbours were quite similar (table 9.1). This is in clear contrast to several other indigenous populations described elsewhere in this book for which the mortality statistics are largely unfavourable in comparison to that of the national populations. The similarities between the Sami and the non-Sami are probably a result of centuries of close interaction, mixed marriages, lifestyle similarities, and equal access to health care and social services.

In an international comparison, the overall health status of the Sami population appears to be good. Many of the health problems that Native populations in the circumpolar region and elsewhere face are not prevalent among the Sami, such as dramatic elevated risks for diabetes, cardiovascular disease, lung cancer, and various infectious diseases. There are generally small differences in risk for the major diseases and causes of death.

In Sweden, the mortality due to diseases of the circulatory system was significantly higher among Sami women than among their non-Sami neighbours. Sami men, however, showed the same risk of dying from cardiovascular diseases as non-Sami men (table 9.1). In Norway and Finland a lower risk for cardiovascular diseases among Sami has been observed.[14]

Among Swedish Sami, the mortality risk for acute myocardial infarction (AMI) was elevated among women, not men. In terms of

Table 9.1   Comparison of mortality rates for selected causes between Swedish Sami and non-Sami

Causes of death	SMR (Men)	SMR (Women)
All causes	0.99	1.09*
All circulatory diseases	1.00	1.12*
ischemic heart disease	1.01	1.17*
cerebrovascular disease	1.02	1.06
subarachnoid hemorrhage	1.60*	1.54*
Cancer	0.87*	1.06
Diabetes	1.17	1.23
Respiratory diseases	1.03	1.25*
Digestive diseases	0.89	1.15
All injuries	1.24*	0.89
vehicle accidents	1.31*	0.98
suicide	1.17	0.76

*95% confidence interval excluding 1.0 (i.e., 'statistically significant'); SMR >1.0 indicates risk of death among Sami higher than among non-Sami.
Note: SMR – standardized mortality ratio, comparing members of Sami cohort with a demographically matched non-Sami cohort (described in box 9.1); computed by the indirect method of age standardization with the non-Sami cohort as standard; deaths during 1961–2000.
Source: Hassler et al. (2005).

incidence, neither Sami men nor women showed an excess risk relative to non-Sami (fig. 9.2). The discrepancy between the mortality and incidence risks suggests that AMI may be underdiagnosed among Sami women or that the mortality is elevated due to long distances to hospitals. The latter seems less likely, since a similar discrepancy would also exist for Sami men. Moreover, if long delays between the occurrence of the AMI and hospital care is the main reason for the excess mortality one would expect higher mortality rates for the reindeer-herding Sami, who spend a considerable amount of time far from roads. Other studies have shown that long distances to hospitals are poorly associated with coronary mortality in Sweden.[15]

While the Sami were at similar risk of dying from stroke overall compared with non-Sami, for subarachnoid hemorrhage (SAH), a subtype of stroke, the mortality was 50–60 per cent higher among Sami (table 9.1). As none of the known risk factors for SAH such as alcohol, smoking, and hypertension were more common among the Sami, it is possible that genetic factors may play a role.

Figure 9.2   Incidence and mortality of cardiovascular diseases among
Swedish Sami compared with non-Sami

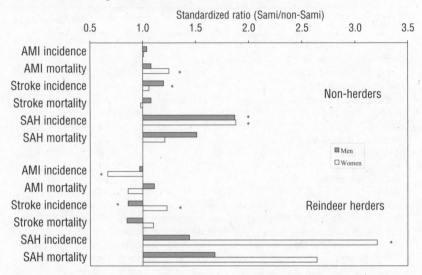

Notes: AMI – acute myocardial infarction; SAH – subarachnoid hemorrhage
Ratio refers to standardized incidence ratio (SIR) or standardized mortality
ratio (SMR), computed by the indirect method of age standardization with
the non-Sami cohort as standard.
Source: Based on data in Hassler (2005).

While the reindeer-herding Sami men had a reduced risk of developing stroke, non-herders displayed an increased incidence rate relative to their non-Sami neighbours. The reason for the higher incidence
rate of the Swedish non-herding Sami is obscure since they appear to
be similarly exposed to behavioural and biomedical risk factors (see
below). The explanation is perhaps related to the acculturation
process, which has affected the non-herding Sami differently from the
herding Sami. Nineteenth-century government policy restricted the
privilege of using the mountain areas for reindeer herding, fishing,
and hunting to a rather small group of Sami, while the majority was
expected to assimilate into the Swedish society. This segregation
policy left the non-herding Sami without possibilities of practising a
traditional lifestyle and culture despite their Sami origin. Whether
this discrimination has created psychosocial conditions that con-

tribute to the increased risk for cardiovascular diseases remains to be elucidated.

Other health problems among the Sami are discussed in further details elsewhere in this book: cancer in chapter 17 (box 17.1); injuries and accidents in chapter 18 (box 18.1); and suicide and mental health in chapter 19.

A possible interpretation of the Sami health situation in terms of acculturation could be that gradual integration of a traditional and modern life style and high living standards compared with other indigenous groups have helped to preserve protective factors for good health. Also, a high educational level among the Sami has contributed to a high level of accessing services and participating in public health promotion activities comparable to that of the general population.

Health Behaviours and Lifestyles

The Sami have undergone a dietary transition that accelerated during the second half of the twentieth century. The consumption of meat and fish has decreased while the intake of fruit and vegetables, and also sugar, has increased. Among Swedish reindeer herders, the modern diet contains less protein, zinc, phosphate, vitamin B12, and selenium and more carbohydrates than before. A Norwegian study, while also showing a similar trend in the intake of fruit, vegetables, and sugar, indicates that the Sami still consume a relatively large amount of meat, fat, and coffee. Reindeer meat contains large quantities of selenium but very little beta-carotene and vitamin C, factors which together could reduce the cancer risk; thus, a high intake of reindeer meat could contribute to the low cancer risk among the Sami. High consumption of wild fish and meat, rich in omega-3 fat, could also contribute to the reduced cancer risk (see box 17.1). The positive effect of a traditional diet is also found among young Sami. In a study comparing the diets of young Sami living in an inland community and a coastal community, the inland adolescents had larger iron stores, higher dietary intake of meat and protein, and lower intake of sugar than their coastal peers. The iron density in the diet may serve as an indicator of positive food habits and lifestyle in general.[16]

The National Health Screening Services of Norway observed that in the 1970s the prevalence of daily smokers was lower among the Sami than among the Norwegians in the same region. However, subsequent studies in the 1980s and 1990s, based on self-reported information, have not shown any difference in smoking habits between the Sami and the non-Sami.[17] (See also chapter 12.)

Small to no differences were observed in the alcohol consumption of Sami and non-Sami adults, even though reindeer herders in Finland of Sami origin were reported to drink more than their Finnish counterparts in the late 1980s. This reflects the common notion that a high consumption of alcohol is a characteristic of most men in the northern parts of Scandinavia, regardless of ethnicity and occupation. In a Norwegian study, it was indicated that adult Sami might have different drinking habits with a more episodic intake of alcohol compared with Norwegians. However, young Sami today appear to show less risk-taking behaviour as far as substances and drugs are concerned, in comparison with other young people in northern Norway. Young Sami also report their parents as less-frequent substance users compared with Norwegian peers. This was particularly the case for Sami mothers living in the inland areas where the Sami are the majority. Attachment to the Læstadian movement was one of the factors contributing to Sami adolescents' limited substance use.[18]

Although the reindeer-herding industry has been mechanized in recent decades, it is still a physically demanding occupation. In the past, most of the herding activities were done on foot or on skies, whereas today, they are carried out with motorbikes, snowmobiles, cars, helicopters, and airplanes. It is reasonable to suspect that the physical demands have changed during the last decades, possibly affecting the health condition of reindeer herders negatively.

Self-reported data from non-herding Norwegian Sami show that both men and women are more physically active during work, and report a higher level of overall physical activity, than non-Sami in the same region. However, Sami women were found to be less active during leisure time than non-Sami women. According to self-reported data, there seems to be no major differences in the level of physical activity between Swedish Sami and non-Sami.[19]

Among the Sami of Russia, smoking and alcohol use are very common. In a survey of fifteen-to-eighteen-year-old Sami in Lovozero in the Kola Peninsula, 59 per cent identified as regular or episodic smokers. Girls tended to smoke more heavily than boys – the average daily cigarette consumption was 8.4 for girls, compared with 6.4 among boys. Alcohol consumption in Murmansk Oblast was among the worst in Russia. In the same survey, half of Sami teens in that age group reported having used alcohol – 14 per cent at least four times in a month, and 3 per cent, five times or more.[20]

A Gender Perspective

An intriguing finding from studies on Sami health in Sweden is the differences between Sami men and women regarding cardiovascular diseases, particularly the risk for stroke, that could not be explained on the basis of the prevalence of traditional biomedical risk factors. This gender difference can be viewed in terms of a differential response to the acculturative process. Different effects of coping with the acculturation process could have influenced the health of men and women in different ways.

The reindeer-herding Sami women show lower intellectual discretion, decision latitude and social support at work, together with lower levels of physical activity. Such psychosocial and behavioural risk factors are related to increased risk for cardiovascular diseases, and women are known to be more sensitive than men to psychosocial risk factors related to unhealthy working conditions. Reindeer-herding women may have a more stressful working situation than the men, and they are more likely to report their quality of life as low. While the reindeer-herding men are responsible for the daily management of the reindeers, the women are typically responsible for service functions related to the reindeer business (e.g., providing food supplement to the reindeers, the vehicle transportation of reindeers, and meat management during slaughter), along with the responsibility for the household and the family's social network. To guarantee a reasonable family income in response to an insecure and variable profit from the reindeer-breeding business, it has become common for the women to also hold a regular part-time job. It seems conceivable that the increased responsibility for the household finances has further added to the unfavourable-risk-factor pattern among herding Sami women.[21]

Box 9.2 The Sami population in the Kola Peninsula, Russia

The Kildin (Kola) Sami population has been slowly growing since the 1930s (see table 5.4). In the 2002 Russian Census, there were 1,991 Sami in the country, 89 per cent of whom resided in Murmansk Oblast. However, the share of the total population of the region has drastically declined. Towards the end of the nineteenth century, the Sami constituted 20 per cent of the population of the Kola Peninsula. At the beginning of the twenty-first century, they were only 0.2 per cent. The reduction is partly a result of the heavy influx of non-Sami migrants from other parts of the Soviet Union whose labour was needed in the

mining developments of the 1920s, the nationalization and collectivization of reindeer herding, purges for alleged secessionist conspir-
acies, and forced relocations of Sami who stood in the way of hydroelectric power projects or military installations.[22]

According to the 2002 Census, about 38 per cent of Sami live in
towns and cities, a higher proportion than the average 28 per cent for
indigenous peoples of northern Russia. Despite the high level of
urbanization, there are no indications of ethnic assimilation in this
group. Since the dissolution of the Soviet Union, the Sami population
has been augmented by an increasing number of the offspring of
interethnic marriages identifying themselves as Sami.

A more detailed analysis of the population changes during
1969–2005 among the Sami living in Lovozero, the major centre of
Sami settlement, revealed the following:

Figure 9.3   Change in age–sex structure of Kola Sami, 1969–2005

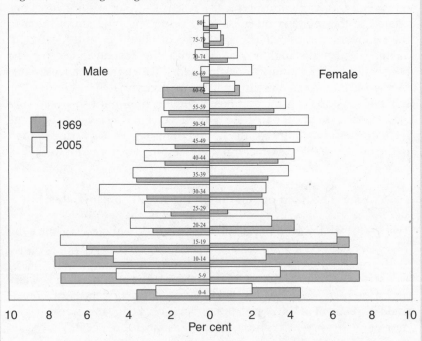

- At the end of the 1960s the age structure of the population showed a high proportion (38 per cent) of the population in the prerepro-ductive (0–14) age range. The high birth rate is characteristic of people in traditional societies.
- In the mid-1970s, the population structure began to transform, with a declining proportion of children and a corresponding increase in the proportion of the postreproductive cohort. By the end of 1985 this trend became more prominent. Net reproduction rate had decreased and the age structure of the population took on the rhomboid shape with a narrow bottom instead of a wide-base pyramid. By 2005, the proportion of children below fifteen was reduced to 20 per cent. The number of Sami over sixty years old has reduced sharply as a result of high mortality rate among males.
- The total Sami population in Russia between Census years 1989 and 2002 increased from 1,835 to 1,991 despite the number of deaths exceeding the number of births. Such a 'non-demographic' increase resulted from the addition of new members who had pre-viously not identified themselves as Sami. Note that this phenome-non is also seen in thirteen of twenty-six northern indigenous peoples of Russia, although not as pronounced as in the Sami (see chapter 5). However, the potential of such non-demographic gain is likely exhausted. A continuing low birth rate and a high death rate may lead to a sharp population decline of this ethnic group in the near future.

Socio-economic Conditions

Studies on Sami health indicate that traditional measures of socio-economic status do not correlate strongly with health outcomes.[23] Reindeer-herding Sami men do not appear to be disadvantaged with regard to cardiovascular risk, despite their having generally lower income and educational levels than their non-herding kin or non-Sami neighbours. However, Sami women show higher cardiovascular risks than their non-Sami counterparts, despite similar levels of education and income. Within reindeer-herding communities, socio-economic status is determined by occupational skills and family relations. The kind of apprenticeship used in the reindeer-herding management,

whereby elders teach the young skills of breeding and herding reindeers, is not part of the state educational system and therefore not
'counted' in official statistics. Furthermore, dietary habits are not much
influenced by the level of income since the basic elements of the Sami
diet, reindeer meat and fish, are the main products of their reindeer-
breeding businesses. The reindeer-associated lifestyle also contains
factors that could have positive effects on health, such as a high level
of physical activity, fresh air, and a high intake of dietary selenium,
zinc, and vitamin B.

It is increasingly recognized that community-level measures of social
well-being are important determinants of health. In a study in northern
Sweden, it was found that support of the Sami language in areas such
as Kiruna corresponded to an increased cultural production and thus
the building of social capital. Former discriminatory language policies
have most likely hampered development of civil society in the multi-
lingual region with negative effects on employment and well-being.
There are indications that revitalisation of the minority language has
positively affected socio-economic conditions.[24] In Norway, the Sami-
dominated Karasjok municipality, with its strong support of indigenous culture and language, has one of the nation's highest educational
level for women twenty-five to forty years of age.

The economic transition of reindeer herding into a modern industry
has created new stress, with its associated psychosocial effects, and
may also play a role in the high rates of work-related accidents. Box 6.1
provides a more in-depth analysis of Sami/non-Sami socio-economic
differences in northern Sweden.

Health Care Delivery

Norway is the only Nordic country which has a specific Sami focus on
public health for the Sami population, acknowledging the need for culturally and linguistically adapted health services. Although health and
social services for the Sami had been established in the 1980s, the first
national plan for health and social services for the Sami population
was made in 1995. As far as the Swedish and Finnish health care
system and public health policies are concerned, the Sami seem to be
nothing less than fully assimilated. A main reason for Norway being a
leading country can be explained by the considerable number of Sami
health and social services workers compared with the other Nordic
countries who advocated for an ethnic-specific health service.

In Norway during the 1980s, the first outpatient psychiatric clinic was funded in the Sami core area with Sami-speaking therapists. Several years later, an outpatient clinic with Sami clinicians provided services in internal medicine, rheumatology, and other specialties. These services are available to both Norwegian and Sami patients and are well used by both ethnic groups.

A Norwegian study on access to health care for minorities found that Sami women used the available drug and alcohol treatment facilities in northern Norway to a lower extent than other groups. In an effort to reduce the high suicide rates in the Karsjok region of northern Norway, a youth office was opened in the early 1990s where children and adolescents could meet and receive professional help and therapy. When the project was evaluated it was noted that the youth office was used mostly by girls. Whether the youth office actually reduced the number of suicides in the region could not be confirmed in the study. Another study compared treatment satisfaction and recovery in Sami and Norwegian patients treated in a psychiatric hospital. It concluded that Sami patients showed less satisfaction in terms of contact with staff, and the quality of information and treatment received. There was also less agreement between the ratings of the therapists and the Sami patients.

In another study of mental health service in the multi-ethnic population in northern Norway, it was recognized that therapists prescribed more sessions and more socially focused interventions when the clients were Sami, although the groups were similar in demographic and psychosocial characteristics. It was also concluded that clinics located in the high-Sami-density areas offered their clients more therapy sessions than in clinics in the low-Sami-density areas and that verbal therapy more often was used by the non-Sami therapists. In a survey of health care among 15,600 Sami and non-Sami aged thirty-five to seventy-nine in Northern Norway, the unilingual Sami participants were less satisfied with the primary health care than the Norwegians and also less satisfied with the physicians' language skills. Although frequent misunderstandings between the physician and the patient due to language difficulties were reported, approximately only two-thirds of Sami patients wanted to use an interpreter in the consultation.[25]

Preventive occupational health measures are critically important components of any Sami-focused health service in the major reindeer-herding regions. A Swedish study showed that the frequency and severity of musculoskeletal pain could be reduced through physio-therapeutic treatment, individual training, information dissemination, and technical improvements of the vehicles. In Finland, written guidelines aimed at preventing accidents and injuries in the reindeer-herding industry were found to be effective in almost halving the number of work-related injuries over a two-year period.[26]

NOTES

1 'Sami' is the preferred spelling over 'Saami' or other variants. In this book, the acute accent on the *a* is generally omitted but is retained in Sami words such as Sápmi or when referring to the proper names of Sami institutions. The Roman historian Tacitus refered to Sami as 'Fenni.' Some etymologists consider the Finnish term for Finland – 'Suomi' – as derived from 'Sami.'

2 Information on Sami history and culture in English is limited. Particularly useful are *The Sámi People* published by the Nordic Sami Institute (Solbakk 2006) and the English translation of Veli-Pekka Lehtola's *The Sámi People* (2nd rev. ed. 2004).

3 There is no single source of data on the Sami population in Scandinavia. The various Sami parliaments maintain voter lists based on linguistic, self-identity, and ancestry criteria. Box 9.1 describes a Swedish research project that combined electoral, kinship, and occupational databases. No similar efforts have been undertaken for the Norwegian and Finnish Sami populations.

4 Cavalli-Sforza, Menozzi, and Piazza (1994) computed and mapped genetic distances based on classical genetic markers (e.g., blood groups, enzymes, immunoglobulins, etc). For studies on the Sami involving DNA markers, see Kaessmann et al. (2002) and Tambets et al. (2004).

5 For an introduction to Sami languages (in English), see Sammallahti (1998).

6 See Hoffecker's (2005) primer on Arctic archaeology.

7 Much of the contents of this section on Sami history and settlement of the North is based on Swedish sources: Sjölin (2004), Ruong (1982), and Sköld (1998).

8 The Swedish policy during this period was discussed in Lundmark (2002) and Lantto (2000, 2004).

9 Information relating to Norway in this section is derived from the essay 'The Sami of Norway' by Wenke Brenna (1997). See also Helander (1992).

10 Berry (1985, 1990) applied the concept of acculturation to the health of circumpolar indigenous peoples.

11 See, for example, Socialstyrelsens 2000:3 and 11. Available online at www.sos.se/sosfs/2003_11/2003_11.pdf.

12 Socialdepartementet, 2000:91, available online from www.regeringen.se/ sb/d/108/a/2822; and Socialstyrelsen, (2005), available online from www.socialstyrelsen.se/Publicerat/2005/8707/2005-111-2.htm.

13 The methods of the database creation were described in detail, as well as two validation studies, in Hassler, Sjölander, and Ericcsson (2004), and in shorter form in Hassler's doctoral dissertation (2005) and in the study on causes of death (Hassler, Johansson, et al. 2005).

14 For data on studies in Finnmark, Norway, see Njølstad, Arnesen, and Lund-Larsen (1998), Tverdal (1997), Utsi and Bønaa (1998), and Thelle and Forde (1979). Studies on Finnish Sami were reported by Luoma, Näyhä, and Hassi (1995), Näyhä (1997), and Näyhä and Järvelin (1998).

15 Gyllerup et al. (1992) did find that mortality increased as distance from hospital increased, but the association was confounded by cold climate.

16 See Håglin (1991, 1999) for data on Swedish Sami dietary data and Nilsen, Arnesen, and Lund-Larsen (1999) for Norwegian data. Serum selenium levels were measured by Ringstad et al. (1991) and Luoma et al. (1992). Brox, Bjornstad, and Olaussen (2003) compared the nutritional status of adolescents in coastal and inland communities in northern Norway.

17 Spein, Kvernmo, and Sexton (2002) and Spein, Sexton, and Kvernmo (2006) reported on youth smoking behaviours from the North Norwegian Youth Study. Edin-Liljegren et al. (2004) obtained risk factor information from among Sami and non-Sami participants of a regional cardiovascular disease prevention program who were included in Hassler's Sami population registry described in box 9.1. Smoking data on Finnish reindeer herders are available from Reijula et al. (1990).

18 Alcohol consumption data are available for Finland from Poikolainen, Näyhä, and Hassi (1992); Norway from Larsen and Nergård (1990); and Sweden from Edin-Liljegren et al. (2004). Kvernmo (2004), and Spein, Kvernmo, and Sexton (2002) and Spein, Sexton, and Kvernmo (2006) discussed risk-taking behaviour among Sami youths in Norway. The Læstadian movement, which advocated strict abstinence, originated in the mid-nineteenth century and was founded by the Swedish Sami priest Lars Levi Læstadius.

19 Hermansen et al. (2002) provided physical activity data from the Finnmark Study. Swedish data are available from Edin-Liljegren et al. (2004).

20 Unpublished data by Kozlov.

21 See survey data reported by Edin-Liljegren et al. (2004). Amft (2000) described the living and working conditions of Sami herders. Hallman et al. (2001) reviewed gender differences in psychosocial risk factors.

22 A brief history of the Kola Sami in English was provided in Lehtola (2004). Demographic data are from the Russian Census and field surveys by Kozlov in Lovozero, reviewing the 'household books,' a type of population register kept by local authorities with detailed information on household members, including their ethnicity, family relationships, housing condition, occupation, and property owned, among other data.

23 See Salonen (1982) and Silventoinen et al. (2005) on the relationship between socio-economic differences and cardiovascuar disease risk.

24 The study by Winsa (2005) also included a minority Finnish dialect prevalent in some municipalities in the Swedish Torne valley.

25 The mental health care initiatives in northern Norway were reported and evaluated by Larsen (1992), Kvernmo (1995), Sorlie and Nergård (2005), and Mollersen, Sexton, and Holte (2005).

26 See Daerga, Edin-Liljegren, and Sjölander (2004) for the Swedish pilot study on musculoskeletal symptoms and Pekkarinen, Anttonen, and Hassi (1992) for injury prevention in Finnish herders.

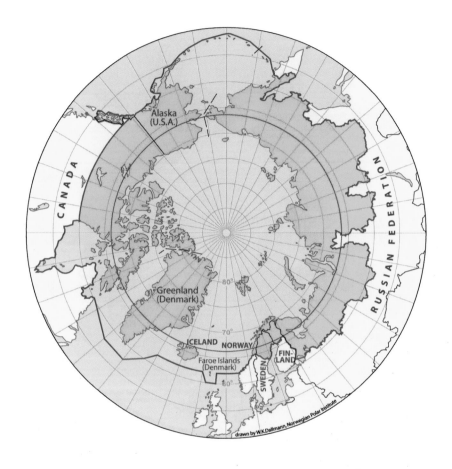

Map 1 Northern regions within countries bordering the Arctic Ocean

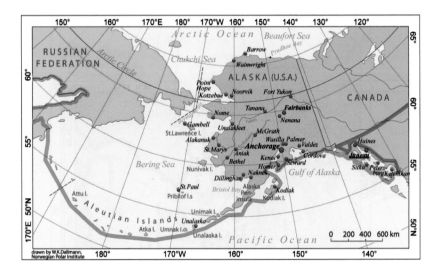

Map 6 Alaska

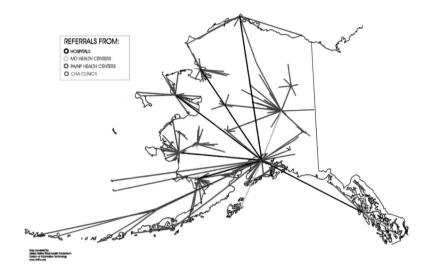

Map 7 Medical care referral patterns for Alaska Natives
Source: Reproduced with permission from the Alaska Native Tribal Health
Consortium, Anchorage, Alaska

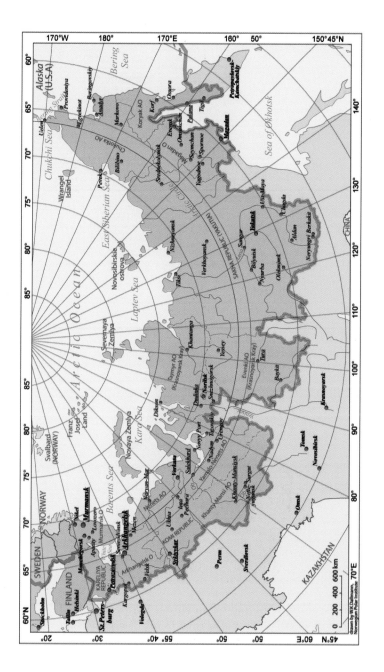

Map 8 Russia, showing northern territorial-administrative divisions

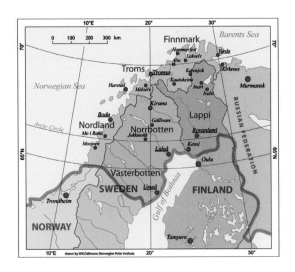

Map 9 Northern Scandinavia

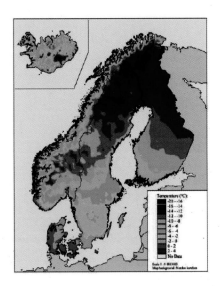

Map 10 Fennoscandia, showing mean winter temperatures
Source: Tveito et al. (2000). Reproduced from *Nordic Temperature Maps*, DNMI
Report 09/00 KLIMA, with permission from the Norwegian Meteorological
Institute, Oslo, Norway

PART THREE

Determinants

10 Environment and Living Conditions

PETER BJERREGAARD, JAMES BERNER,
AND JON ØYVIND ODLAND

As a health determinant, 'environment' is usually conceived of separately from 'biology' and encompasses all that is external to the human body. It is often further divided into the 'physical and social,' spreading out in expanding concentric circles that represent the home, the workplace, the community, and ultimately the entire planet. The influence of the environment on health has long been recognized, from Hippocrates' book *Airs, Waters, and Places* to the 1992 WHO Commission on Health and Environment and the 2007 report of the Intergovernmental Panel on Climate Change. The distinction between physical and social environment is arbitrary, as there are close interrelationships between human activity in all spheres and the integrity of the natural environment, which interact to influence the health of populations.[1]

The Arctic is often assumed to be a pristine, unpolluted area. It is true that there are few major industries in the sparsely populated Arctic, but scattered mining, oil, and gas projects under development may have a serious effect on the immediate environment. In the Russian Arctic, large-scale industrialization powered by coal has resulted in substantial pollution. One legacy of the Cold War is the abandoned Distant Early Warning (DEW) radar stations in Canada and the nuclear waste disposal sites in Russia. Also posing a threat to human health is invisible contamination by synthetic chemical substances, which are produced far from the Arctic but transported to the region by ocean and atmospheric currents and which are biomagnified in the marine food chain and bioaccumulated in humans.

Socio-economic Conditions

The association between socio-economic factors and health has been observed for a long time. A gradient across different socio-economic classes, no matter how such classes are defined, has been consistently demonstrated for various measures of mortality and morbidity, for individual diseases and all causes combined. This gradient exists in many countries around the world, and has persisted despite major improvements in the overall health and wealth of the population. The disparity in health status between indigenous peoples and the larger national population to which they belong has often been attributed to their poor socio-economic status or position.

The measurement of socio-economic status (SES) is not an easy task, as there are many unresolved theoretical and methodological issues that are beyond the scope of this book. It is, however, relatively simple to examine and compare various components of SES derived from the census or special surveys, even if we shy away from creating an all-encompassing SES index. In the early chapters of this book that discuss each Arctic region and specific population groups such as the Inuit, Dene, and Sami, extensive socio-economic data have been presented. In this chapter, specific studies in the Arctic that demonstrate the association between SES and health are reviewed. Among circumpolar populations as elsewhere there is a lack of knowledge about the mechanisms of how SES affects health.

The association of some of these SES indicators with self-reported health status can be demonstrated in many surveys. For example, in the Aboriginal Peoples Survey of 1991, Canadian Inuit, who reported excellent or very good health, tend to have a higher level of education. Those in the highest-income category are also more likely to report excellent health than others in lower-income categories. The association of education with good self-reported health was also found in the Greenland Health Interview Survey and it remained after controlling for age and sex. In all age groups, self-rated health was better among those with the longest schooling, and few reported long-standing illness.

In an ecologic study of forty-nine Inuit and Dene communities in the NWT, based on community-level data from the 1992 NWT Housing Survey and routinely reported health and social service agency data, there was a correlation between most housing and SES indicators with the rate of health centre visits used as a measure of morbidity.[2]

Concerning infectious diseases, it is well known from numerous studies from all over the world that poor socio-economic conditions are associated with high morbidity and mortality. Studies from the Arctic support these findings.[3] In Europe, the incidence and mortality from tuberculosis began to decline long before effective medical prevention (vaccination) or treatment (drugs) was available, and this decline can be attributed to improvements in housing and nutrition among other things. In the Arctic much of the decline in infectious diseases can also be explained by a general improvement in living conditions during the latter part of the twentieth century. The quality of the houses being built is superior to the stone-and-turf houses, heating is no longer by blubber lamps or coal stoves, and housing density, that is, the number of persons per room, is decreasing. This leads to less intense transmission of airborne diseases such as respiratory infections and tuberculosis. Improved sanitation and water supply is likely to reduce the number of gastrointestinal infections, hepatitis A, and skin infections. Periods of starvation will weaken a population's resistance to infections and their complications, and these previously common periods have disappeared altogether in Inuit communities.

Obesity, one of the more important risk factors for a variety of chronic diseases, including ischemic heart disease, diabetes, and hypertension, varies according to education level among Canadian Inuit. However, this relationship differs between men and women. In men, the more highly educated are more likely to be obese, while in women those who are less educated are more obese. Similar results were found in Greenland.

In general, Inuit men tend to show the pattern observed in developing societies, where obesity is more prevalent among those with higher SES. Inuit women are more characteristic of developed societies, where obesity is associated with a lower SES. The different sex roles in a rapidly modernizing population are most likely responsible for this phenomenon.[4]

At the population or ecologic level, social change or transition is also a powerful health determinant. During the second half of the twentieth century, Arctic regions and peoples were transformed into a modern society and thoroughly integrated into the global political and economic systems. This change is concurrent with observable secular trends in dietary patterns and levels of physical activity, the incidence and mortality rates of infectious diseases, chronic diseases, and injuries, and overall measures of mental and psychosocial health.

Inequalities and Discrimination

Studies have shown a significant impact of inequalities in income on health irrespective of the absolute income level. In Greenland, the distribution of income is becoming increasingly unequal, but there are no studies that relate this to health. Discrimination is another example of a social factor with a likely negative impact on health in the indigenous communities in the circumpolar north. During the latter half of the twentieth century, the influx of non-indigenous people into the northern communities was intense. The newcomers were skilled or professional people, who often stayed for a few years and never became integrated into the local communities. The general ideology was to help the indigenous people to develop a modern (i.e., Western) society, which placed the non-indigenous people in control and cast the indigenous peoples as humble recipients. Ethnic discrimination and mistrust was the inevitable result. It is possible but not proven that discrimination and lack of respect are causally related to the high suicide rates and alcohol and drug abuse in many circumpolar communities. This area is largely unstudied.

Health inequalities and disparities are also apparent among regions within the Arctic. The northern regions in the Scandinavian countries generally fare better in a variety of health indicators than those in North America and Russia. Within each country in Scandinavia, the 'north-south' disparity is also much less marked, or absent altogether. The health of the Sami (discussed in chapter 9) is substantially better than indigenous peoples in Alaska, northern Canada, Greenland, and Arctic Russia, which can largely be attributed to their similar socioeconomic positions relative to the non-indigenous population in the same regions. In Alaska and northern Canada, the non-indigenous population, in fact, has health status that is very similar to the total population of the country.

Work and Health

The psychological as well as the physical work environment exert a major influence on health. Classical work exposures like chemical substances, dust, cold, noise, and repeated movements are all present in the indigenous communities in the North along with lack of job control and high job demands. Yet few studies have been conducted there.

A major work-related factor in the indigenous populations is unemployment and underemployment. There are few jobs available, especially for unskilled workers. Among the Inuit, women tend to be more successful than men in their adjustment to the rapid societal changes. While many women were able to both continue their traditional roles as caregivers in the family and enter the labour market, the transition from hunter and sole breadwinner to wage earner in a subordinate position (or even as unemployed worker) was hard for men.

Reindeer herding among the Sami is associated with many hazards and a range of health problems, from musculoskeletal symptoms to fatal injuries, making it one of the most hazardous occupations in Sweden (see box 18.1). The industry is also increasingly mechanized, with the associated increased risk in vehicular accidents and decreased level of physical activity, both of which can have a negative impact on health.

Cultural Influences

While many indigenous peoples are economically less well off than their fellow citizens nationally, a fact which accounts partially for the disparity in health status, they are also 'protected' in some sense by the resilience of their culture. Culture affects health in many different ways. Among traditional cultures, there are many examples of how cultural beliefs and practices expose people to, or protect them from, diseases and injuries, including dietary customs, childcare practices, religious rituals, migration patterns, kinship relations, and medical therapies. In populations undergoing cultural change, health becomes affected when there is discrepancy between modern and traditional values. Conflicts at the cultural level can reinforce individual vulnerability and provoke disease among those already susceptible. When groups of people belonging to different cultures come into contact, one or both groups may undergo cultural change, a process often referred to as acculturation. This is particularly acute in the case of traditional cultures coming into contact with modern cosmopolitan culture, the experience of the Inuit in the circumpolar countries being a prime example. In responses to the stresses of acculturation, individuals and groups may develop coping strategies, building on their cultural repertoire. However, these stresses may be so strong and novel that the protection of traditional culture can be overtaken. The degree to which cultural identity has been retained by an individual or group during the process of cultural change can be measured in terms of variables such as proficiency in the Aboriginal language, participation in traditional cultural activities, and the consumption of foods 'from the land.'

The strength and viability of the Inuit language in Canada and Greenland is in stark contrast to the state of indigenous languages in Alaska and Chukotka and Athabaskan languages in Canada (see chapters 7 and 8). According to the Survey of Living Conditions in the Arctic (SLiCA), more than 70 per cent of Inuit in Canada and Greenland speak the indigenous language very well compared with only 40 per cent in Alaska and Chukotka. In Greenland, Greenlandic is the official language, and it is the primary vehicle of instruction in schools. In all age groups the majority speak Greenlandic, while Danish is spoken as a second language by 63 per cent of those below the age of sixty and by 22 per cent of those above.

The results of SLiCA indicate that the Inuit generally have a high participation rate in traditional activities, in particular subsistence hunting and fishing. In Canada and Greenland, 69 per cent of the adult population participated in fishing, while the proportion was even higher in Alaska and Chukotka. The high cost of imported foods and inadequate income mean that the nutritional value of country foods cannot easily be substituted and compensated in full. Subsistence and living off the land, besides the immediate nutritional benefits, promotes physical activity and enhances spiritual health. SLiCA results show that for about two-thirds of the surveyed households, locally harvested meat and fish make up at least half of the total meat and fish consumed, most in Alaska and least in Chukotka. The Inuit diet is covered in more detail in chapter 11. Note that country foods are also increasingly becoming expensive, in terms of capital expenditures on boats, snowmobiles, and guns, and the recurrent costs of fuel and ammunition.[5]

A survey of Yupik residents in six villages in the Yukon-Kuskokwim delta of Alaska found that those who reported living a more American lifestyle (called 'Kass'aq') reported experiencing greater psychosocial stress, less happiness, and greater use of drugs and alcohol to cope with the stress. The opposite was true for those who identified more with a traditional Yupik way of life and who tended to rely on religion and spirituality to cope with stress.[6]

Healthy Communities

Besides individual socio-economic and cultural factors, attributes of aggregates of individuals, that is, the community, are also important determinants of health. Studies have shown the influences of social relations, social capital, and social vitality of communities on individual health status. A healthy community can be characterized as a safe environment that provides opportunities for social integration and is neither conflictual, abusive, nor violent. Health promotion research has shown that community members' involvement in the social life and their shared pursuit of broader social goals through psychosocial processes can positively affect health. Research specific to the Arctic using such concepts and methods is only just beginning.[7]

The quality of communal life can be measured by such indicators as crimes reported to the police. However, such data are not often not available by ethnic group. The quality of community life is also a matter of perception. Public security as perceived by members of the community may not necessarily correspond to actual crime rates reported by the police. In the Aboriginal Peoples Survey, 21 per cent of Inuit claimed that they did not 'feel safe' in their community, and 9 per cent actually reported being physically assaulted. A variety of problems are identified as afflicting the community: alcohol abuse (58 per cent), drug abuse (49 per cent), suicide (41 per cent), family violence (44 per cent), sexual abuse (35 per cent), and rape (25 per cent).

On the positive side, the existence of a personal support network in the community was reported by 96 per cent of Inuit. A network is the web of social relationships which surround an individual. Members of a network provide emotional, financial, and other support to one another. In the epidemiologic literature, the relationship between social networks and chronic diseases, especially ischemic heart disease, is well established. Data specific to the Inuit or other Arctic populations, however, are not available. In remains to be seen if the concept of social network, based on work done in non-indigenous communities, can indeed be applied to Arctic indigenous peoples.

Housing Conditions

The indigenous peoples of the Arctic no longer live in the traditional houses of stone, turf, and whalebone, in skin tents or temporary shelters of snow or ice. In the towns, the majority live in apartment blocks or single houses with running water, electricity, and flush toilets, while housing conditions are generally considerably poorer in the villages. Historically, houses have been small and households large in order to strike a reasonable balance between comfort and the need for fuel for heating. Studies from the colonial period in Greenland estimated a housing density of 1–2 square metres per person, that is, households with on average seven to eight persons in houses of 10–15 square metres. In 1935–55, the houses had increased in size and the households decreased, resulting in an average of 3.5–4 square metres per person, and the development continued: 7.6 square metres in 1965 and 12.6 square metres in 1976, according to the official censuses of dwellings. These figures are for the Inuit; in 1976 the houses of Danes in Greenland offered 25 square metres per person, which was twice as much as for Inuit but still only half of the average space available per person in Denmark.[8]

By 2006 the housing situation had further improved in Greenland. Including both Inuit and Danes, the average size of dwellings had increased to 65 square metres and the household size decreased to 2.6 persons, or 25 square metres per person. This average, however, covers noticeable differences among towns and especially between towns and villages. The number of persons per room is another indicator for crowding; in Greenland there were 0.91 persons per room and in northern Canada the average size of an Inuit household was 4.3 with 0.8 persons per room.

The size of the dwelling relative to the number of inhabitants is, of course, only one aspect of housing quality. In Greenland, surveys in the 1990s showed that in towns about 50 per cent – and in villages, 72 per cent – of those interviewed complained of cold or cold floors. Furthermore, a technical review showed that about 20 per cent of all houses in villages in Greenland were in need of major repair, and that another 20 per cent were beyond repair. Waiting lists for dwellings are long.[9]

Among the Inuit, traditional heating was by burning blubber in a soapstone lamp. In Greenland, the introduction of stoves fired by shrubs, driftwood, and coal took place in the nineteenth century. In 1870, 38 per cent of houses in Greenland were furnished with a stove while the rest were heated by the traditional lamp, and by 1935 almost all houses were heated by a stove. After 1950, the coal-fired stoves were increasingly replaced by central heating.

All towns in Greenland and almost all of the villages have their own municipal electricity plant. Four towns are supplied with electricity and heat from hydroelectric plants and the potential for development is large. Currently, about half of the total energy produced in Greenland comes from these hydroelectric plants. The municipal power plants supply virtually all private households with electricity and a significant number with heat. The reliability of the power supply is very high in the towns – in the arctic climate a power breakdown of even a few hours will seriously affect public health and safety. The fuel for the power plant will quickly freeze, resulting in a permanent interruption of electricity supply, breakdown of heating and water supply, and a potentially disastrous situation. Almost all Inuit (95 per cent) households in northern Canada have electricity.

In Canada, during the 1950s, the Canadian government began experimenting with various forms of prefabricated houses that could be shipped to the arctic communities. In 1969 the last family in Igloolik in the Northwest Territories moved from a traditional house into one of these housing units. By 1990 all had central heating. Other Inuit communities in Canada and Alaska underwent similar housing development.

Homes in the Arctic are fully modernized in terms of telecommunications. Access to telephone services, including access to the Internet, and television reception have improved vastly. In Greenland, more than 98 per cent of the population now have full telephone services, including Internet access and GSM mobile phones.

Indoor air quality is an important health issue in the Arctic as elsewhere, and likely responsible for a high burden of respiratory illnesses. A housing and health survey in Cape Dorset, Nunavut, found that 25 per cent of children had been hospitalized at some time for respiratory illnesses. While NO_2 concentrations were within acceptable limits, there were reduced air change rates, overcrowding (with a median of six occupants per house), and passive smoking was present in 90 per cent of the homes. Particulates were found to be correlated with nicotine but not NO_2 concentrations, implicating tobacco smoking rather than leaky furnaces as the source.[10]

Water Supply, Sanitation, and Waste Management

To most inhabitants of Arctic towns, piped water is available all year round, flush toilets are present, and waste is removed and disposed of in the same way as in the south. In the villages, the situation is often very different. Freshwater may have to be carried a long way from lakes or may have to be melted from snow or ice, the 'honeybucket' is emptied outside and its contents removed by the dogs, which similarly dispose of (or rather, scatter) other types of waste. In Greenland, all towns and most villages have municipal water supplies all year. In the villages, water can be tapped at central locations all year round. The water comes from a nearby lake, a large tank which is filled regularly, or from desalination of sea water.

In Greenland, waste disposal and incineration appear not to be well controlled in towns and particularly in villages. It is possible that some town and village dumps cause significant contamination of the environment. The traditional way of waste disposal is an increasing problem as the population increases and as more and more non-biodegradable waste is produced.

Box 10.1 Freshwater in Canadian Inuit communities

There is an abundance of freshwater in the Arctic, contained in its rivers, lakes and icefields. The Canadian Arctic can boast of the longest river in the country (the 4,240 kilometre-long Mackenzie) and the largest lake that is entirely within its borders (Great Bear Lake, with a surface area of 31,000 square kilometres). Yet, for the inhabitants, this water supply is not readily available in sufficient quantity and quality.

Four systems are used in the delivery of water to individual homes (and also the disposal of sewage). In Inuit communities on the Labrador coast, water is generally obtained untreated from a lake or reservoir situated at high elevation, delivered by gravity via underground pipes to homes. In the large towns of Nunavut and the Northwest Territories, the utilidor system of above-ground pipes deliver water from municipal treatment plants. In most communities, tanker trucks are used to deliver water to storage tanks within buildings. In the smaller, more remote communities, the age-old individual-haul method brings water from surface or public sources. It has been estimated that Inuit consume less than the minimum standard of sixty-five litres per person per day as established by Health Canada. By comparison, the average Canadian consumes more than 300 litres per day. Water supply is a costly business in the North. The cost per 1,000 litres for Canadians nationally was $0.40, compared with almost $50 for Inuit!

In 2004, as part of the Nunavik Health Survey conducted on board the Canadian Coast Guard ship *Amundsen*, a survey of water use found that almost 30 per cent of the water consumed was 'raw' water obtained directly from rivers and lakes, and while the water itself may not be contaminated, the plastic containers in which they were carried often were.

Water issues are foremost environmental concerns in the communities, and many Inuit residents have reported personal experience within their lifetimes in dealing with changes in the availability of fresh water and their impact on health and well-being.[11]

Improved water supply and sanitation has been an important factor for the decrease in the incidence of a number of waterborne diseases such as gastroenteritis and dysentery. A general improvement of the housing conditions further contributed towards the reduced transmission of tuberculosis and acute respiratory infections. In the Northwest Territories in the 1980s, communities with low level of per capita water consumption, up to about 60–70 litres per person per day, reported high rates of skin and intestinal infections. There was also a linear (inverse) relationship between the rates of intestinal and skin infection and water tank size, another measure of the quantity of water used. These diseases occur more frequently among individuals served by a truck-and-honeybag system than those served by a truck-pumpout system (see box 10.1). In one community where a pipe/sewer system was in place, individuals served by the system had the lowest rate compared with the other methods involving trucking. For housing, rates of respiratory, skin and eye diseases were found to be higher in crowded houses (as indicated by household size and number of persons per bedroom). No relation was found with housing type (detached, movable homes, etc.) or tenure (government, private, rental). In a cohort of infants followed from birth for the first year of life, such housing and sanitation factors as public water supply, household size, persons/bedroom, and cleanliness of house were found to be associated with infant mortality, morbidity score, and the incidence of respiratory, intestinal, and skin infections.[12]

Environmental Contaminants

A number of persistent toxic substances (PTSs) are recognized as being responsible for adverse development and health effects in humans (see box 10.2). Examples of important substances relevant for the Arctic include pesticides such as the DDT-group, the HCH-group, and chlordane, and polychlorinated substances such as PCB-congeners. Focus has also been directed towards newer groups of contaminants because of their even stronger toxicity in laboratory models, for example the brominated flame retardants.PBDE, HBCD, and the PFAS-group.[13]

Box 10.2 Chemical abbreviations and names

To non-specialists in the field, the names and abbreviations of numerous chemical substances can be bewildering, but they are essential for communication. In fact, many have already entered into common everyday speech.

There are three groups of persistent toxic substances based on their origins, functions, and chemical structure. Those that are organic compounds are also referred to as persistent organic pollutants (POPs):

1 industrial compounds and by-products (each group or family may itself be comprised of up to several hundred 'congeners' or chemically related compounds):
   • PCBs: polychlorinated biphenyls, with 209 congeners
   • PCDDs: polychlorinated dibenzo-p-dioxins, or dioxins, with 75 congeners (i.e., closely related compounds yet with different properties)
   • PCDFs: polychlorinated dibenzofurans, or furans, with 135 congeners
   • PCNs: polychlorinated naphthalenes, with 75 congeners
   • PBDEs: polybrominated diphenylethers
   • PBBs: polybrominated biphenyls
   • PAHs: polycyclic aromatic hydrocarbons
   • PFAS group: perfluorinated alkylated substances
   • HBCD: hexabromocyclododecane
2 pesticides:
   • HCHs: hexachlorocyclohexanes
   • HCB: hexochlorobenzene
   • DDT group: dichloro-diphenyl-trichloroethane
   • Cyclodienes: include chlordanes, heptachlor, aldrin, dieldrin, and endrin
   • Toxaphene: a mixture of chlorinated bornanes (CHBs) and others

3 heavy metals:
- Hg: mercury
- Pb: lead
- Cd: cadmium
- As: Arsenic

The fetus and newborn child are especially sensitive to the toxic effects of many persistent heavy metals and organic pollutants found in the environment. These substances may exert their toxicity for decades because of resistance to degradation. Several of these substances move from mother to fetus via the umbilical cord and to the infant via breast milk. The levels of these contaminants in maternal blood during pregnancy give an indication of the potential risk to the developing fetus. Of special concern are the long-term, subtle effects that might influence reproductive health, pregnancy outcomes, reduced defence against diseases, delayed mental development, and an increased risk of cancer.

Many of the contaminants are accumulating in the Arctic because they are transported by air, ocean and river water, and ice drift. Most of them are lipid soluble and are stored in the fat of marine mammals. Their concentration increases with each step in the food chain and is very high in predatory species like seals, toothed whales, and polar bears. Generally, it is the coastal populations of the Arctic who have the highest concentrations of many contaminants, especially those who obtain a substantial proportion of their diet from marine mammals.

Since the early 1990s, several multidisciplinary international projects have been monitoring levels of PTS in Arctic populations and investigating their impact on human health. The most important is the Arctic Monitoring and Assessment Programme (AMAP) that started in 1991 and includes all Arctic countries (Canada, Denmark, Finland, Iceland, Norway, Russia, Sweden, and the United States). After its first report in 1998, AMAP evolved from mostly monitoring contaminant levels in biota and human biological samples to conducting comprehensive research on the sources of contaminants, especially dietary sources. It has also undertaken epidemiological and molecular effect studies on human reproduction and pregnancy outcomes, which are of special concern because most of the contaminants are 'hormonal mimics' or have carcinogenic potential.

Some effects have been shown but more research is needed to verify observations from the laboratory to human populations. Lead in placenta and maternal blood has a negative impact on birth weight, even at low levels. Lead is probably associated with delayed brain development in some risk groups. Mercury is associated with delayed brain development. High levels of contaminants from the DDT-group are associated with low birth weight. A change in the sex ratio of newborn children in the Russian Far East has been observed, and high maternal levels of PCBs have been implicated.

There are substantial regional differences within the Arctic in terms of human exposure and biological effects. The AMAP PTS Study of the Indigenous Peoples of the Russian Federation has filled in the last 'black holes' of information. The circumpolar blood study by AMAP describes the situation of Greenland and northern Canada as worrying in regard to organic contaminants and mercury. The Russian PTS-study reports high PCB-levels and regionally high concentrations of other contaminants, like the DDT-group, but more moderate levels of mercury. These findings point to possible local sources of contaminants in the Russian Arctic, as well as to long-range transport, while in the Canadian and Greenlandic areas it seems that the bulk of contaminants come from long-range transport.

Action must be implemented at many levels to prevent health damage by contaminants on humans. New epidemiological and laboratory research will increase our knowledge and provide recommendations for critical stages of life. Local contaminant problems, like the PCB-waste left behind in old military installations in the Russian Arctic and the local use of pesticides, must be cleaned up. Communities must balance the risks of contaminants with the nutritional benefits of country foods. A similar problem is connected to breast feeding – some scientists have discovered alarming levels of contaminants in breast milk and have started to recommend reduction in breast feeding without taking the undoubted psychological and nutritional benefits of breastfeeding into consideration. Risk management and communication go beyond the scientific process of risk assessment and involve complex policy decisions and actions that also take into account political, social, and cultural conditions operating within the affected population.

Climate Change and Health

The rapid changes in social factors, living conditions, and lifestyles in the Arctic since the mid-twentieth century have affected the health of its inhabitants. These factors will most likely be modified and their impact accentuated by future climate change. The Arctic is particularly vulnerable to climate change. Its low mean temperature and variations in available daylight have always required adaptive measures that have tested the ability of humans. The links between climate and human welfare may be especially close and clearly visible in Arctic regions where people live on the margins of human habitat. Repeatedly, human habitation has decreased due to climate change, from the disappearance of the first Palaeo-Eskimo cultures to that of the Norse in Greenland (see chapters 2 and 7).[14]

Over the next 100 years the average temperature of the earth is projected to increase significantly, glaciers and inland ice will melt, the extent of permafrost will decrease, the levels of oceans will rise, and heavy precipitation will increase, but at the same time areas affected by droughts will also increase, and the weather will be more extreme. Local and regional climate features are not well represented in the global climate models, but the models do predict higher than average rise in temperatures in most of the Arctic.[15]

Modern human societies have a high degree of resiliency in dealing with climate change, and it is next to impossible to predict health outcomes from macrolevel climate models. However, some likely scenarios can be presented. Impact mechanisms can be divided into direct – those due to the immediate effect of heat, cold, or ultraviolet (UV) radiation – and indirect, where climate change influences intermediate factors such as settlement structure and the availability of game, and the effects on human health come later. The direct effects of cold are discussed in detail in chapter 14.

Examples of indirect effects include the increasing risk of infectious diseases, especially those with insect vectors and animal or aquatic reservoirs, that is, zoonotic diseases. These diseases are threats within the Arctic as well. Unique to the Arctic are permafrost-dependent village sites, airfield runways, and sanitation infrastructures. Melting permafrost in these locations can destroy public health infrastructures and homes. Arctic wildlife, including animal species dependent on sea ice, form a significant part of some regional diets, and are often a critical part of traditional culture. Retreat of shore-bound sea ice makes hunting dangerous or sometimes impossible, and species survival may be threatened. Local knowledge, such as when a frozen river is safe to cross, may provide poor guidance as rapid Arctic warming makes later freezing and thinner ice a major cause of drowning in winter. Worldwide climate warming has the potential to increase transport of contaminants into, and in some cases, out of the Arctic. Research in contaminant transport pathways, and in rates and mechanisms of deposition and removal from the Arctic, are in progress. As yet these pathways are poorly understood.[16]

General warming and the disappearance of ice may also open new areas for hunting and fishing and introduce new species. Alaska Natives have noted Pacific salmon spawning in growing numbers farther north along the Bering and Beaufort Seas, and they can harvest these previously unavailable species. Moose have continued to extend their range northwards in Alaska as have beavers, whose damming of streams has attracted many more migratory waterfowl that are harvested by interior Alaska Arctic Natives.[17] The example in box 10.3 illustrates how climate change, through the appearance and disappearance of important species, has affected the socio-economic development of a local community.

Box 10.3 Fishing, migration, and climate change in a Greenland community

In Greenland, the shift from a traditional Inuit to a modern society started in the beginning of the twentieth century. Due to a warming climate, cod appeared in great shoals off the west coast. The traditional subsistence based on hunting of seals and whales began to make way for a modern cash economy based on the fishing industry. As a result, the population began to be concentrated in fewer and larger towns and the number of villages decreased. In the 1960s, however, a cooling climate along with overfishing resulted in the disappearance of the cod from the west coast of Greenland, but then at the same time, large numbers of shrimp were detected in Disko Bay. The shift from cod to shrimp fishing further changed Greenlandic society, which may be illustrated by the example of the village of Qasigiannguit.

From a population in 1955 of only 343, the village developed into a lively town centred around the shrimp factory. In 1982, when the population was at its maximum, it numbered 1,800 inhabitants. During the 1990s, the shrimp disappeared from the coastal waters and the factory had to be closed. People started moving away from the town and, in 2004, the population of Qasigiannguit was only 1,341, with an unemployment rate that was among the highest in Greenland: 14 per cent compared with 7 per cent in the towns in general.[18]

It is important to recognize that climate change is only one of the many factors influencing health and social change in the Arctic. Population movements from small villages to larger towns is as much the result of conscious political forces encouraging the population to move to towns with schools, health care, shops, and so on, as are changes in the physical environment.

The impending warming climate over much of the Arctic will result in many threats to the health of Arctic residents by different mechanisms. A critical component of public health practice in a warming Arctic is regional- and community-based environmental monitoring. A monitoring infrastructure can be based in observations of key environmental variables, both physical and biological, that monitors the threats, detects sentinel events (such as wildlife mortality rates), and monitors trends in wildlife population numbers and ranges. It should include locally critical measures, such as permafrost temperature and ice thickness in rivers. Regional authorities should collate, analyse, and disseminate local monitoring input. Village monitoring should be configured to meet local, regional, and national concerns and objectives.

NOTES

1 See the commission's report *Our Planet, Our Health* (WHO, Commission on Health and the Environment 1992). The third (2001) and fourth (2007) reports of the Intergovernmental Panel on Climate Change (IPCC) and associated documents can be found on its website, www.ipcc.ch.

2 Young and Mollins (1996) also used factor analysis to construct composite housing and SES indicators. SES, but not housing, was strongly correlated with health centre visits. When both housing and SES indices were included in multiple regression models to predict the rate of health centre visits, SES emerged as the stronger factor.

3 See, for example, Hobart (1975); Bjerregaard and Bjerregaard (1985); and Bjerregaard (1990).

4 The sociocultural correlates of obesity were investigated using data from the Keewatin health survey (Young 1996a).

5 The Survey of Living Conditions in the Arctic (SLiCA) is a circumpolar interview study of more than 7,000 indigenous people predominantly

from Inuit/Inupiat communities in Alaska, Canada, Greenland, and Chukotka. A summary of the results and over 500 tables are available online from www.arcticlivingconditions.org (Poppel et al. 2007).

6 The survey among Yupiks was reported by Wolsko et al. (2007).

7 For overviews of this rapidly growing field, see Taylor and Repetti (1997) and the text on social epidemiology by Berkman and Kawachi (2000). Data on Canadian Inuit from the Aboriginal Peoples Survey in Canada were originally presented in Bjerregaard and Young (1998:178).

8 Historical sources on housing in Greenland include Ryberg (1894), Bertelsen (1937), and Svendsen (1930). Contemporary data were cited in Bjerregaard and Bjerregaard (1985).

9 Housing surveys are regularly conducted by Statistics Greenland, see for example the 2005 report (Grønlands Statistik 2006). Reports from the 1990s are also available on the website, www.statgreen.gl.

10 The pilot study by Kovesi et al. (2006) involved a structured housing inspection, sampling and measurement of air quality, and administering a respiratory health questionnaire.

11 Information in this box is based on the *Environment Bulletin*, no. 3 (2005), published by the Inuit Tapariit Kanatami (ITK), especially articles on water management by Fandrick and the Nunavik water survey by Martin. ITK, the national Inuit organization, held a Sectoral Roundtable on the Environment in March 2005, which was devoted to discussion of water issues.

12 Michael (1984) conducted two studies, an ecologic one involving all communities in the NWT using official statistics, and a field study in three communities where more detailed information on individuals was obtained. The Perinatal and Infant Mortality and Morbidity Study (PIMMS) followed a cohort of 1,191 infants born during 1973–4 for twelve months (Spady 1991).

13 Much of the content of this section is derived from various AMAP reports, especially *Arctic Pollution Issues* (AMAP 1998), *Human Health in the Arctic* (AMAP 2003), and the Russian PTS-Report (AMAP 2004), all available on the AMAP website, www.amap.no. See also Odland et al. (2003), Odland, Sandanger, and Heimstad (2005), and the review by van Oostdam et al. (2005).

14 See McGhee (1996) on the probable effects of climate on Palaeo-Eskimo and historic arctic cultures.

15 The massive *Arctic Climate Impact Assessment* (ACIA) report released in 2005 (available online from www.acia.uaf.edu) summarizes the complex technical and scientific issues of climate change as they relate specifically to the Arctic.

16 See the special issue on climate change and health in the *International Journal of Circumpolar Health*, especially Parkinson and Butler (2005) on the impact on infectious diseases, Warren, Berner, and Curtis (2005) on infrastructure, and Kraemer, Berner, and Furgal (2005) on contaminants.

17 Welch, Ishida, and Nagasawa (1998) studied the northward shift of Pacific salmon. Other animal-related information and Native concerns about climate change is available from the Alaska Traditional Knowledge and Native Foods Database maintained by the Alaska Native Science Commission (www.nativeknowledge.org). Canadian Inuit's observations and views on climate change were reported by Nickels et al. (2005).

18 The case study was highlighted in Curtis, Kvernmo, and Bjerregaard (2005).

11 Diet, Nutrition, and Physical Activity

PETER BJERREGAARD AND MARIT JØRGENSEN

Considerable lifestyle changes have occurred over the past decades among indigenous peoples in the circumpolar region. Parallel to this has been a change in disease patterns, with an increase, for example, in cardiovascular disease and diabetes (see chapter 16). Among the main causes of such adverse transitions are alterations to the diet and levels of habitual physical activity, as the population shifts from their traditional hunting and fishing economy to more Westernized living conditions.

Diet and Nutrition

For many indigenous peoples in the Arctic, the traditional diet is not only a way of obtaining the necessary nutrients but it is also a social and cultural issue. For example, many Inuit feel that it is only the traditional diet of sea mammals and caribou that is sufficiently filling and able to keep them warm. More important, eating traditional food creates a sense of being Inuit and of adhering to the old values. Furthermore, it is a social act to eat traditional food together, which is comparable to having a cup of coffee at the office or a beer at the pub in Western societies. Strangers are sometimes judged by their willingness to eat traditional dishes and by how well they like the traditional food. A 'real' Inuk eats and appreciates traditional food, and asking Inuit about their food preferences is, therefore, more than merely a question of taste. It is probably more like asking whether people are proud of being Inuit.

In the Greenland Health Interview Survey in the early 1990s, participants were asked about their food preferences and to rate thirteen traditional Greenlandic food items and eleven store-bought items. The top quartile included four traditional items (muktuk, dried cod, guillemot, and crowberries) and two store-bought items (rye bread and potatoes), while the lowest quartile included one traditional item (seal liver) and five store-bought items – hamburger, pork chops, Danish pastry, chicken, and *medisterpølse* (pork sausage). Men and women agreed on their preferences, but the elderly were more fond of traditional food and less fond of store-bought food than the younger. In the eighteen to twenty-four year age group the preference for store-bought food was in fact similar to that of traditional food.[1]

A similar study among the Inuvialuit of the Mackenzie River delta shows that food preferences reflect the available species. The best liked food included dried caribou meat, bannock, caribou tongue, arctic char, beluga muktuk, and caribou meat, while the least liked food included white bread, wieners, canned luncheon meat, and meat balls with macaroni, but also seal and moose. For most food items there was little difference between adults and children, but children rated several store-bought food items higher than their adult counterparts.[2]

The species consumed by various Inuit groups show a wide variation according to the locally available resources. In Greenland, the eastern Canadian Arctic, and along the arctic coastline, marine mammals and in particular seal are the traditional staple. For some Inuit groups who live inland, caribou make up the greater part of the traditional diet, while the Yupik of the Yukon-Kuskokwim delta rely on salmon. In all regions the staple is supplemented with a variety of other mammals, fish, bird, and plant food such as berries and seaweed, although the plant food makes up a very small proportion in much of the Arctic.

The amounts of traditional food consumed varies considerably among population groups. In one Inuit community on Baffin Island, traditional food accounts for 33 per cent of the total energy intake. The species most frequently used on an annual basis in Baffin Island are ringed seal, caribou, and arctic char, followed by narwhal, shellfish, and walrus. Similarly, in another Inuit community, the species most frequently used are ringed seal, blue mussels, eiderduck, and arctic char.[3]

Recent dietary surveys have shown a sustained but decreasing consumption of locally harvested food. Men usually consume local food more frequently than women, and there is a marked age trend with young people consuming considerably less than older people. In

Nunavut, the Keewatin Survey in the early 1990s showed that the rate of daily consumption of meat from the land goes from 47 per cent in teenagers and 45 per cent in young adults to 65 per cent in middle-aged adults and 81 per cent in the older age group. The change from a traditional to a mixed diet is not a recent development. In Greenland, an estimated 83 per cent of the diet was traditional around 1900, a proportion that had decreased to 37 per cent by 1930, although this estimate is based on a questionable, indirect assessment. Since 1955 a gradual decrease has taken place with the most recent dietary surveys estimating the proportion of traditional food at less than 20 per cent. The ongoing Inuit Health in Transition Study will give detailed and comparable information about the diet of Inuit in Greenland, Nunavik, and Nunavut.[4]

Several studies of traditional Inuit food in Canada show that the density of most nutrients is superior to that of store-bought food. Calcium and vitamin A are the only two nutrients that occur in the traditional food in concentrations below the desired level. Special attention must be paid to dietary fat. The fat content of store-bought food is generally rich in saturated fatty acids, which are considered harmful to cardiovascular health while the fat of marine mammals and fish, which in most areas make up a substantial part of the traditional Inuit food, is believed to counteract the development of cardiovascular disease. It should also be mentioned that traditional food in contrast to store-bought food does not contain refined sugar and therefore beneficial for dental health.[5]

Among Yupik adults in western Alaska, traditional foods account for 22 per cent of energy intake overall, which varies by age, education, and geographic location. Those in the highest quintile of traditional-food intake consume significantly more vitamin A, D and E, iron, and omega-3 fatty acids compared with those in the lowest quintile, whereas vitamin C, calcium, and total dietary fibre has decreased.[6]

The discourse on traditional food is closely related to the contaminant issue (dealt with in chapter 10) and with the cultural issue. While there is no doubt that traditional food is important in a cultural and social context, the commonly expressed notion that traditional food is healthy and imported food is unhealthy is an over-simplification of matters. It is highly probable, although far from proven, that the fat of marine species is beneficial for cardiovascular health, but there is hardly convincing evidence that the large amounts of these fats in the contemporary average diet of the Inuit carries additional benefits compared with the modest amounts used in intervention trials. It is, furthermore, highly probable that mercury and other contaminants, which are part of the traditional 'dietary package,' are harmful especially to the unborn child. Imported food also has healthy and unhealthy aspects. While it is true that many Arctic residents favour refined sugar in junk food and beverages, and consume lard and fatty meat instead of vegetables, fruit, and pulses, to be unhealthy is not an inherent property of imported food but rather a result of dietary habits that can be changed.

In the Greenland Health Interview Survey in 1993–4, participants who did not eat traditional food on a daily basis were asked why. The most frequent reasons were a wish for dietary variation and that it was difficult and expensive to obtain traditional food. Only 1 per cent abstained from eating traditional food more often because of fear of pollution. In a separate study, qualitative analyses showed that Greenlanders know about a number of aspects of the risk of contamination of locally harvested food. However, this does not seem to have any great influence on their intentions towards choice of food because the positive perception of local food seems to outbalance the possible health-damaging effects of the pollution.

A high level of reliance on traditional foods is not restricted to the Inuit. In the mid-1990s, a major survey in eighteen Dene communities in the Yukon and the Mackenzie basin of the Northwest Territories was conducted in the summer and winter seasons to reflect the different seasonal foods available. On any given day, over 90 per cent of the participants in the Northwest Territories and 50 per cent of those in the Yukon consumed some land animal meats.[7]

It can be seen from table 11.1 that intake of specific species varies according to the season and is generally higher in the summer than in the winter. There are also gender differences, as men tend to consume more traditional fish, land animals, and birds than women. Intake is higher in the Yukon during the summer and in the Northwest Territories in the winter.

Dene children consume much less traditional foods than adults. In a survey of ten- to twelve-year-olds, traditional foods contributed on average less than 5 per cent of energy in their diets, most of which came from land animal meats. More than half of the energy intake

Table 11.1   Per capita traditional food use among Dene in Yukon and the Northwest Territories

	Summer		Winter	
	Female	Male	Female	Male
Northwest Territories				
Fish	113	109	64	91
Land animals	168	185	204	242
Birds	17	34	6	17
Plants	19	10	8	5
Total traditional foods	317	338	282	355
Yukon				
Fish	137	156	36	42
Land animals	230	256	136	150
Birds	9	14	3	4
Plants	19	13	8	4
Total traditional foods	395	439	183	200

Note: Per capita intake (in grams per person per day), derived from frequency of consumption over all participants (from food frequency questionnaire multiplied by median daily serving from 24-hour recall).
Source: Batal et al. (2005).

from market foods came from less nutrient-dense foods ('junk foods'). Overall, 50 per cent of children were below the estimated average requirement for vitamins A and E, phosphorus, and magnesium, while mean intakes were below the adequate levels for vitamin D, calcium, dietary fibre, and omega-6 and omega-3 fatty acides. Compared with those who did not, children who consumed traditional foods had significantly more protein, iron, trace elements (zinc, copper, magnesium, phosphorus) and vitamins (E, riboflavin, and B6) in their diet.[8]

Participants of focus groups conducted in two Dene communities in the Yukon and Northwest Territories reported witnessing variable changes in the climate that have affected their traditional food harvest. (The impact of climate change on health is discussed in chapter 10.) The appearance of new species and changes in migration routes have altered the food supply and changes in water levels have affected access to harvest areas.[9]

· Box 11.1 Food insecurity in northern Canada

A disturbing but increasingly common phenomenon in affluent, developed countries such as Canada is the appearance of food banks and breakfast clubs to cater to families and children without basic access to food, let alone a healthy diet. Food security, according to the Food and Agriculture Organization, 'exists when all people, at all times, have access to sufficient, safe and nutritious food to meet their dietary needs and food preferences for an active and healthy life.'

In the Canadian Community Health Survey, households were asked specific questions on whether members of the household in the past year, because of a lack of money, (a) did not eat the quality or variety of foods they wanted; (b) worried that there would not be enough to eat; and (c) did not have enought to eat. Those who responded 'often' or 'sometimes' to at least one of these questions were considered to have experienced food insecurity.

As expected, food insecurity is income-dependent. However, regional disparities are pronounced, even when stratified by income (see table 11.2). Nationally, food insecurity affects the young more than old and Aboriginal people more than non-aboriginal.

Table 11.2   Prevalence of food insecurity in northern Canada

	Total food insecurity (%)			Not enough to eat (%)		
	Total	Low income	Middle/high income	Total	Low income	Middle/high income
Canada	15	42	12	7	28	5
Yukon	21	58	18	10	30	7
Northwest Territories	28	61	22	18	49	12
Nunavut	56	74	47	49	68	40

Source: Canadian Community Health Survey 2000–1 (Ledron and Gervais 2005).

A survey of indigenous women in forty-four communities across northern Canada found considerable regional variation, with 40–70 per cent reporting that they could not afford enough food. Up to 50 per cent indicated they had inadequate access to hunting and fishing equipment and could not afford to go hunting or fishing.

Focus groups conducted in Nunavut identified the high costs of hunting and changes in lifestyle and cultural practices as barriers to food security and the consumption of traditional foods. Participants suggested increased economic support for local community hunts, the installation of communal freezers, and better access to cheaper and higher quality market foods.[10]

As a high proportion of daily energy requirements are obtained from non-traditional sources, the quality of the overall diet in the North is far from ideal. In northern Canada, the Canadian Community Health Survey investigated dietary practices. One indicator was whether respondents consumed fruits and vegetables less than five times a day. The norm for all Canadians was 55 per cent, but the proportion was much higher in Nunavut (67 per cent) and the Northwest Territories (63 per cent). The Yukon (53 per cent) was actually lower than the rest of Canada, reflecting the generally higher socio-economic status (see chapter 3) of this ethnically mixed territory.[11]

Physical Activity

The traditional circumpolar lifestyle was characterized by physical demands that included subsistence hunting and fishing, dog sledging, transporting water by hand, and carrying young children on the back. Among the Sami populations, reindeer herding was a labour-intensive occupation, often carried out in hostile environmental conditions and requiring a nomadic lifestyle. Since the 1950s, modernization has produced major shifts in subsistence patterns followed by greater mechanization of equipment and processing techniques.

Today Western ways of exercising have become a part of the modern Arctic societies. Typical sports include skiing, soccer, jogging, bicycling, softball, aerobics, and so on. However, many of the traditional activities still exist as leisure-time activities such as hunting, fishing, berry picking, camping, and boating. The degree to which physical activity is a natural part of one's occupation or one's leisure time varies from region to region.

Considering the connection between physical activity and health status, relatively little has been done to find out about the physical activity of peoples in the Arctic region. In the Greenland Population

Figure 11.1   Prevalence of leisure-time physical inactivity in Alaska

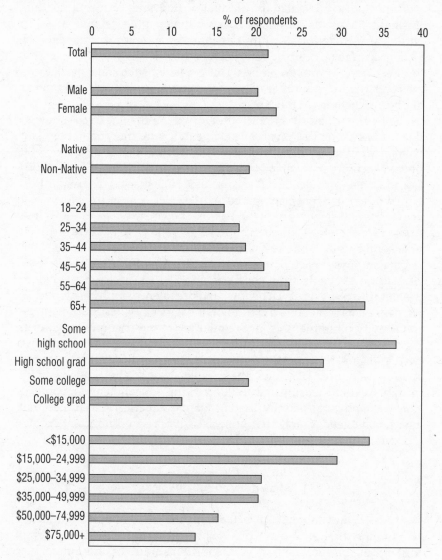

Note: Data aggregated for the four years 2002–5.
Source: Alaska Department of Health and Social Services, *Annual Report of the Behavioral Risk Factor Surveillance System*, 2002–3 and 2004–5.

Study of Inuit from 1999–2002, 15 per cent of men and 16 per cent of women reported a sedentary lifestyle during their leisure time. Surprisingly, there was a trend towards a higher physical activity level with Westernization within Greenland, and Inuit migrants in Denmark were significantly more physically active than the residents in Greenland. However, as box 11.2 explains, such data need to be interpreted with caution because of the very different cultural context of physical activity in the North.

The Finnmark Study in northern Norway in the late 1980s showed that despite being less physically active in leisure time, Sami men and women were more physically active at work and had a higher total physical activity score than Norwegian men and women.[12] In northern Canada, the prevalence of leisure-time inactivity was highest in Nunavut (56 per cent), compared with 47 per cent in the Northwest Territories and 40 per cent in the Yukon. The latter two results are close to or lower than the Canadian national average of 48 per cent. Women in general tend to be more inactive than men.[13]

Data on physical activity among Native and non-Native residents of Alaska are available from the Behavioural Risk Factor Surveillance System (BRFSS). Figure 11.1 shows the prevalence of physical inactivity, defined as someone who did not engage in any leisure-time physical activity other than his/her regular job in the past month, according to age, sex, ethnicity, education, and income. Associations with and barriers against physical activity have been studied in Canada and Alaska. As figure 11.1 shows, the prevalence of leisure-time inactivity is higher with increasing age and decreasing education and income. A review of physical activity among Native Americans indicates that age, female gender, and lack of social support are important factors associated with physical inactivity.[14]

Box 11.2 Measurement of physical activity

In most studies of physical activity in the circumpolar region, the measurement of physical activity is based on questionnaires about leisure-time physical activity adopted from studies of non-indigenous populations. The focus on leisure-time physical activity, rather than total activity, may be less useful in these populations where leisure time and occupation time are not necessarily clearly separated, and organized sports are not always available. Tools used for the measurement of physical activity may not necessarily assess culturally based forms of physical activity and may underestimate activities spent in domestic care. Women tend to engage in lower-intensity activities like walking, childcare, and housework – all of which are relatively more difficult to assess and less reproducible than higher-intensity activities such as those found in many organized sports. This reinforces the need to validate existing measurement tools or develop new tools to use in these populations.

Physical activity surveys tend to group respondents into various categories (usually as 'vigorously active,' 'moderately active,' or 'inactive,' sometimes also dichotomized into 'active' versus 'inactive') based on their responses to specific questions. On the basis of the duration, frequency, and intensity, numerical values of daily energy expenditures can also be calculated (kilocalories or kilojoules of energy per kilogram of body weight per day).

A few efforts have been done to modify and validate questionnaires on physical activity for use in indigenous populations. A modified version of the Modifiable Activity Questionnaire (MAQ) (originally designed for the Pima Study in the southwestern United States) was used in the study of residents of a subarctic Native community in Canada. The MAQ was designed for easy modification to maximize feasibility and appropriateness in a variety of minority populations.[15]

In Greenland, as part of the international Inuit Health in Transition Study, the International Physical Activity Questionnaire (IPQA) was modified and translated into Greenlandic. The questionnaire was validated against a combined measurement of heart rate and movement accelerometry and showed a high correlation with physiologic measurements, both for low- and high-intensity activities.

Intervention Programs

Only a few intervention programs have been developed that target diet and physical activity among indigenous peoples in the circumpolar region.[16] A pilot study was conducted among Alaska Native women in 2000–1 by the Southcentral Foundation as part of the WISE-WOMAN study, a randomized controlled heart disease prevention program. The intervention consisted of twelve weekly two-hour educational sessions taught by a multidisciplinary team (nutritionist, exercise specialist, health educator, and traditional wellness coordinator). At twelve weeks, significant improvements were noted in moderate walking and physical activity self-efficacy. Also observed was substantial movement from the contemplation and preparation stages to the action stage regarding physical activity and heart-healthy eating.

In the Bering Sea region of Alaska, a four-year diabetes prevention program consisted of risk-factor screening and personal counselling that focused on increasing the consumption of traditional foods and decreasing specific store-bought foods high in palmitic acid. It reported significant reductions in plasma cholesterol and improved glucose tolerance, although no weight change was detected.

Over the past decade in the Northwest Territories, a joint initiative of various government departments (from health, education, culture, employment, and municipal affairs), called Get Active Community Challenge, encourages individuals and organizations to register and log their physical activities online. Each year they are tallied and the top-ranking communities receive prizes that enable them to purchase recreation equipment. Another program using a similar challenge concept, called Drop the Pop, is a tri-territorial school-based health-promotion campaign that raises awareness about healthy eating and encourages students to not consume soft drinks for one full week.

Improving health promotion knowledge and skills of front-line health workers is difficult in the North because of great distances and limited access to educational programs. In Nunavut, an Internet-based nutrition and healthy living course was developed as a partnership of university-based nutrition experts, local health professionals, and community health workers. It has proven to be feasible and well accepted, and could potentially serve as a model for other remote areas.[17] Another good model is the Greenland prevention program, Inuuneritta, that focuses on intervention against poor diet and a sedentary lifestyle. It is more fully discussed in chapter 21.

NOTES

1 Dietary data from the Greenland Health Interview Survey of 1993–4 are reported in Pars, Osler, and Bjerregaard (2001).
2 See Wein and Freeman (1992).
3 The studies were conducted in Broughton Island (Kuhnlein, Kubow, and Soueida 1991) and Sanikiluaq on the Belcher Islands (Wein, Freeman, and Makus 1996).

4 The Keewatin (since renamed Kivalliq) Study was reported by Moffatt, O'Neil and Young (1994). The historical Greenland estimates were based on a subtraction of the total amount of imported food from the calculated energy expenditure of the population (Bertelsen 1937). The Inuit Health in Transition Study is a multinational collaborative cohort study, with baseline surveys to be completed in Nunavik and west Greenland by 2007. Other parts of the Arctic will be surveyed by the end of the decade.

5 Nutrient quality of traditional foods was analysed by Kuhnlein (1995), Kuhnlein, Soueida, and Receveur (1996), and Godel et al. (1996).

6 The CANHR Study was conducted in seven Yupik communities among 241 men and 307 women aged 15 to 94, using twenty-four-hour recall. See Mohatt et al. (2007) for further details.

7 The survey (Batal et al. 2005) of a representative sample of 1,356 subjects involved both food frequency and twenty-four-hour recall question-naires.

8 Nakano, Fediuk, Kassi, and Kuhnlein (2005) and Nakano, Fediuk, Kassi, Egeland, et al. (2005) interviewed 222 children in five communities during 2000–1 using twenty-four-hour recall.

9 Guyot et al. (2006) conducted the focus groups in Beaver Creek, the Yukon and Fort Providence, Northwest Territories.

10 Data from the 2000–1 Canadian Community Health Survey was reported by Ledrou and Gervais (2005). Lambden et al. (2006) surveyed 1,771 Dene and Inuit women in forty-four communities. The focus groups were conducted by Chan et al. (2006) in six communities in Nunavut in 2004.

11 Data are from the 2003 Canadian Community Health Survey conducted by Statistics Canada and covered respondents aged twelve and over.

12. Greenland data were reported by Jørgensen, Borch-Johnsen, and Bjerre-gaard (2006), and Norwegian Sami data by Hermansen, Njølstad, and Fonnebo (2002).

13 Data are obtained by combining the 2003 and 2005 Canadian Community Health Surveys. Physical inactivity is defined as energy expenditure of less than 1.5 kcal/kg/day.

14 Coble and Rhodes (2006) reviewed twenty-eight studies on physical activity among indigenous peoples in Canada and the United States, but none from the Arctic. Wilcox et al. (2000) identified Native ethnicity as one of the determinants of inactivity among rural American women.

15 The instrument was developed by Kriska et al. (2001) for use in the subarctic Cree community of Sandy Lake in northwestern Ontario, modi-fied from the one used in the Pima Study in the southwestern United States, a well-known long-term cohort study of diabetes. Background

on the International Physical Activity Questionnaire can be found on
www.ipaq.ki.se.

16 Witmer et al. (2004) reported on the Alaska WISEWOMAN trial and
Ebbesson et al. (2005) on the diabetes prevention program in the Alaska
Siberia Project.

17 Hamilton et al. (2004) described the Nunavut internet-based training
course. Further information about the Northwest Territories challenge
programs can be found at the NWT government websites, www.hlthss
.gov.nt.ca/features/programs_and_services/getactivenwt/2006/
getactive.htm and www.hlthss.gov.nt.ca/features/programs_and_
services/ drop_the_pop/default.asp.

12 Smoking, Alcohol, and Substance Use

ANNA RITA SPEIN

Many personal behaviours or lifestyles are associated with the development of a variety of diseases and health conditions. Smoking and alcohol use are among the most important of such lifestyle determinants of health. As forms of addiction, they can be considered 'diseases' in their own right and not just risk factors for other diseases. The modification of such behaviours has become the mainstay of public health programs in most jurisdictions. In this chapter, the patterns, determinants, and consequences of smoking, alcohol, and substance use in the circumpolar region are discussed, with particular focus on the Sami in Scandinavia and other indigenous peoples in the Arctic.

Historical Perspective

Tobacco is indigenous to the Americas, where it was cultivated and also gathered wild. Its use was ceremonial and medicinal, and it was widely traded among tribes but probably not into the Arctic. It was introduced into Europe in the sixteenth century. Tobacco has been popular with the Inuit since it was introduced by European whalers and traders at the time of first contact. Among the Sami, a few reports indicated that tobacco was used as offerings to the spirits by shamans (*noaide*) as part of their pre-Christian religion.[1]

Alcohol was introduced into Alaska during the Russian period and, by the nineteenth century, its use and misuse was widespread among the indigenous population. As elsewhere in North America, alcohol was an important trading good. In Greenland, under the tight control of the Royal Greenland Trade Department, alcohol was not sold to the Inuit during colonial times. After the Second World War, the sale of alcohol was liberalized and consumption steadily increased.

Box 12.1 Importation of cigarettes and alcohol into Greenland

Because of its isolation, the importation of cigarettes and alcohol into Greenland provides a useful estimate of the populations exposure to these substances and the increase in the magnitude of the problem over time.

Figure 12.1   Trend in per capita consumption of cigarettes and alcohol in Greenland

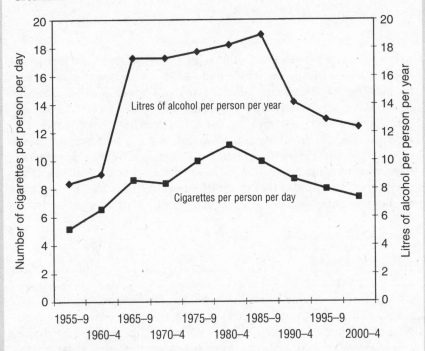

Note: Units of beer, wine, and spirits have been converted into equivalent litres of 100% alcohol.
Sources: Updated from Bjerregaard and Young (1998: figs. 11.1 and 8.3); data from 1995 onwards from Statistics Greenland (www.statgreen.gl).

In the 1950s, shortly after it was 'opened up' to external influences, import statistics indicated that per capita cigarette consumption was about five cigarettes per day among persons aged fifteen years and above. This rapidly increased to double that amount throughout the 1980s, after which it declined to the level of 7.4 during 2000–4 (fig. 12.1). Note that 'consumption' was derived from dividing import and sales figures by the entire population, smokers and non-smokers alike. The level among smokers was therefore much higher. It also does not tell what proportion of the population actually smoked, how often and for how long.

Similarly for alcohol, per capita consumption soared and reached a maximum of the equivalent of twenty litres of pure alcohol per adult per year in the 1980s. Note that this amount also includes alcohol consumed by Danes living in Greenland whose per capita consumption of alcohol has generally been much higher than the Greenlanders'.

From 1979 to 1982 there was a general restriction on the amount of alcohol that each person could purchase. Every month on the date corresponding to their birthdays, those adult residents were issued coupons good for the purchase of seventy-two beers, twelve bottles of wine, or an equivalent amount of liquor. The administration of the restriction policy created problems and was discontinued when it resulted in a thriving trade in both authentic and counterfeit coupons. The decrease since the late 1980s was likely the combined effect of an increased alcohol tax, a general weakening of the economy, and a decrease in the proportion of (well-salaried) Danes in the population (see fig. 2.3).

Among the Sami, scattered reports indicated that the shamans used alcoholic beverages as a way of altering their consciousness. Similar to indigenous peoples in North America, there has been a stereotypical view in Scandinavia historically about the 'drunken Sami,' assuming the Sami to be heavier users of alcohol than their majority counterparts. A study of Jokkmokk parish in north Sweden during the eighteenth and nineteenth centuries found that the Sami did not use alcohol more frequently than other Swedes living in the parish. Similar observations were noted among the Sami in Norway. Alcohol use among the Sami mostly took place for a short period during market days. There were restrictions and, later on, there were prohibitions on liquor sales in Swedish Lapland. The Swedish claimed that the Sami needed protection from the negative effects of alcohol. The prevailing view considered the Sami to be more vulnerable to the effects of alcohol. Undoubtedly, alcohol use contributed to severe social and economical problems among the Sami in the 1840s.[2]

By the latter half of the nineteenth century, there was less observed drinking among the Sami, particularly the reindeer-herding Sami, as a result of the influence of the Swedish priest Lars Levi Laestadius (1800–60) and the Laestadian movement that he founded. Laestadius himself was of Sami heritage, and he encouraged the Sami way of life and the use of the Sami language, which he considered to be a holy language. Laestadius experienced alcohol problems within his family, having a drinking father. Moreover, Laestadius considered alcohol use as an unchristian act as well as being a cause of severe social problems. It was clearly a threat to the Sami nomadic lifestyle and therefore had to be opposed. Laestadius and his movement, Laestadianism, initiated temperance organizations, with missionaries serving as temperance 'agents.' The goal was total abstinence. The Laestadian movement soon became widespread among several Sami subgroups or tribes in northern Scandinavia. Its rise corresponded to a simultaneous decline in the sale and use of alcohol among the Sami.

In contrast, Laestadianism did not advocate against smoking, and Laestadius himself was a smoker. However, towards the end of the twentieth century, anti-smoking norms were also promoted by the Laestadian movements leadership because of the severe health consequences of smoking.[3]

Patterns of Smoking among Adults

Smoking is widespread in all Inuit regions and the proportion of the population who smoke is higher than in most other populations in the world. In most areas, it was particularly during the latter decades of the twentieth century that cigarette smoking reached the level of 60–80 per cent among both men and women. In contrast, studies of smoking among the Sami indicate that the prevalence generally differs little from their fellow citizens in the same regions.

Box 12.2 Measuring smoking and alcohol use in populations

A convenient and relatively inexpensive way to determine the prevalence and pattern of smoking is by asking people about their habits in a survey. Based on responses to questions about smoking initiation and cessation, respondents can be divided into 'never' and 'ever' smokers, the latter into 'former' and 'current' smokers, who can be further divided into 'regular' (or daily) and 'occasional' smokers. Current smokers differ in terms of the number of cigarettes they smoke per day, and can be designated as heavy, moderate, or light smokers. The duration of smoking can also be incorporated into an index of lifetime exposure with pack-years as the unit. In comparing populations, it is important to be clear if the same indicators are being used.

Survey questions can also be designed to determine the frequency, quantity, and type of alcohol use. In the Greenland Health Interview Survey, the reported per capita consumption of alcohol was only about 56 per cent of the consumption calculated on the basis of import statistics (see box 12.1), which in the absence of widespread home-brewing is believed to give a reasonably true estimate of the total consumption.[4]

Surveys clearly must rely on recall, which may be faulty or even untruthful. For smoking, there are biochemical methods which measure nicotine, its metabolite cotinine, or thiocyanate (a metabolite of cyanide) in various body fluids such as blood, saliva, and urine. Carbon monoxide can also be measured in the breath. Such studies have not been done in the Arctic. For alcohol, biomarkers such as serum levels of the liver enzymes glutamyl transferase and aspartate aminotrasferase can also be used to complement and validate responses to questionnaires.

Various studies on cardiovascular risk factors have indicated high smoking rates (as much as 60 per cent) among adult men in the ethnically diverse population of Finnmark county in Norway, with only minor differences between Sami and non-Sami residents. The prevalence among adult Sami women varied from 6 per cent to 43 per cent in these studies, consistently lower than among their non-Sami counterparts, particularly in the Sami highlands. Pooled data from 1999 to 2003 of sixteen to seventy-four year-olds indicated that 37 per cent men and 36 per cent women in Finnmark county were daily smokers – among the highest rates reported in Norway.[5]

In Sweden, risk-factor information obtained from participants of a regional cardiovascular disease prevention program in Västerbotten county during 1990–2001 indicated that 22 per cent were daily smokers, with little difference between Sami and non-Sami, or between reindeer-herding and non-reindeer-herding Sami. That smoking prevalence

Table 12.1 Prevalence of smoking among adults in Alaska, northern Canada, and Greenland.

	Proportion of adults (%)			Mean number of cigarettes per day among smokers
	Current smokers		Former smokers	
	Daily/regular	Occasional		
Alaska[a]				
Natives (1991–3)	42(M), 36(F)		–	
Natives (2000–2)	44 (M,F)		–	13.5(M,F)
Non-Natives (1991–3)	27(M), 23(F)		–	
Non-Natives (2000–2)	24(M,F)		–	18.1(M,F)
Canada				
Canadian Inuit (1991)[b]	64(M,F)	8(M,F)	–	
Inuit in Kivalliq region, Nunavut (1990–1)[c]	69(M),66 (F)		20(M), 19(F)	17.7(M), 14.7(F)
Inuit in Nunavik region, northern Quebec (1992)[d]	65(M) 71(F)	5 (M,F)	16(M,F)	–
Yukon (2003)[e]	23(M) 20(F)	6(M,F)	37(M) 41(F)	–
Northwest Territories (2003)[e]	29(M) 31(F)	7(M,F)	32(M) 38(F)	–
Nunavut (2003)[e]	56(M) 60(F)	7(M,F)	21(M) 19(F)	–
Greenland				
Health Interview Survey (1993–4)[f]	82(M) 78(F)	8(M,F)	12(M,F)	12.8(M) 9.7(F)

[a]Alaska data are from Behavioral Risk Factors Surveillance System 1991–3 and 2000–2; age 18+ (Kaplan et al. 1997; Alaska Native Health Board 2004).
[b]Canadian Inuit data from Aboriginal Peoples Survey, 1991, from Statistics Canada (1993); age 15+.
[c]Keewatin Health Survey, 1990–1, from Young, Moffatt, and O'Neil (1993); age 25–64.
[d]Santé Québec Inuit Survey, 1992, from Jetté (1994); age 18–74.
[e]Canadian Community Health Survey 2003, from Statistics Canada (CANSIM Table 105-0227); age 12+.
[f]Greenland Health Interview Survey 1993–4, from Bjerregaard, Mulvad, and Pedersen (1997); age 18+.

among Swedish Sami, especially men, tends to be lower than Norwegian Sami may partly reflect the generally lower rates of smoking in Sweden, the lowest in Scandinavia. Futhermore, a study of male reindeer herders in Finland found that 58 per cent of Sami were regular

smokers, compared with 27 per cent of ethnic Finns, while the proportion who had quit did not differ between the two groups.[6]

Elsewhere in the Arctic, the prevalence of current smokers is very
high in all regions and population groups surveyed. Table 12.1 summarizes survey data from the 1990s and 2000s in Alaska, northern
Canada, and Greenland. These data compare with rates of current
smoking of 25 per cent (male) and 21 per cent (female) among all Canadians in 2003. The prevalence among Inuit had changed little since the
1990s.[7]

Heavy smokers, smoking more than ten cigarettes per day, make up
28 per cent of adult Greenlanders, while 40 per cent of Inuit in Canada
(both nationally and in Nunavik region) smoke more than ten cigarettes per day. In Greenland, the average age of smoking initiation was
fifteen years among the eighteen to twenty-four year age group, but
increased with age to twenty-one years among those aged sixty and
above.

Smoking among Adolescents and Youths

The only available data on cigarette smoking among indigenous Sami
adolescents are from Norway. Among young people aged fifteen to
twenty years, national Norwegian data from the mid-1990s indicated
that Finnmark county had the highest rates of daily smokers, averaging 27 per cent. This trend continues, as 8 per cent of tenth graders in
Finnmark were daily smokers in 2005, still the highest in the country.
There has been a decline in daily smoking rates for adolescents since
2000 for both genders and also at a regional north Norwegian level.
Whether this decline is equally distributed across ethnic groups has so
far not been investigated.[8]

Smoking behaviour was investigated in the Youth, Well-being and
Behaviour Study in 1990 in central Finnmark. As seen in table 12.2, sig-
nificanly more Sami junior high school students reported current
smoking than their non-Sami peers, and they also initiated smoking at
earlier ages. However, a higher proportion of Sami adolescents
reported that their mothers were non-smokers, while no ethnic differences in smoking rates were found among the fathers. These findings
corroborate earlier studies on adult smoking behaviour conducted in
Finnmark that show lower smoking rates among adult Sami women as
compared with non-Sami.[9]

The North Norwegian Youth Study followed some 3,000 youths
aged fifteen to nineteen years for three years during the mid-1990s. At

Table 12.2   Smoking and drinking status by ethnicity among 13- to 16-year-old students in central Finnmark, Norway

	Sami (n=249)	Non-Sami (n=210)	Effect of ethnicity
Smoking			
Among respondents			
% non-smokers	67	81	p≤.01
% light smokers[a]	24	14	
% heavy smokers[b]	9	5	
Mean debut age in years			
(standard deviation)	12.3 (2.70)	13.2 (0.90)	p≤.05
Respondents' mothers			
% non-smokers	52	38	p≤.01
% light smokers	27	33	
% heavy smokers	21	29	
Respondents' fathers			
% non-smokers	44	47	NS[c]
% light smokers	28	32	
% heavy smokers	28	21	
Drinking			
% who drank past 30 days			
– Beer	48	43	NS
– Wine	44	38	NS
– Hard liquor	46	42	NS
% who have been intoxicated			
– Never	59	65	NS
– Occasionally (≤ 10 times)	30	25	
– Frequently (>10 times)	11	10	
Mean debut age in years (SD)			
– Beer	12.4 (2.43)	13.0 (2.10)	NS
– Wine	13.0 (2.21)	13.5 (1.19)	NS
– Hard liquor	13.2 (2.17)	13.7 (1.06)	NS
% paternal drinking	62	82	p≤.001
% maternal drinking	30	29	NS

[a]Light smokers: occasional smoker or smoke less than 10 cigarettes per day.
[b]Heavy smokers: ≥ 10 cigarettes per day.
[c]NS: Non-significant (p>0.05).
Source: Youth, Well-being and Behavior Study (Kvernmo 2000).

baseline, 38 per cent were never smokers, 29 per cent were regular (daily) smokers, 11 per cent were occasional ('party') smokers, and 23 per cent were former smokers. At follow-up there was little change in

Table 12.3   Prevalence of smoking among adolescents and youths in Alaska and northern Canada

	% youths	
	Current smokers	Former smokers
Alaska[a]		
Native (1995)	63 (M), 61 (F)	–
Native (2003)	40 (M), 49 (F)	–
Non-Native (1995)	33 (M), 32 (F)	
Non-Native (2003)	13 (M), 11 (F)	
Canada[b]		
Yukon (2005)	13 (M), 18 (F)	9 (M,F)
Northwest Territories (2005)	20 (M), 15 (F)	16 (M,F)
Nunavut (2005)	35 (M), 51 (F)	29 (M),18 (F)
Northwest Territories (2002)		
Aboriginal	36 (M,F)	20 (M,F)
Non-Aboriginal	13 (M,F)	14 (M,F)

[a]Alaska Youth Risk Behavior Survey 1995 and 2003, from Peterson, Fenaughty, and Eberhart-Phillips (2004). A smoker is defined as someone who has smoked at least one cigarette in the past 30 days. High school students in Grades 9–12 were surveyed.
[b]Canada, 2005: Canadian Community Health Survey, 2005, from Statistics Canada. A smoker is defined as either a daily or occasional smoker. Ages are from 12 to 19 (CANSIM Table 105-0427). Northwest Territories, 2002: NWT School Tobacco Survey 2002, from Northwest Territories Health and Social Services (2004). Ages are from 10 to 17.

the prevalence of current smokers. Ethnic differences in cigarette smoking were minor. Sami students reported a significantly lower proportion of occasional smokers (8 per cent) and a higher rate of former smokers (26 per cent) than their non-Sami peers. No ethnic differences in the proportion of heavy smokers were found, as 32 per cent of daily smokers in both groups reported smoking fifteen or more cigarettes per day. Generally, girls were more involved in cigarette smoking than boys.[10]

In Alaska and northern Canada, smoking among adolescents and youths is a serious problem, and its prevalence tends to follow that of adults in the same region. Where data are available, a much higher proportion of indigenous people smoke than the rest of the population (see table 12.3).

Smokeless and Other Forms of Tobacco

The vast majority of smokers (>95 per cent) in Greenland smoke cigarettes, the remainder smoke mainly pipe. The use of smokeless
tobacco, that is, snuff and chewing tobacco, is widespread in Canada
and Alaska, especially among Inuit children and adolescents. It is non-
existent among adolescents and adults in Greenland. In the Northwest
Territories, 18 per cent of Inuit boys aged fifteen to nineteen used
chewing tobacco and 19 per cent used snuff, while only 1 per cent of
girls used one or the other. In the Kivalliq region of Nunavut during
the early 1990s, 11 per cent of adolescents and 7 per cent of adults used
chewing tobacco. In Alaska, even among preschool children, there is a
high prevalence of smokeless tobacco: 10 per cent of boys and 18 per
cent of girls aged five used chewing tobacco or snuff. Among adults, it
was 6 per cent during 2000–2. However, among Alaska Natives, the
prevalence was 16 per cent, four times that of non-Natives.

Little data on snuff are available specifically for Sami residing in
Norway. National figures from 2005 indicate that both rates of occasional (19 per cent) and daily snuff users (11 per cent) were highest
among tenth-grade students living in northern Norway.[11]

Determinants of Smoking

Smoking patterns differ according to geographic regions, ethnic
groups, age, sex, and socio-economic status. In most countries, the
prevalence of smoking tends to be higher among people with less education and a lower income. Among the Inuit, sex differences tend not
to be large, although women generally smoke fewer cigarettes per day
than men (see table 12.1). Most studies show that smoking prevalence
decreases with age, suggestive of an increasing secular trend. In
Greenland, the prevalence of smoking is lower in Nuuk than in the rest
of the country. Among socio-economic groups, hunters and fishers and
those not working smoke more often than other persons of similar age.

The reasons why people smoke are varied and complex, including
the pharmacologic action of nicotine, individual personality, social
interactions, market forces, and the legislative and regulatory environment. Knowledge of the health consequences of smoking plays only a
minor role in deterring people from smoking.[12]

The availability of cigarettes, especially their retail price, has a major
influence on smoking behaviour, notably among adolescents. In

Greenland, young smokers smoke fewer cigarettes than did the older age groups. As tobacco is heavily taxed in Greenland, this may reflect the differences in buying power between age groups. Globally, the tobacco industry devotes massive resources towards sales promotions that are highly targeted at specific sociodemographic groups.

Among the Sami, substance use (intoxication and illicit drug use), externalizing problems, sexual activity, and attending vocational training are associated with regular smoking both in late adolescence and in young adulthood, similar to their non-Sami peers. That daily smoking among youth is strongly associated with the co-occurrence of other risk-taking behaviours is observed in other populations also. Laestadian affiliation or background and having parents engaged in primary industries are associated with experimental smoking among Sami during late adolescence. Furthermore, fifteen-to-nineteen-year-old Sami who reported frequent truancy (>10 times/year) have higher rates of daily smoking (53 per cent), cannabis use (11 per cent), and illicit substance use (6 per cent).[13]

Young Sami with weaker cultural ties are more likely to be current smokers, when simultaneously controlling for potentially confounding sociodemographic factors such as gender, age, family structure, parental socio-economic status, Laestadian affiliation or background, and ethnic context (regions based on number of indigenous Sami). For example, Sami residing in assimilated contexts with few ethnic members are more likely to be current smokers. Prospectively, favouring assimilation in late adolescence predicted current smoking in young adulthood. These findings may be related to acculturation stress, as the young Sami residing in assimilated contexts may experience less structural ethnic or cultural support. Moreover, strong ethnic group identification has been associated with current smoking in late adolescence. One possible explanation for this paradoxical finding is that fifteen to nineteen year old Sami who currently smoke and who have strong ethnic-group identification may represent a subgroup of more separated or 'traditional' Sami, and smoking may partly be due to a lack of bicultural competence.

Why are Sami different from other indigenous peoples of the Arctic in their pattern of smoking, especially in having a prevalence that is often similar to that of the majority population? There are several potential explanatory factors. First, compared with indigenous people elsewhere in the Arctic, Sami are less socially and economically disadvantaged relative to their majority peers. Secondly, Sami youths are much less exposed to environmental (passive) smoking as smoking rates among adult Sami – the 'parental generation' – tend to be much lower than among Greenlanders, Canadian Inuit, and Alaska Natives (table 12.1). Thirdly, Sami have lower school dropout rates when compared with indigenous groups elsewhere. Finally, the Sami have no history of the cultural use of tobacco, unlike some North American Native groups. Both the tradition of cultural use of tobacco and frequent use of smokeless tobacco may enhance the socialization into cigarette smoking among Native American youths, and may increase their vulnerability to smoke. However, it does not explain the high smoking rates found among Greenlanders, among whom smokeless-tobacco use is extremely uncommon.[14]

Consequences of Smoking

Over 4,000 chemicals have been identified in tobacco smoke in the vapour phase and as particulates. While nicotine is the addictive substance, at least forty known carcinogens and/or mutagens are present, including carbon monoxide, hydrogen cyanide, arsenic, nickel, cadmium, lead, benzene, vinyl chloride, polycyclic aromatic hydrocarbons, N-nitrosamines, aldehydes, aromatic amines, aza-arenes, and others.

Smoking causes a variety of cancers, especially in the respiratory tract from the mouth to the lungs, and also the eosphagus, urinary tract, and cervix. It causes chronic bronchitis and emphysema, ischemic heart disease, and stroke. In addition, smoking is associated with complications of pregnancy, perinatal and neonatal mortality, sudden infant death syndrome, and child growth retardation.

As shown in chapter 17, smoking-related cancers are particularly high in the Inuit populations of Alaska, Greenland, and northern Canada. There are few estimates of population attributable risk for smoking-associated diseases in the Arctic. United States Indian Health Service data indicate that infant mortality attributable to maternal smoking was about 16 per cent among Alaska Natives. As discussed in chapter 9, the Sami do not appear to suffer from elevated rates of lung cancer or ischemic heart disease, although they are at higher risk for a subtype of stroke.

Even when not causing overt disease, smoking compromises physiological function. Lung function tests in one Canadian Inuit community over three decades showed gradual deterioration, which was attributed to a combination of cold air and near universal smoking. Smoking may also potentiate other risk factors, such as environmental contaminants. In the Nunavik region, Quebec Inuit smokers had blood cadmium levels ten to twenty times those of non-smokers, even in the absence of any occupational exposure.[15]

Intervention Programs

Control of smoking requires behavioural change, which can be induced through both individual education and broader societal measures that enact and enforce laws to regulate sales and promotion, prohibit smoking in public places and the workplace, and increase taxation of tobacco products. Such measures reflect the growing social unacceptability of smoking, and they in turn reinforce and promote non-smoking as a social norm. It is noteworthy that both Nunavut and the Northwest Territories of Canada have passed comprehensive tobacco control acts that prohibit the sale of tobacco products to youths under the age of eighteen, advertising and public displays of tobacco, and smoking in public places.

Few smoking control programs in the Arctic have been evaluated. A smoking cessation program in the early 1990s at the Alaska Native Medical Center in Anchorage, involving behavioural modification and transdermal nicotine patches, resulted in a quit rate of 20 per cent at twelve months. The fact that smoking prevalence among adults has hardly changed for decades reflects the lack of success of public health efforts. However, at least among Alaskan teens, both Native and non-Native, substantial reductions in smoking prevalence has been observed (see table 12.3).[16]

Alcohol Use among Adults

There are many parallels between smoking and alcohol use. At one point, both are considered 'vices' and many jurisdictions have attempted the official prohibition of alcohol. One can view tobacco and alcohol as examples of an array of pharmacologic agents human societies have discovered through the ages which are capable of producing pleasurable effects, but unfortunately also unwelcome health consequences.

Box 12.3 Terminology of alcohol and substance use

There is considerable confusion in the terminology denoting the use and abuse of alcohol and other psychoactive substances. 'Harmful use' or 'substance abuse' needs to be distinguished from 'dependence.' The former refers to use which causes damage to health. Dependence develops after repeated use and is associated with a variety of behavioural, cognitive, and physiological phenomena. The American Psychiatric Association's *Diagnostic and Statistical Manual*, the 1994 edition of which is referred to as DSM-IV, recognizes both substance abuse and substance dependence. Both refer to a maladaptive pattern of use leading to clinically significant impairment or distress, although for a patient to be designated as dependent, the criteria of tolerance, withdrawal, and compulsive use need to be present, whereas abuse refers only to the consequences of repeated use. Abuse and dependence can be applied to alcohol and a host of other substances. Widely used terms such as alcoholism and addiction, however, do not appear in DSM-IV.

The term 'alcoholism,' however, continues to be favoured by some specialists in the field. The National Council on Alcoholism and Drug Dependence and the American Society of Addiction Medicine proposed a definition of alcoholism:

a primary, chronic disease with genetic, psychosocial, and environmental factors influencing its development and manifestations ... often progressive and fatal ... characterized by impaired control over drinking, preoccupation with the drug alcohol, use of alcohol despite adverse consequences, and distortions in thinking, most notably denial.

The public health approach to smoking, alcohol, and substance use focuses more on the pattern of use and abuse and their health consequences, and less on the more individual, clinical concerns of addictions and alcoholism.

Different national health and statistical agencies tend to quantify alcohol consumption differently. The Behavioural Risk Factor Surveillance System (BRFSS) in Alaska (and the rest of the United States), for example, uses these operational definitions:

- 'heavy drinking': having one or more drinks (for women) or two or more drinks (for men) per day in the past thirty days

- 'binge drinking': having five or more drinks on one or more occasions in the past thirty days

A commonly used instrument to detect harmful drinking is the CAGE test, which is a four-item questionnaire. It was modified in the Greenland Population Study of 1999 and expanded to six questions, covering topics such as feeling the need to reduce drinking, being annoyed by criticism about drinking, guilt feeling, practices such as drinking first thing in the morning and outside mealtimes, and the number of drinking days per week.[17]

In Alaska during 2001–5, the proportion of adults who had at least one drink in the past month was lower among Alaska Natives (47 per cent) than either the state or national all-race average (about 60 per cent). The proportion of heavy drinkers was not different between Alaska Natives and the state or national average (about 5 per cent). Only in the prevalence of binge drinking was the Native rate (20 per cent) slightly higher than the state (18 per cent) and national (15 per cent) rates.

In northern Canada, among persons twelve years and over, the proportion who consumed five or more drinks on one occasion, more than twelve times a year (equivalent to the 'binge drinking' definition of BRFSS in box 12.3) was higher in the Yukon, Nunavut (both 31 per cent), and the Northwest Territories (40 per cent) than in Canada nationally (21 per cent). As expected, the proportion was higher in men than in women.[18]

According to the Greenland Health Survey in the early 1990s, 17 per cent of adults (22 per cent of men and 12 per cent of women) reported never drinking alcohol, and 5 per cent drank alcohol three times per week or more. Those aged sixty and above were most often never to drink alcohol, while those aged thirty-five to fifty-nine were most likely to drink three or more times per week.

In Siberia, the indigenous people of Chukotka drink only once or twice per month, but their consumption per episode is high: typically 129 to 246 grams of pure alcohol for males, equivalent to between half a bottle and a bottle of vodka or ten to eighteen drinks, and 44 to 101 grams for females. These doses are twice as high as those reported from western Siberia. In a comparative study between indigenous inhabitants in north-eastern Siberia (Chukotka and Kamchatka) and those of north-western Alaska and the Aleutians, the proportion of ever-drinkers among Russian Natives was much higher than that of Alaska Natives.[19]

The few studies documenting alcohol use among adult Sami in Norway do not indicate higher drinking rates compared with the majority population. In Finnmark county, self-reported annual alcohol consumption level among inhabitants in the Sami highland (including the five main Sami municipalities) was lower than in two 'non-Sami' areas (i.e., those with a low Sami population). A comprehensive review of data from 1976–7 was undertaken in the Sami highland on alcohol sales at state and commercial outlets, alcohol-related admissions to the regional alcohol treatment centre and local county hospitals, and police records of arrests for drunken and disorderly conduct. The Sami bought less alcohol and had fewer alcohol-related health problems, but they were arrested more often. This may reflect local law enforcement practices and the low tolerance of the majority Norwegian society towards public intoxication.[20]

A Finnish study in the late 1980s among male reindeer herders found that, while the mean daily intake of alcohol and proportion of heavy drinkers were higher among Sami than those of Finnish origin, there was no difference in the mean annual frequency of intoxication, thus not justifying the stereotypic view of the 'drunken Sami.' In Sweden, similar alcohol consumption levels were observed among Sami and non-Sami, or between reindeer-herding and non-herding Sami. However, Swedish Sami men consumed more alcohol than Swedish Sami women. Among the Sami people living on the Russian Kola Peninsula, the Sami made up about 6 per cent of the population in Lovozero district during the mid and late 1990s, but contributed to 20 per cent of the diagnosed alcoholics in the district, and alcoholism was in particular a male problem.[21]

Alcohol Use among Youths and Adolescents

The Youth, Well-being and Behaviour Study in central Finnmark (table 12.2) indicated no ethnic differences in mid-adolescence drinking rates. The only difference was in paternal drinking, as Sami adolescents reported higher abstainer rates among their fathers. Longitudinal findings from the North Norwegian Youth Study during the 1990s indicated significantly lower drinking rates among Sami for all drinking measures. Among Sami, rates of current drinkers increased from 46 per cent by late adolescence to 71 per cent by young adulthood.

A higher proportion of Sami aged fifteen to nineteen years (53 per cent) drank in public gathering places than among non-Sami (44 per cent). This 'drinking style' may contribute to maintaining the existence of the long-standing stereotype of 'the drunken Sami.'

A Norwegian government report on Sami health issues based on data from the community of Kautokeino indicated that only 4 per cent of thirteen to sixteen year olds reported weekly alcohol use. Moreover, Sami seem to initiate drinking at an early age, on average at twelve years old. Among older adolescents and young adults (sixteen to thirty), 27 per cent reported alcohol abuse, predominantly a male problem. However, an episodic drinking pattern with long periods of abstinence was commonly observed.[22]

Determinants of Drinking

Whether alcohol abuse or alcoholism has any genetic basis has been the subject of much controversy. There is widespread acceptance among biologically oriented researchers that there is a genetically inheritable predisposition to the development of alcohol abuse. There appears to be ethnic differences in the metabolism of alcohol, and certain Asiatic peoples (and also some indigenous North Americans) may react with physical symptoms such as facial flushing, headaches, and tachycardia to even relatively small amounts of alcohol. Regardless of the presence of ethnic differences in alcohol metabolism, social and cultural conditions are without any reasonable doubt more important explanatory factors. Furthermore, interventions can only be directed at modifiable risk factors.[23]

Regardless of ethnic background, youth drinking is a social behaviour and occurs in multiple social contexts in north Norway, as elsewhere. The overwhelming majority of fifteen to nineteen year olds reported drinking with friends and at parties. Sami were significantly more likely to report having worries about drinking among family and friends than non-Sami. The negative attitudes towards drinking among Sami youths may be moulded by their upbringing by parents, among whom a high proportion were abstainers, and the influence of the strongly anti-alcohol Laestadian movement in the Sami areas.

Generally, less Sami orientated individuals showed higher involvement with alcohol. Older adolescents who favoured assimilation were more likely to report current drinking and annual intoxication; those who resided in assimilated contexts and showed weaker ethnic identity were more likely to report binge drinking, regardless of gender, age, parental socio-economic status, family structure, Laestadian affiliation, or background. Prospectively, favouring assimilation in late adolescence predicted the respondents perception of excessive drinking in young adulthood. The findings indicate that although Sami as a group generally show less alcohol involvement than non-Sami peers, Sami with weaker cultural ties to their native culture manifest higher 'intraethnic' drinking rates during late adolescence.

As with smoking, Sami are unlike other indigenous people in the Arctic in not showing excessive alcohol use relative to non-indigenous people. Possible reasons include the less-acute social inequalities between Sami and non-Sami, exposure to abstaining parents serving as positive role models, higher educational attainment, and the anti-alcohol norms espoused by the Laestadian movement.

The Greenland Population Study of 1999 investigated the effect of urbanization and migration on alcohol intake and drinking patterns. In Greenland, there was generally little difference in alcohol intake between residents of large and small communities. Greenlanders who had migrated to Denmark, however, had higher mean alcohol intake, but a lower proportion of abstainers, binge drinkers, and those showing problem drinking based on the CAGE questionnaire. Among Greenlanders living in Denmark, the duration of stay was associated with a decrease in the prevalence of binge drinking, though not in other indicators.[24]

Health Effects of Alcohol Use

Alcohol use leads to acute mental, cognitive, and behavioural disturbances, and severe intoxication is a form of poisoning, sometimes even with fatal consequences. Alcohol is an etiologic agent in a variety of diseases, such as alcoholic hepatitis and cirrhosis, alcoholic cardiomyopathy, alcoholic gastritis, and alcoholic pancreatitis. Alcohol also plays a contributory role in many injuries, various gastrointestinal cancers, infectious diseases and nutritional deficiencies. The impact of alcohol extends into the second generation in the form of fetal alcohol syndrome. Beyond disease and injury, alcohol disrupts the social and economic well-being of families and communities.

In Alaska, data from the late 1990s indicated that 'alcohol-related' deaths (based on specific causes-of-death codes) accounted for 7 per cent of all deaths among Alaska Natives, but <1 per cent in the United States nationally. The age-standardized mortality rate for this group of causes was ten times higher among Alaska Natives.

In Greenland, during the period with restriction on the sale of alcohol, alcohol-related mortality dropped to 70 per cent of the level of a control period, but this was counterbalanced by a significant rise in mortality from non-alcohol-related marine accidents. This might have been caused by more time and resources for potentially dangerous outdoor activities being available when alcohol was restricted. In a comparison of Alaska villages with and without restrictive alcohol laws, overall mortality from injuries during 1990–3 was 1.6 times higher among Alaska Natives from villages without restriction than among those from villages with restriction. Mortality from alcohol-related injuries was 2.5 times higher. In Greenland, the mortality rate was significantly higher among infants and children whose mothers had had an alcohol-related contact with the health care services during the past five years.[25]

Substance Use

Other drugs (prescribed and non-prescribed, legal and illegal) that have an impact on health include opioids, cannabinoids, sedatives and hypnotics, cocaine, stimulants, hallucinogens, and volatile solvents. Different populations 'favour' certain drugs over others, depending on availability, social preferences, law enforcement practices, and cultural beliefs.

In the Greenland Health Interview Survey, 64 per cent of the eighteen to thirty-four year olds and 25 per cent of those thirty-five years old or more reported having smoked marijuana at least once, while 21 per cent and 6 per cent, respectively, were current users of marijuana. In Nunavik, 55 per cent had smoked marijuana at least once and 38 per cent had done so within the last year, while in the Kivalliq region of Nunavut only 10 per cent reported ever having smoked marijuana. The NWT survey of alcohol and drug use had a 33 per cent rate of marijuana use during the past year among the Inuit of Nunavut, more than four times the national average. In Greenland the use of marijuana is considerably higher on the southern and central west coast than in the more remote parts of the country.[26]

Solvent abuse (sniffing of gasoline, nail polish remover, glue, etc.) is common in many Aboriginal communities in Canada. In the Kivalliq region, 8 per cent of adolescents reported solvent abuse, while in a survey of Inuit youth in one community in Quebec, 21 per cent reported having used solvents at one time, and 5 per cent had used them within the last month. In the Nunavik survey, 19 per cent of the population had tried sniffing solvents and 9 per cent of adolescents were current users, and the use decreased steeply with age. In Nunavut, 26 per cent of Inuit had sniffed solvents at some time compared with less than 1 per cent for Canada as a whole. Finally, in Greenland, a similar proportion of eleven-to-seventeen-year-old school children (19 per cent) had tried sniffing.

In Norway, Finnmark county had the highest national rates of lifetime sniffing, averaging 12 per cent. Among thirteen to sixteen year olds in the Youth, Well-Being and Behaviour Study in Finnmark, 15 per cent of Sami youths, compared with 7 per cent of non-Sami, reported having been sniffing. There was no gender difference. In the North Norwegian Youth Study of fifteen to nineteen year olds, the prevalence of use in the previous year was lower among Sami (3 per cent) than non-Sami (5 per cent). However, those living in assimilated environments reported significantly higher rates (6 per cent) than their peers residing in the Sami highlands (0.5 per cent).

The use of other illicit drugs (cocaine, heroin, etc.) has not been reported from Greenland. This is contrary to the situation in Canada and Alaska. In Kivalliq only 1 per cent reported having tried these drugs, while in Nunavik 10 per cent had tried cocaine and half of these were current users. In Nunavut, 7 per cent of Inuit reported the use of other illicit drugs during the past year, more than four times the national average. In Alaska as a whole and among Alaska Natives in particular there is a high rate of use of cocaine and injection drugs. Chapter 20 (table 20.4) presents drug use data from the Alaska Youth Risk Behaviors Survey of 2003.

In north Norway, significantly fewer fifteen-to-nineteen-year-old Sami high school students than non-Sami peers reported ever having used cannabis (4 per cent vs. 10 per cent) and ever being offered cannabis (20 per cent vs. 27 per cent) during the mid-1990s. Generally higher cannabis rates are found in Tromsø, the largest city in northern Norway, averaging 10 per cent compared with the regional average of about 6 per cent. The increase in cannabis use observed among Sami during the follow-up period may be due to increasing age and to changes in attitudes. On a national Norwegian level, the proportion reporting that cannabis should be sold freely increased from about 2 per cent to about 10 per cent, while the proportion reporting that they would try cannabis if there were no danger of being arrested increased from about 5 per cent to about 13 per cent during the 1990s. These trends may also have reached young Sami residing in rural and semi-rural areas, although no studies have explored this issue in this population.

Like cannabis, the use of other illicit substances has become geographically concentrated in the larger centres throughout the country. In north Norway, illicit substance use was reported by 2 per cent of fifteen to nineteen year olds, with no ethnic differences. Among those using illicit drugs other than cannabis, two-thirds had been in contact with the police at least once during the year prior to the survey, although the reason for this contact may have involved incidents other than drug use. National figures indicate that <1 per cent of fifteen-to-twenty-year-old Norwegians have ever used illicit drugs during the mid-1990s.

Among fifteen-to-nineteen-year-old Sami high school students in the mid-1990s, alcohol and illicit substance use was significantly associated with various types of problem behaviours such as frequent truancy (more than ten times a year) and most types of minor and major delinquency. The risk of daily smoking among this age group reporting frequent truancy was doubled (53 per cent), while the risk of cannabis use (11 per cent) and illicit substance use (6 per cent) were increased by threefold.[27]

The Social Transitions in the North Study of indigenous peoples in north-eastern Siberia and north-western Alaska found that the prevalence of ever use of marijuana, cocaine, and inhalants was much lower in the Russia group, compared with Alaska.[28]

NOTES

1 See Pego et al. (1995) and Jones and Dunavan (2006) on the historical and cultural aspects of tobacco use among North American Indians, and Pollan (1993) on Sami shamanism.
2 See Kvist (1986) and Sköld and Kvist (1988) for the series of studies on Jokkmokk from 1760 to 1910. Alcohol use among Norwegian Sami was discussed in Zorgdrager (1997).
3 Laestadianism and alcohol use among Sami was discussed by Boreman

(1953) and Larsen (1993). Additional information was also provided by Roald E. Kristiansen, University of Tromsø.

4 Rehm (1998) reviewed the measurement of alcohol consumption. Findings of the Greenland Health Interview Survey can be found in Bjerregaard and Young (1998:159).

5 Results of the Finnmark studies can be found in Abildsnes, Søgaard, and Hafstad (1998); Njølstad, Arnesen, and Lund-Larsen (1996); and Utsi and Bønaa (1998). Norwegian regional smoking statistics are also available from Lund and Lindbak (2004).

6 See Edin-Liljegren et al. (2004) for Swedish Sami data and Näyhä and Hassi (1993) for Finnish data. The construction of the Sami cohort was described in detail in box 9.1.

7 For further details and earlier data in Alaska, see Lanier, Bulkow, et al. (1990) and Kaplan et al. (1997); Millar (1990a) on the Northwest Territories; and Bjerregaard, Mulvad, and Pedersen (1997) on Greenland.

8 Norwegian smoking data among youth are available from Skretting (1996) and also on the Norwegian Institute for Public Health website, www.fhi.no.

9 See the doctoral thesis of Kvernmo (2000). The study included 249 Sami and 210 non-Sami junior high school students from eight municipalities, ranging in ages from thirteen to sixteen years old.

10 A school-based sample was assembled in 1994–5. About 1,500 respondents were followed up in 1997–8 by postal questionnaires (Spein, Kvernmo, and Sexton, 2002).

11 Norwegian data are available from the National Institute for Public Health website, www.fhi.no. Trend data for smokeless tobacco use in Alaska are available from BRFSS; for earlier data, see Schlife (1987). Canadian data are reviewed in Millar (1990b).

12 There is a substantial literature on the determinants of smoking: see the reviews by Fisher et al. (1990) and Logan and Spencer (1996).

13 See Spein, Sexton, and Kvernmo (2004) and Kvernmo et al. (2003) for data on Sami. For other populations, see the study by Osler and Kjær (1996) in Greenland; and Blum et al. (1992) and Pothoff et al. (1998) on American Indians and Alaska Natives.

14 These differences are discussed in detail in Spein, Kvernmo, and Sexton (2002). Socioeconomic data on Norwegian Sami can be found in Sosial-og helsedepartementet (1998–9). The cultural use of tobacco among Native Americans was discussed in U.S. Department of Health and Human Services (1998).

15 Bulterys et al. (1990) used IHS data to calculate PAR. Rode and Shephard

(1994) performed extensive physiological measurements among Inuit in Igloolik, Nunavut, from the 1970s to the 1990s. Benedetti et al. (1994) measured the body burden of cadmium in Nunavik region.

16 Hensel et al. (1995) presented the evaluation of the Alaska Native Medical Center program.

17 Various definitions of these terms can be found in manuals of ICD-10 (WHO 1992) and DSM-IV (American Psychiatric Association 2000). Note that the BRFSS introduced 'heavy' drinking in 2001, with different criteria for men and women, replacing 'chronic' drinking, defined as two drinks per day averaging 60 drinks or more in the past month for either sex. The modified CAGE test was described in Madsen et al. (2005).

18 Canadian data cited are from the 2003 Canadian Community Health Survey, which is repeated every two years, and unlike many other national surveys, do not exclude the remotely located and sparsely populated northern territories. Brems (1996) reviewed alcohol use data among Alaska Natives. The 2001–5 data were extracted from the BRFSS interactive website, www.cdc.gov/brfss.

19 Greenland data are from Bjerregaard and Young (1998:159). Russian data are from Kurilovitsch et al. (1994) and Segal and Saylor (2007).

20 Alcohol use among the Sami was documented by Larsen and Nergård (1990), and Larsen and Saglie (1996). Hetta et al. (1978) review medical, official, and crime statistics.

21 Poikolainen, Näyhä, and Hassi (1992) conducted the Finnish Sami study; Edin-Liljegren et al. (2004) used the Swedish Sami conduct; and Snellman (1998) reported on the situation among the Kola Sami in Russia.

22 Results of the two studies on Sami youth were reported by Kvernmo (2000), Kvernmo et al. (2003), and Spein, Sexton, and Kvernmo (2006). The Norwegian governments Sami health and social plan (Sosial-og helsedepartementet 1995) included a section on 'risk groups.'

23 There is a substantial literature on the genetics of alcohol abuse. For a recent review, see Quickfall and el-Guebaly (2006).

24 See Madsen et al. (2005). Greenlanders in Denmark refer to persons born in Greenland sampled from the Danish Central Population Registry. In Greenland, the survey was conducted in Nuuk, Sisimiut, Qasigiannguit, and four villages in Uummannaq municipality.

25 Alcohol-related mortality data in Alaska are for the period 1996–8, as reported in the U.S. Indian Health Services *Regional Differences in Indian Health, 2000–2001*. Studies on injury mortality in 'dry' versus 'wet' communities in Alaska, impact of alcohol sale restriction in Greenland, and

association between child mortality and maternal alcohol use were reviewed in Bjerregaard and Young (1998:162).

26 Data on drug use in Greenland in the mid-1990s were reported in Bjerregaard and Young (1998:162–3); Nunavik by Jétte (1994); and Alaska by Brems (1996).

27 Sami youth data in north Norway are from Kvernmo et al. (2003). Norwegian national and regional drug use trends were presented in Skretting (1996), Bye (2003), and Hordvin (2005).

28 Mason (2004) provided an overview of the Social Transition in the North Project, a unique binational collaborative research effort between Siberia and Alaska. Data on alcohol and drug use were presented by Segal and Saylor (2007).

13 Genetic Susceptibility

ROBERT HEGELE AND REBECCA POLLEX

The Genetic Basis of Disease

It has been known for centuries that children tend to look like their parents, that certain diseases run in families, and that there is an intangible inherent factor that dictates present and future health. In the present scientific age, with our ability to read DNA sequences and manipulate the human genome in vitro, we have shifted from largely observational studies, such as the work carried out by Mendel with his pea plants, to direct investigations into the precise molecular basis of many human traits and disorders. It is now clearly understood that genetics can play the lead role in disease, such as in the case of rare inherited monogenic disorders that involve mutations in a single gene, which are inherited in a Mendelian fashion (i.e., autosomal dominant, autosomal recessive or X-linked dominant), or in the case of disorders resulting from chromosomal aberrations or mitochondrial DNA defects. Spontaneous genomic mutations may also occur and some of these contribute to the development of cancer, disorders of the immune system, and the aging process.

Least understood are the genetic factors involved in the more common disorders that, to varying degrees, affect all populations. Rather than being caused by a mutation in a single gene or by the presence of extra chromosomal material, these complex disorders, such as obesity, hypertension, diabetes, and cancer, arise from the interplay of several genetic factors together with environmental factors. Subtle, single nucleotide changes, termed single nucleotide polymorphisms (SNPs), are the most common type of genetic variation that determine susceptibility, resistance, and severity of complex diseases. SNP variations are like single letter 'misprints' in the genetic 'instruction manual' and occur when a single nucleotide, such as an adenine, is replaced by one of the other three nucleotides – cytosine, guanine, or thymine. SNPs span the entire human genome; current genomic databases contain information on more than 12 million human SNPs.[1] Most SNPs occur outside coding regions and have no obvious impact on the structure or function of a protein; these presumably 'silent' SNPs may still serve as biological markers for pinpointing a disease on the human genome map. Others, however, are of great interest to researchers as they code for functional changes that affect the amino acid sequence of the protein product and thus display a more direct potential association with disease.

An additional source of variation in the human genome was identified with the discovery that duplications or gaps in the human genome quite commonly exist, with, on average, twelve large-scale copy number variations (gains or losses of several kilobases to hundreds of kilobases) present in healthy individuals.[2] The impact of such large-scale heterogeneity of human genome structure on disease susceptibility has yet to be fully appreciated.

For complex traits, one's genetic background is often insufficient to be the sole cause of the disorder. Instead, the genetic background creates a 'fertile soil' for susceptibility to environmental factors, and it is the interaction of genetic susceptibility with environmental factors that increases the risk of disease. Potential environmental triggers include diet, lifestyle, and/or activity level. The concept of underlying genetic susceptibility accounts, at least in part, for individual differences in response to the same environmental factors, such as diet or even medication. Given the complexities of such interactions, simple patterns of inheritance do not apply to common diseases; however, the tendency for them to cluster within families is often observed.

Gene Identification Strategies

Identifying causative genes for monogenic traits and 'susceptibility genes' for complex traits has become more feasible because of the recent advances made in the mapping of the human genome coincident with the wide availability of millions of DNA markers together with powerful genomic technologies and bioinformatic tools. The two main contrasting strategies to identify disease genes have been broadly characterized as the 'positional cloning approach' and the 'candidate gene approach,' as discussed in a landmark article by

Lander and Schork.[3] Briefly, the positional cloning approach is undertaken without any a priori understanding of the gene products involved in the disease process. The genome is screened using a set of evenly spaced DNA markers to identify chromosomal regions that bear a statistical relationship with a disease in a test sample. A genome-wide 'association study' evaluates these patterns in an unrelated cohort of affected and/or unaffected populations, while a genome-wide 'linkage study' evaluates the relationships in a collection of large or small family units. After significant phenotype-genotype associations or linkages have been found, the genomic region containing the disease gene can be further narrowed using additional genetic markers, or the genomic DNA sequence can be directly interrogated to find the culprit change that was underlying the statistical signal. A genomic DNA variant that is found within the linked region can be argued as being causative for a phenotype based upon the predicted change in protein structure and/or function, or again with statistics. Functional studies at the laboratory bench then follow in an attempt to prove causation mechanistically in vitro, or sometimes in vivo in an animal model. While non-geneticists might regard this to be a 'backward approach' for identifying molecules, positional cloning moves forward from the geneticist's perspective and has an excellent track record in disease gene identification, especially for monogenic diseases.

In contrast, the candidate gene approach typically utilizes information from prior cellular, biochemical or physiological functional studies to target a gene of interest. Molecular markers are developed and the relationship of the gene of interest with the disease phenotype is evaluated typically using statistical correlation or regression analysis. Non-geneticists regard this as a 'forward' approach for identifying disease genes, since the evidence for a functional role of the protein has already been derived from other lines of experimentation. However, the applicability of this approach, when defined strictly, is limited to genes whose products have already been functionally evaluated. Thus, traditional candidate genes are those whose dysfunction might reasonably be expected to cause a disease because of evidence from non-genetic experiments. In cardiovascular disease (CVD) for instance, candidate genes may be selected because the proteins they encode, such as lipid metabolic enzymes or blood clotting factors, are involved in pathways that lead to the development of an atherosclerotic plaque. Candidate genes can be evaluated for their relationship with disease phenotypes using either association studies in unrelated individuals or linkage studies in family units.

Identifying the causative genes for Mendelian diseases and the susceptibility genes for complex diseases are priorities for several reasons. First, bioanalytical assays based on genomic information will probably add value to clinical decision-making algorithms for diagnosis, prognosis, early prediction of disease susceptibility and/or patient stratification to maximize the efficacy of therapies. Also, genomic science broadens the spectrum of experimental approaches available for the discovery of biological pathways and mechanisms in health and disease. This information should help to specify new molecular targets for either classical pharmacological or novel molecular interventions.

Genetics Studies among the Inuit

Historically, Inuit have had a shorter duration of sustained exposure to European individuals and influences compared with other Aboriginal peoples. For the most part, Inuit even today still live in relative geographical isolation from other populations, and the numbers of individuals from European or other ethnic backgrounds living in their communities are relatively few. Thus, the Inuit can be considered to constitute a genetic isolate, with relatively few accumulated genetic influences from other populations. This isolation has resulted in some genetic differences, observed in a previous era for such genetically determined serological and biochemical markers as blood groups, the human leukocyte antigen system, and erythrocyte enzymes (discussed in chapter 7).[4] From a human genomic perspective, it also appears that such differences are seen at the DNA level, with distinctive patterns of distributions of SNP genotypes among the Inuit. In turn, there may be differences in the distribution of the subset of functional SNP genotypes that determine susceptibility to complex traits. This has been the hypothesis underlying the fledgling field of genetic studies of disease susceptibility in the Inuit – how does this population differ from others at the genomic level and do such differences influence disease susceptibility?

As mentioned above, there are two basic strategies used to pinpoint genes that might play a role in disease, namely, genome-wide scanning of families to find a linked chromosomal segment with positional target genes or the direct evaluation of polymorphisms within functional candidate genes whose identity has already been established.

One genome-wide linkage study – the Genetics of Coronary Artery Disease in Alaska Natives (GOCADAN) Study – enrolled 1,214 Inuit from several coastal villages in the Norton Sound region of western Alaska to identify loci influencing CVD-related traits.[5]

Thus, the majority of studies about the Inuit so far have been association studies involving a functional candidate, such as a SNP in a candidate gene, which is then evaluated for its relationship with disease phenotypes (tables 13.1–13.3). At least twenty-six common polymorphisms have been examined in the Inuit to date. These investigations in the Canadian, Greenland, and Alaskan populations have revolved primarily around cardiovascular and metabolic diseases.

Cardiovascular Diseases

The genetic component of atherosclerosis is complex, with the contributions of numerous genes interacting with environmental determinants.[6] Alleles of many different candidate genes, such as those involved in lipid metabolism (*APOE, APOB, APOC3, CETP, LPL,* and *PON* genes), homocysteine metabolism (*MTHFR* gene), blood viscosity (*FGA* and *F5* genes), platelet aggregation (*GP3A* gene), leukocyte adhesion (*SELE* gene), and the renin-angiotensin system (*ACE* and *AGT* genes), have been variably shown to be associated with atherosclerosis and its intermediate traits in various populations.

Inuit have long been considered to have a lower CVD burden than the general population.[7] Studies of CVD in the Canadian Inuit found lower age-adjusted mortality rates for coronary heart disease (CHD), fewer hospitalizations due to vascular disease, and an overall ~40 per cent reduction in CVD mortality for the Inuit in comparison to the general Canadian population. However, a more recent review has questioned such observations and has shown that the mortality from CHD was similar or just slightly lower among the Inuit of Alaska, northern Canada, and Greenland compared with white control populations (see chapter 16).

Part of putative health advantage for Inuit people might be attributable to protective environmental or lifestyle factors, such as dietary omega-3 fatty acids in Arctic fish (see chapter 11). The Inuit have also been noted to have fewer CVD risk factors, with generally lower levels of hypertension, except among young men, and favourable plasma concentrations of lipids. However, a high level of obesity among Inuit women has also been observed (see chapter 16). Genetic studies have attempted to determine whether Inuit have some endogenous protection against CVD. The studies have included examining the prevalence of common disease-associated alleles, and also testing associations between candidate genes and intermediate quantitative traits related to vascular disease (tables 13.1–13.3).

Box 13.2 *APOE* gene encoding apolipoprotein E

One of the most commonly studied candidates in atherosclerosis is the *APOE* gene encoding apolipoprotein (apo) E, a protein constituent of plasma lipoproteins, specifically very low-density lipoproteins (VLDLs), high-density lipoproteins (HDLs) and chylomicrons. Functionally, apo E participates in the transport and exchange of cholesterol and other lipids among various cells of the body, playing a key role in the uptake of remnant lipoprotein particles through its ability to mediate high-affinity binding to specific lipoprotein receptors. There are three circulating isoforms of apo E, designated E2, E3, and E4 (Mendelian Inheritance in Man [MIM] database numbers 107741.0001, 107741.0015, 107741.0016), that are the result of SNPs that encode arginine to cysteine substitutions at codons 112 and 158. The circulating protein isoforms of apo E have varying degrees of binding affinity for cell surface receptors in turn affecting circulating lipid and lipoprotein concentrations (12). The E4 allele has consistently been associated with increased plasma concentrations of low-density lipoprotein (LDL) cholesterol, increased susceptibility to coronary artery disease and increased carotid arterial wall intima-medial thickness, thus making it a prime candidate as a risk factor for atherosclerosis and CVD.[8]

In three Inuit communities studied – from Greenland,[9] northern Canada,[10] and Alaska[11] – the E4 allele frequency ranged from 0.19–0.23, which was notably higher than in European individuals and much higher than in individuals of South Asian or Pacific Rim ancestry. Among Greenland Inuit, carriers of the E4 allele also had a trend towards an increasing extent of atherosclerotic lesions in the aorta and coronary arteries. Among Alaskan Inuit, *APOE* genotype was associated with coronary artery atherosclerosis, but somewhat paradoxically, while the E4 allele correlated with increased atherosclerosis risk within the Inuit population, its high frequency in the Inuit seems to be out of keeping with the apparent absence of obvious increased CVD and CHD risk in Inuit compared with other populations. The results suggest that other factors – genetic and/or environmental – might modulate the effects of this 'deleterious allele' upon atherogenesis and CVD risk in the Inuit.

In studies that evaluated a larger set of candidate gene markers for CVD in Canadian Inuit, it was found that, of fifteen alleles examined, five were significantly less frequent among Inuit than among individuals of European descent, five were significantly more frequent, and five were not different in frequency. These results then were consistent with, respectively, decreased, increased, and no difference in CVD risk among Inuit compared with individuals of European descent (table 13.1). The particular alleles whose frequency was significantly higher among Inuit than among individuals of European descent were *ADRB3* R64, *AGT* T235, *APOE* E4, *FABP2* T54, and *PON1* R192. Similarly, among Greenland Inuit, alleles of six candidate genes were found to be significantly less frequent than in Caucasians, consistent with decreased risk, while the *AGT* T235 and *APOE* E4 alleles had increased frequencies, as in Canadian Inuit (table 13.2). Among Alaska Inuit, significantly higher frequencies for both the *APOE* E4 and *ADRB3* R64 alleles were observed (table 13.3).

At the very least, these limited, preliminary studies confirmed a significant difference in genetic architecture based on SNP genotypes among Inuit compared with individuals of European descent. However, these differences could not be directly translated into population risk of CVD outcomes. The genetic variants tested might have had little biological association with disease in the Inuit, while unmeasured genomic variants could have played a more important role. In addition, genetic associations might have been 'context dependent' – that is, their effect on risk depended on background genetic and environmental factors – and their direct role, if any, on CVD risk could not be determined without understanding these contextual influences. For example the *ACE* deletion, *F5* Q506, and *MTHFR* 677T alleles might have been relatively more important determinants of CVD susceptibility among Inuit than in other groups, and their lower frequency would thus impart greater protection from disease. A full understanding of the genetic component of CVD in the Inuit will require more effort because of confounding factors such as context-dependency, small

Table 13.1 Genetic studies in Canadian Inuit

Gene		Allele	Frequency	Comparison
ACE	angiotensin converting enzyme	deletion	0.31[a]	low frequency in comparison with Europeans* protective role against atherosclerosis?
F5	factor V Leiden	Q506	0[b]	
HFE	hemochromatosis	Y282	0[a]	
MBL	mannose-binding lectin	non-A	0.09[c]	
MTHFR	methylenetetrahydrofolate reductase	677T	0.061[d]	
ADRB	β-3 adrenergic receptor	R64	0.30[a]	high frequency in comparison with Europeans* increased risk for atherosclerosis?
AGT	angiotensinogen	T235	0.82[e]	
APOE	apolipoprotein E	E4	0.23[e]	
FABP2	fatty acid binding protein	T54	0.35[e]	
PON1	paraoxonase-1	R192	0.70[e]	
APOC3	apolipoprotein CIII	-455C	0.47[a]	similar frequency to Europeans no difference in risk for atherosclerosis
GNB3	G protein 3 subunit	825T	0.50[f]	
LIPC	hepatic lipase	-480C	0.60[g]	
PON2	paraoxonase-2	G148	0.29[a]	
PPP1R3	protein phosphatase-1 regulatory subunit 3A	deletion	0.33[a]	

Table 13.1 (continued)

Gene		Allele	Frequency	Association
ABCA1	ATP-binding cassette A1	M823	0.29[h]	elevated HDL cholesterol 21
APOC3	apolipoprotein CII	-455C	0.47	metabolic syndrome (for women only) low HDL cholesterol (for women only)
APOE	apolipoprotein E	E4	0.23[a]	elevated LDL cholesterol
CRP	C-reactive protein	1059C	0.0[i]	CRP and CTSS haplotype – variation in CRP
CTSS	cathepsin S	-25A	0.404[i]	elevated serum CRP
CYP7	cholesterol 7-α hydroxylase	-278A	0.49[j]	elevated total and LDL cholesterol
FABP2	fatty acid-binding protein	T54	0.35[e]	low 2-h post prandial glucose
GNB3	G protein β3 subunit	825T	0.50[f]	elevated weight, BMI, waist girth, hip girth, skinfold thickness (subscapular and triceps)
LMNA	lamin A/C	1908T	0.48[k]	elevated weight, BMI, waist girth, waist to hip circumference, skinfold thickness (subscapular and triceps)
PON1	paraoxonase-1	M55	0.097[l]	elevated total and LDL cholesterol

*Allele frequency is significantly different (p<0.05).

[a]Hegele (1999).
[b]Mandelcorn et al. (1998).
[c]Hegele, Busch et al. (1999).
[d]Hegele, Tully, et al. (1997).
[e]Hegele, Young, and Connelly (1997).
[f]Hegele, Anderson, et al. (1999).
[g]Hegele, Harris, et al. (1999).
[h]Wang et al. (2000).
[i]Hegele, Ban, and Young (2001).
[j]Hegele, Wang, et al. (2001).
[k]Hegele, Huff, and Young (2001).
[l]Fanella et al. (2000).

Table 13.2 Genetic studies in Greenland Inuit

Gene		Allele	Frequency	Comparison
ACE	angiotensin converting enzyme	deletion	0.40[a]	
F7	factor VII	promoter	0.68[b]	
		P0	0.38	
		HVR4 (H6)	0.71	low frequency in comparison with Europeans - protective role against atherosclerosis?
		R353		
FGA	α-fibrinogen	T1	0.53[c]	
FGB	β-fibrinogen	-455A	0.11[c]	
		B2	0.12	
GP3A	glycoprotein IIIa	Pl(A2)	0.037[d]	
PLAT	tissue-type plasminogen activator	insertion	0.37[a]	
AGT	angiotensinogen	T235	0.70[a]	
APOE	apolipoprotein E	E4	0.21[e]	
PAI1	plasminogen activator inhibitor 1	deletion	0.88[a]	high frequency in comparison with Europeans - increased risk for atherosclerosis?

Gene		Allele	Frequency	Association
FGB	β-fibrinogen	-455A	0.11[c]	higher plasma fibrinogen (for males only)

[a] de Maat, Bladbjerg, Johansen, de Knijff, et al. (1999).
[b] de Maat, Green, et al. (1997).
[c] de Maat, de Knijff, et al. (1995).
[d] de Maat, Bladbjerg, Johansen, Bentzen, et al. (1997).
[e] Boudreau et al. (1999).

Table 13.3 Genetic studies in Alaskan Inuit

Gene		Allele	Frequency	Comparison
APOE	apolipoprotein E	E4	0.19[a]	increased total surface lesion involvement for both right and left coronary arteries; frequency significantly higher than American white population
ADRB3	β-3 adrenergic receptor	R64	0.38[b]	no associations found; highest frequency to date, increased risk for atherosclerosis?

[a]Scheer et al. (1995).
[b]Biery et al. (1997).

genetic effects, non-Mendelian inheritance, gene-gene interactions, and gene-environment interactions. Even with more understanding of the meaning of the Inuit 'genetic profile' as conferring either suscepti-bility or resistance to atherosclerosis, it is possible that lifestyle factors could further attenuate or amplify any genetic influence(s).

Hypertension

An important risk factor for CVD is hypertension, a complex trait with a heritable component. A recent study found that mean blood pressure in Inuit ranks intermediate on a global scale but low in comparison with most European populations. Furthermore it was observed that the Inuit population itself is heterogeneous, with differences observed between regional subgroups, likely influenced by differences in diet, lifestyle, and underlying genetic factors.[12]

Some potential candidate genes for blood pressure include two that encode key participants in the renin-angiotensinogen system of blood pressure control, namely ACE encoding angiotensin converting enzyme and AGT encoding angiotensinogen, and also a component of autonomic nervous signalling pathways, namely GNB3 encoding the G-protein beta-3 subunit. All three candidates have been studied in Canadian Inuit, and ACE and AGT have been examined in the Green-land Inuit (tables 13.1 and 13.2). As no significant associations were found between the selected genes and blood pressure, their relation-ship with hypertension for the Inuit is unclear. Interestingly, the observed allele frequencies for the AGT T235 'risk' allele were high among the Inuit, with Canadian Inuit notably having one of the highest frequencies of the AGT T235 allele of any population in the world. This suggests either that variation in AGT is not an important genetic determinant of blood pressure in the Inuit, or that other factors – genetic or environmental – attenuate the possible relationship between blood pressure and AGT variation. One such genetic factor might be the impact of a 'favourable' lower frequency of the ACE dele-tion allele among Inuit.

Metabolic Syndrome

The metabolic syndrome (MetS) is another complex clinical entity with multiple genetic determinants. MetS is associated with an increased risk of developing type 2 diabetes and CVD, and is characterized by abdominal obesity, hypertension, hypertriglyceridemia, low plasma concentration of HDL cholesterol, and elevated plasma concentration of glucose, with underlying insulin resistance. MetS is a very common trait and will likely become even more pervasive, considering the poor lifestyle habits prevalent in many societies today. While the increased prevalence in MetS is primarily related to an imbalance between caloric intake and expenditure, genetic factors are also likely to be important. Each of the defining components has been previously linked to genetic modifiers, indicating that there are numerous possibilities for genetic players in the overall MetS – both independently and in more complex interactive pathways.[13]

A potential candidate underlying genetic susceptibility to MetS is apolipoprotein C-III (*APOC3*), one of the most studied genes in lipoprotein metabolism. *APOC3* encodes a 79-amino-acid glycoprotein produced mainly in the liver, which acts as a constituent of triglyceride-rich lipoprotein particles, inhibiting the action of lipoprotein lipase and interfering with receptor-mediated lipoprotein uptake. Within an insulin-response element of the *APOC3* promoter region lies two SNPs, -455T>C and -482C>T, which are hypothesized to hinder regular insulin-mediated down-regulation, leaving the gene constitutively active. Consequently, when considering the role of apoC-III in lipoprotein metabolism, overexpression may promote the development of hypertriglyceridemia, as has been observed in other studies previously, and, more recently, *APOC3* promoter SNPs have been associated with MetS in both South Asians and Aboriginal Canadian females.[14]

While examining the –455T>C *APOC3* promoter polymorphism as a candidate gene for MetS in Canada Inuit, it was found that female –455C allele carriers had an unfavorable lipid phenotype with elevated plasma triglyceride and depressed HDL cholesterol concentrations and, furthermore, female –455C allele carriers also had an increased risk of MetS (OR 5.74, 95% CI 1.05, 31.4; $P=0.044$) (Hegele, unpublished data). In contrast to the females, *APOC3* –455T>C had no association with MetS among Inuit males. Any underlying genetic associations may have been concealed by the lower prevalence of MetS among male Inuit and certainly there may have been additional untested genes that played a greater role in the risk of MetS for males. This association between the –455T>C *APOC3* promoter polymorphism and MetS for Inuit females was likely mediated, at least in part, through associations with some intermediate quantitative traits that are used in the definition of the syndrome (i.e., triglycerides and HDL cholesterol).

Since abdominal obesity is a key component of the MetS – probably the cornerstone for its development – understanding the genetic determinants of obesity among the Inuit might help illuminate the genetic basis of MetS. In this regard, the 1908C>T SNP genotype of *LMNA*, which encodes nuclear lamins A and C and is a genetic determinant of fat distribution in some families, was associated with increased body mass index, waist circumference, waist to hip circumference ratio, subscapular skinfold thickness, and subscapular to triceps skinfold thickness ratio among Canadian Inuit. For each significantly associated obesity-related trait, the *LMNA* 1908C>T SNP genotype accounted for between approximately 10 to 100 per cent of the attributable variation of these obesity-related traits.[15] Also, the *GNB3* 825T allele was associated with increased body weight, body mass index, waist girth, hip girth, subscapular skinfold thickness, and triceps skinfold thickness among Canadian Inuit. The *GNB3* 825C>T genotype accounted for approximately 10 per cent of attributable variation of the obesity-related traits.[16] These two examples indicate that common genomic variation may be an important determinant of obesity-related quantitative traits in Inuit, and perhaps even with the MetS itself, creating opportunities for future studies in the Inuit, not just to confirm the associations, but also to examine prospectively the influence of interventions and relationships between genotypes and long-term complications of obesity and MetS.

Conclusion

The biological pathways, intermediate biochemical and physiological subsystems, and clinical endpoints of atherosclerosis and CVD among the Inuit are complex. This will likely cloud the assessment of the genetically determined risk of atherosclerosis among Inuit. However, even if more advanced analytical approaches are applied, it may be impossible to predict the clinical onset of atherosclerosis in a particular individual because the factors at the instant of acute luminal occlusion may not be influenced by predictable determinants. At best, any probability statements of risk for an individual must be derived from large numbers of observations and the totality of experimental evidence, which may be sometimes conflicting. Probability statements would be approximate and might serve only to reduce uncertainty about risk rather than to predict the onset of disease.

Finally, the modern revolution in molecular genetics and biology has focused our attention on the genetic component of disease, at the expense of the environmental component. This is true not only for atherosclerosis but also for cancer, diabetes, obesity, and neuropsychological disorders. The implication that genetics is of prime importance in the etiology of disease is reminiscent of a similar situation a century ago. At that time, just after the discovery of bacteria, the appealing power of the fledgling field of microbiology led overzealous investigators to naively attribute many diseases to microbial causes. Subsequent scientific progress helped to define strict criteria for attributing causation to infectious agents. This imposed a satisfying rigour on the concept of disease etiology and more importantly permitted the development of rational interventional strategies. The current obsession with genetic etiologies can be viewed as part of a general societal trend in which external, uncontrollable deterministic factors are seen to be of primary importance in any adverse outcome, at the expense of the component of personal responsibility. It is likely that personal decisions and actions will be shown to mitigate the impact of unfavourable genetics. Thus, even the individual who carries genes that predispose to atherosclerosis and CVD can take personal responsibility for actions to avoid victimization by her/his genetic endowment. For a population like the Inuit that is experiencing profound changes in lifestyle and environment, the likely primacy of environment over genetics as a determinant of CVD risk should be appreciated in design of public health or preventive strategies.

NOTES

1 For a discussion of SNPs in the human genome, see Ireland et al. (2006).
2 Iafrate et al. (2004).
3 Lander and Schork (1994).
4 See Eriksson, Lehman, and Simpson (1980) for a review of genetic studies among circumpolar populations, and also Bjerregaard and Young (1998:216–17) for a summary of some of the older studies relating to rare genetic disorders that have been identified among Inuit.
5 The design and methods of the GOCADAN Study were presented by Howard et al. (2005).
6 Summary tables of gene frequency tables can be found in Hegele (1999).
7 See Bjerregaard and Dyerberg (1988) for data from Greenland; Middaugh (1990) for Alaska; and Young, Moffatt, and O'Neil (1993) for Canada.

Bjerregaard, Young, and Hegele (2003) came to the conclusion that the reputed low risk of cardiovascular disease among Inuit lacks evidence.

8 For a general review of the biology of APOE, see Mahley (1988) and Sing and Davignon (1985).
9 Boudreau et al. (1999).
10 Hegele, Young, and Connelly (1997).
11 Scheer et al. (1995).
12 Bjerregaard et al. (2003b).
13 The definition of the metabolic syndrome is provided in the summary report of the National Cholesterol Education Program Expert Panel on Detection, Evaluation, and Treatment of High Blood Cholesterol in Adults (2001). Since then, other definitions and criteria have been developed.
14 Data on South Asians were provided by Guettier et al. (2005) and on Aboriginal Canadians by Pollex et al. (2006).
15 Hegele, Huff, and Young (2001).
16 Hegele, Anderson, et al. (1999).

14 Cold Exposure, Adaptation, and Performance

TIINA MÄKINEN AND MIKA RYTKÖNEN

Circumpolar residents are exposed to cold during their occupational activities, while commuting to work, and/or during their leisure time. Circumpolar environmental conditions are characterized by marked fluctuations in temperature and sunlight, with long, cold, and dark winters and short, cool, bright summers. In these northern areas, winter is the longest season. For example, in Finland, the number of days when the mean daily temperature drops below 0°C range between 90 and 220. Most often, the coldest days occur in January and February, and temperatures as low as –50°C have been recorded in Fennoscandia (map 10). The cold conditions in winter are often further aggravated by wind and precipitation. The reduced amount of daylight and the presence of snow and ice are factors that modify the environment and the hazards associated with it. Cold affects the performance of a variety of tasks, and directly and indirectly affects human health (fig. 14.1). In response, humans have developed anatomical, physiological, and behavioural adaptations to enable them to cope, survive, and thrive in the Arctic.

Extent of Cold Exposure

The type of cold exposure people encounter in their everyday life includes exposure to cold air, immersion in water, and contact with cold surfaces (from sitting, lying, or standing on them). Accordingly, cooling may target different parts of the body. Prolonged exposure to cold, often associated with insufficient clothing or physical inactivity, may result in whole-body cooling and a decrease in core temperature. This type of cooling is further enhanced by exposure to wind or cold water, which increases the convective heat loss from the body to the

Figure 14.1   Effects of cold on humans

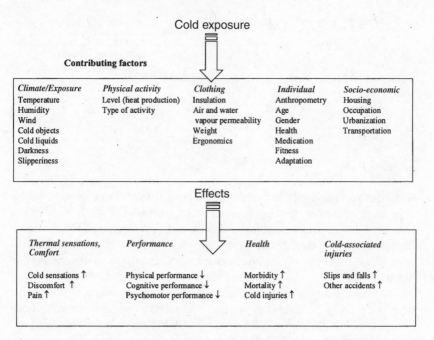

Source: Reprinted from *American Journal of Human Biology* 19, no. 2 (2007), with permission of Wiley-Liss, a subsidiary of Wiley and Sons, Inc.

environment. Cooling can also be restricted to the extremities (head, hands, and feet), and is often exacerbated by touching or handling cold objects. This type of cooling is common both in occupational and leisure-time activities. In some cases, cooling may also involve specific body regions, such as the respiratory tract. Respiratory tract cooling from oronasal breathing can be pronounced during heavy exercise in cold weather.[1]

Exposure to cold in our modern society tends to occur for repeated but relatively short periods. A population survey conducted in Finland demonstrated that the average self-reported cold exposure time in winter is approximately 4 per cent of the total time.[2] The degree of exposure to cold is dependent on several factors, such as occupation, gender, age, health, exercise activity, and education. Also, motivational or personality factors may affect an individual's decision to be exposed to cold. Circumpolar residents are commonly confronted with cold during their outdoor leisure-time activities. Work-related cold exposure in industrialized countries is relatively short or absent altogether. However, it may be substantial in some industries such as agriculture, forestry, mining, factory work, construction, and related occupations[2] where thermal strain and different adverse performance effects are likely to occur.[3] For indigenous people who still pursue their traditional activities such as reindeer herding, hunting or fishing, cold exposure can be significant. One population group that is also exposed to cold significantly is military personnel. The duration of outdoor cold exposure in winter during military training can equal or exceed that of other cold outdoor occupations. In these conditions, adverse performance effects and cold injuries are common.[4] Workers employed in a cold indoor environment, especially in the food industry, can be exposed to excessive cold. Fresh foodstuff is often processed at temperatures of −10°C, and frozen goods at temperatures below −20°C. Under such cold indoor conditions, increased muscular strain and different musculoskeletal complaints and symptoms are common, especially with repetitive work tasks.[5]

Although circumpolar residents are commonly exposed to cold in their daily life, there are factors that reduce the potential adverse cold effects. Modern humans live in housing that separates them from the environment and reduces the cold stress. In many northern countries, central heating has enabled high indoor temperatures in homes throughout the year. An additional factor reducing cold stress is modern cold-protective clothing, permitting many activities to be carried out under even harsh environmental conditions. Modern transportation vehicles also allow commuters and employees to travel and work under conditions that minimize cold stress.

Cold Adaptation

Humans can adapt to living in cold environmental temperatures, similar to other stressors. An individual's physiological adaptation denotes a progressive reduction in thermal strain when repeatedly exposed to stress (see definitions in box 14.1). Adaptation to the circumpolar cold climates may partially be genotypic, a result of long-term genetic selection. A study by Piazza and others demonstrated that 60 per cent of the thirty-nine independent alleles of different indigenous populations around the world showed significant associations with climate. Furthermore, latitude, more particularly the distance from the equator, suggested selective pressures for certain genes.[6]

Box 14.1 Definitions of thermal adaptation

Terms such as adaptation, acclimatization, acclimation, and habituation are often used interchangeably in everyday speech. The International Union of Physiological Sciences (2001) published a glossary of terms for thermal physiology, which are reproduced here:

Adaptation: Changes that reduce the physiological strain produced by stressful components of the total environment. This change may occur within the lifetime of an organism (phenotypic) or be the result of genetic selection in a species of subspecies (genotypic).
Acclimation: Adaptation that occurs within an organism in response to experimentally induced changes in particular climatic factors.
Acclimatization: Adaptive changes that occur within an organism in response to changes in the natural climate.
Habituation: Reduction of responses to, or perception of, a repeated stimulation.

One example of genotypic adaptation to northern climates is the ecological generalizations of the nineteenth-century biologists Allen and Bergmann, who showed that northern animal species had a larger body mass and lower surface area to mass ratio (i.e., shorter extremities), which favoured heat conservation.[7] Among humans an inverse relationship between body mass and environmental temperature was demonstrated by Roberts, who studied 116 different indigenous populations around the world, and by Newman, who studied Native American populations in the western hemisphere. Although climatic factors affect body size and morphology, changes in nutrition have moderated their influence. Maintaining homeostasis and a high body temperature are energetically expensive and may have been conflicting selection pressures influencing the variability of thermogenesis in humans.[8] The observed different thermal responses and cold adaptation patterns between different indigenous populations residing in both northern and southern latitudes could also suggest phylogenetic differences in cold tolerance.[9] However, the evidence of genotypic adaptation is not consistent, and the results of these studies may have been confounded by the diversity of lifestyles and environments.

Much of the observed adaptation to cold is phenotypic, that is, occurring rapidly and within a lifetime of an individual human being. In fact, the majority of thermal changes related to repeated exposures to cold occur within a couple of weeks. Physiological adaptation due to repeated exposures to cold is a neural process, including changes mainly in the circulation and endocrine organs. Habituation is the most common form of cold adaptation and develops in response to repeated cold exposures where whole-body cooling is not substantial. When becoming habituated to cold, shivering and the vasoconstrictor response are blunted, stress responses are reduced, and the sensations of cold becomes less intense. Cold habituation responses can develop quickly, even after a few repeated cold exposures. Hence, it could be hypothesized that this is the most common form of adaptation in modern circumpolar societies, where on average cold exposure is short, winter clothing and housing adequate, and where repetitive marked whole-body cooling is unlikely to occur. If a more substantial whole-body cooling occurs repeatedly, the main cold adaptation responses are either to allow a drop in core temperature before heat production mechanisms are initiated (hypothermic response), increase the amount of insulation (insulative response due to more subcutaneous fat and/or enhanced vasoconstriction), or increase the level of heat production (metabolic response due to shivering or non-shivering thermogenesis). Mixtures of the previous types, for example insulative-hypothermic or metabolic-insulative responses, have also been detected and, in general, large interindividual variation in these reactions is observed. Factors affecting the thermal responses include, for example, age, gender, amount of subcutaneous fat, general health, fitness, medication, and previous adaptation. In addition to the individual characteristics, the resultant cold adaptation strategy depends on the type (air, water) and intensity of the cold exposure.[10]

Physiological cold acclimatization responses among the circumpolar indigenous populations were studied mainly in the 1950s and 1960s.[11] Canadian Indians of the Yukon and Inuit were intermittently exposed to cold while hunting and trapping. Furthermore, they were often well protected with arctic clothing. The adaptation to cold was largely restricted to the extremities (e.g., hands) where higher skin temperatures were recorded. The metabolic rate was also higher compared with non-acclimatized people. The pattern of adaptation among the Inuit resembles metabolic acclimatization. In contrast to the Inuit, the nomadic Sami showed no increase in metabolic rate, but a pronounced drop in rectal temperature indicating a hypothermic insulative acclimatization. Since the 1990s there has been a resurgence of interest in the basal metabolic rate (BMR) of northern indigenous populations. A meta-analysis combining data from several circumpolar populations from North America and Siberia implicate that indigenous populations have a higher BMR, which is suggested as being due to both functional and genetic factors (e.g., thyroid function).[12]

What type of thermal adaptation is prevalent among present-day circumpolar residents? The modern lifestyle associated with urban circumpolar areas indicate a lack of typical cold habituation responses. Overall, information of urban seasonal adaptation to cold is scarce, is limited in many cases to mild/moderately cold climates, and has shown divergent results.[13] Moreover, a direct comparison between these studies is difficult due to differences in the study protocols, individual characteristics, as well as climatic factors. In contrast to urban indoor workers, signs of physiological cold acclimatization could probably be detected among people employed in outdoor occupations and those exposed to cold repeatedly and for prolonged periods. It is also unclear whether the seasonal thermal responses of the northern indigenous populations of today resemble those reported in the 1950s and 1960s.

A substantial portion of cold adaptation in circumpolar areas is behavioural, including seeking shelter, using protective clothing, improving housing, transportation and so on. Circumpolar residents' behavioural adaptation to cold may have been more efficient compared with people from more southern latitudes. Support for this hypothesis is found from a study where inhabitants of northern Europe tended to protect their extremities more efficiently compared with residents from southern Europe with a given fall in temperature. In this study, the geographical differences in the use of hats, gloves, and scarves were associated with cold-related mortality. Overall, mortality has been shown to increase to a greater extent with a given fall in temperatures in regions with warm winters, in households with low indoor heating, and among people wearing fewer clothes and being less active outdoors. This observation would support behavioural adaptation to life in northern climates.[14]

Human Performance in the Cold

The prerequisite of maintaining performance in cold is a functional sensory system, as well as proper physical and psychological functions. Manual dexterity is also essential for performing many of the tasks outdoors. Being able to operate in cold conditions also requires adequate functioning of the circulatory, respiratory, and hormonal systems, as well as the maintenance of energy and fluid balance to support the performance functions.

A cold environment is associated with increased energy expenditure. This is due to an increased metabolic rate related to maintaining thermal balance in the cold. In laboratory conditions, a decrease in the environmental temperature from 27°C to 22°C increased energy expenditure on average by 156 kJ·°C^{-1}, and from 22°C to 16°C on average by 116 kJ·°C^{-1}. Cold activates the sympathetic nervous system or pituitary-thyroid axis, affecting the secretion of adrenal and thyroid hormones and altering the metabolic rate. The increased energy expenditure in cold can also be related to a lowered physical performance, as well as the increased energy costs related to wearing winter clothing. Although it protects the body from cooling, winter clothing may sometimes impair sensory functions, decrease dexterity, restrict movements, and increase the energy expenditure. Clothing increases the energy expenditure by approximately 3 per cent per kilogram of clothing which is largely due to the weight, bulkiness, and friction caused by the garments.[15]

Manual Performance

The extremities are likely to be cooled first under cold conditions because of their large surface area-to-mass ratio. A decrease in tissue temperature is known to impair manual performance, leading to a lowered capacity to perform a certain task within a defined time, or to an increased amount of errors in doing the task. Cold affects finger dexterity, pinch and handgrip strength, as well as the abduction/adduction of fingers. A slight lowering of skin temperature below the optimum (33°C) causes decreases in tactile sensations. The critical skin temperature in hands, where after a further drop in temperature rapidly impairs manual performance, is 12–15°C. The extremities become numb when the skin temperature decreases to approximately 7°C. If the cooling of the hands progresses further, there is an increased risk of frostbite. Individuals with peripheral circulatory disorders (e.g., Raynaud's phenomenon) can experience further decrements in sensory perception and manual performance in the cold compared with healthy individuals.[16] However, local adaptation to cold in the hands may restore the impaired performance, though not always. This type of adaptation, where skin temperatures are higher and the cold-induced vasodilatation occurs earlier, has been demonstrated among northern indigenous populations as well as among fishers.[17] The disadvantage of a dampened vasoconstriction in hands is a higher heat loss and increased risk of frostbite, if the cooling is continued.

Physical Performance

Many of the functions of physical performance are impaired in cold. Cooling of the muscle impairs most of its functional properties like power, force production, and velocity. Dynamic exercise (external movements) is more susceptible to cooling than static or isometric exercise. In dynamic work, the maximal force production, power, and time to reach the maximal force level, as well as the relaxation rate of the muscles is increased. Especially fast movements are susceptible to cooling. A dose-dependent relationship between the degree of muscle cooling and decrement in performance has been observed, and already a slight lowering of muscle temperature significantly impairs its performance. For example, performance of dynamic tasks decreases by 2–10 per cent/°C decrease in muscle temperature. Furthermore, a cold exposure commonly observed in winter in the circumpolar areas causes a 5–20 per cent decrement in physical performance.[18] The impaired power and force production of cooled muscles could be a result of changes in their neuromuscular and reflex functioning or altered nerve conduction velocity.[19] Balance may also be impaired because of cold exposure and related cooling effects on sensory, neural, and muscular functions. This finding may be important to recognize during leisure-time or occupational activities performed in cold environmental conditions. Moreover, persons that are at higher risk of falling (e.g., elderly people, persons with a neurological or muscu-losceletal disorder) may be especially susceptible to the effects of cooling because of changes in their postural control.[20]

The above-mentioned deficits in power and coordination related to cooling of muscles and nerves, combined with the complexity of human movements, are likely to result in impaired physical performance and in an increased risk of accidents in the cold. Furthermore, as a result of these changes, more effort has to be put into fulfilling a specific task compared with when performing it in a warm environment.

Psychological Performance

Mental performance plays an important role in the areas of orientation, safety, decision-making, work productivity, and reactions to emergency situations. It is known that both hot and cold environmental temperatures impair cognition. Overall, cold exposure may adversely affect vigilance, concentration, memory, reasoning, and general intelligence.[21] In general, the adverse effects of cold are demonstrated as an increase in errors and in longer response times. The effects are dependent on the type of tasks, as well as the type and duration of the cold exposures.

It is well known that marked whole-body cooling associated with a reduction in core temperature by 2–4°C impairs cognitive functions, such as memory and concentration.[22] If body cooling progresses below the level of hypothermia (35°C) symptoms of confusion, amnesia, and decreased alertness and consciousness are seen. The results of moderate, non-hypothermic cold exposure on cognition are inconsistent, however, so that decreased, unaltered, or even improved cognitive performance has been observed. This type of cooling would be more likely to occur during occupational or recreational activities of circumpolar residents. Two distinct theories on the effects of cold on cognitive performance have been proposed. The distraction hypothesis suggests that the discomfort caused by cold could consume central attention resources, causing a momentary switch of attention from the primary task and leading to impaired performance.[23] Another theory suggests that the general arousal level is increased by mild to moderate cold exposure, which initially leads to improved performance. However, with continued, prolonged, or more severe cooling arousal may increase to a level where performance is degraded.[24] Recent studies have suggested that a moderate cold exposure, involving only cooling of the superficial parts of the body, may affect performance on complex cognitive tasks beneficially through an increase in arousal, while simple tasks are impaired, possibly due to cold-related distraction.[25]

It is also possible that season is associated with changes in cognition. The increased prevalence of depressive symptoms/negative mood states in winter was named seasonal affective disorder (SAD) by Rosenthal in the 1980s. The lack of light is known to trigger SAD and also to increase the occurrence of subclinical depressive symptoms (S-SAD) in winter. The prevalence of winter SAD ranges from 1–10 per cent and winter S-SAD from 2–19 per cent in North America and Europe, and has been suggested to increase with latitude, but the evidence supporting this hypothesis is not entirely conclusive. The negative mood states associated with winter could impair cognitive processes, for example disrupting encoding processes and leading to incomplete learning and memory.[26]

It is possible that a cold season could affect cognition through endocrinological changes as well. Cold exposure and a cold season are known to affect the hypothalamic pituitary-thyroid axis, increasing the secretion of thyroid-stimulating hormone (TSH), leading to increased thyroid hormone production and clearance rates and lower levels of free thyroid hormones.[27] This state is called the polar T_3 syndrome and has been demonstrated in over-wintering personnel in Antarctica, as well as in residents living in northern circumpolar environments and employed in outdoor occupations. The lowered levels of free thyroid hormones can lead to a state of subclinical hypothyroidism and increased anxiousness and depression impairing cognition. Further support for the assumption that cognitive performance is connected to season and decreased levels of thyroid hormones was provided by Reed, who demonstrated that the decline in cognitive performance among personnel over-wintering in Antarctica is reversed with a thyroid hormone supplement.[28]

Effect of Cold on Health

A cold climate may pose significant health risks. Exposure to low environmental temperatures is known to result in increased morbidity and mortality, as well as cold injuries and accidents. The population groups especially susceptible to the adverse health effects of cold are small children, the elderly, individuals with health problems, those with poor physical fitness, and persons who are otherwise poorly prepared.[29]

Cold may be an aetiological factor for certain diseases or aggravate the symptoms of prevailing chronic diseases. Symptoms induced by cold temperatures are diverse and originate from various organs of the human body. They are manifested as symptoms of diseases and illnesses such as cardiovascular, respiratory, peripheral circulatory, musculoskeletal, and skin diseases. The prevalence of different symptoms and complaints in cold is common among the general population, as well as in different outdoor occupational groups. The most common symptoms are respiratory symptoms (shortness of breath, increased extraction of mucus, cough) and white fingers, with a lesser amount of cardiac symptoms. These symptoms become more prevalent during exercise in the cold and with aging. This may limit outdoor activities in the elderly population. Cold-related symptoms start to appear more commonly when the temperature falls below –10ºC. With a decrease in temperature, cardiovascular symptoms are the first to appear, followed by respiratory symptoms, white fingers, and peripheral circulatory, as well as musculoskeletal symptoms. Finally, outdoor activity becomes difficult or even restricted in extreme cold (below –25°C) due to these symptoms and complaints.[30]

Wintertime increases morbidity from cardiovascular and respiratory diseases. The rate of hospital admissions for acute myocardial infarction tends to increase during the cold season.[31] Inhalation of cold air cools and dries the respiratory tract, causing airway narrowing and asthma-like symptoms in cold. These symptoms are aggravated specially among people who have a chronic respiratory disease (e.g., asthma, chronic obstructive pulmonary disease) or who are smokers. However, breathing cold air has been shown to increase the amount of inflammatory cells in the lungs of healthy individuals. The increased prevalence of respiratory symptoms, combined with a reduced respiratory capacity, impairs the performance in cold, especially among persons with a respiratory disease.[32]

Excess winter mortality is a well-reported phenomenon throughout the world, and most countries suffer from 5 per cent to 30 per cent excess winter mortality (fig. 14.2). Mortality generally increases below or above an optimum ambient temperature threshold.[33] This increase in mortality with lowered or increased environmental temperature forms a U- or V-shaped curve. Often, increases in mortality become apparent several days or even a week after a cold spell. The temperature thresholds for minimum mortality vary between populations and geographical areas. In the Mediterranean countries this threshold varies between +22 to +25°C, whereas in Finland the mortality minimum is observed at +14°C. The temperature threshold for the mortality minimum is lower in the north than in the south.[34]

Figure 14.2   Seasonality in daily all-cause mortality in Finland, 1961–97

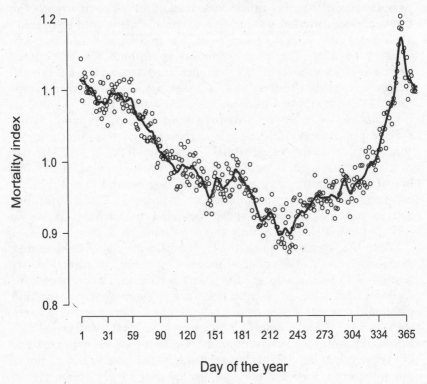

Note: Mortality index based on annual mean mortality = 1.0. Circles represent actual values, line is from smoothing by lowess regression. Day 1 refers to Jan 1.
Source: Näyhä (2005). Figure originally appeared in *Duodecim*, reproduced with permission from the Finnish Medical Society, Helsinki.

Half of the excess winter mortality is due to cerebrovascular diseases (e.g., stroke) and ischemic heart disease, and the other half to respiratory disorders (respiratory infections). The mechanisms are still unknown for the excess winter mortality, but the effects of environmental temperature on human health are most likely multifactorial. An increased sympathetic tone, blood pressure, myocardial oxygen consumption, red blood cell and platelet count, plasma beta-thromboglobulin, platelet factor 4 and plasma fibrinogen, and decreased antithrombin III could be contributing factors. Respiratory and other infections, viral and bacterial, which mostly occur in winter, may trigger attacks of coronary heart disease or stroke, as they affect blood coagulation factors, causing damage to vessel walls, and may promote atherosclerosis.[35] In summary, the available knowledge indicates that cold may be a more important health-risk factor for morbidity and mortality than we have expected so far.

Cold Injuries

Cold injuries (i.e., frostbite) are associated with body cooling, whereas cold-associated injuries are indirectly associated to cold through a more complex pathway (e.g., changed environment). Unsafe behaviour leading to accidents increases when the temperature deviates from 20°C. Cold-associated injuries are commonly strains and sprains resulting from slip-and-fall accidents. The rate of these injuries has been shown to increase markedly when the ambient temperature decrease to or below 0°C. The cold environment is often a contributing cause of injury and not always shown in statistics.[36]

A cold exposure that leads to freezing of the tissues causes frostbite (freezing injury). Frostbite is common in civilian life and can be observed often among young people working or staying continuously in cold environments. Several individual (e.g., peripheral vascular disease, earlier cold injury, psychiatric disorders, use of alcohol, medication, hydration level) and environmental factors (e.g., exposure duration, wind, moisture, contact with cold objects, latitude of residence) affect the frostbite risk. It should be noted that deep frostbite commonly causes different sequelae resulting in long-term symptoms, functional limitations, and disability.[37] Repetitive frostbite in the same individual is also common. The treatment of severe frostbite is difficult, often requiring long hospital treatment periods. Cold may also cause non-freezing injuries (trench foot/immersion foot, hypothermia), which can in severe cases lead to peripheral nerve damage and tissue necrosis. Accidental hypothermia is defined as an unintentional fall in core temperature below 35°C. It is a relatively uncommon problem among active and healthy individuals and occurs primarily among the elderly. Accidental hypothermia may be the result of prolonged exposure to cold air, often associated with attacks of certain diseases or a sudden immersion into cold water.[38]

Management of Cold

Overall, circumpolar residents have learned to cope in harsh environmental conditions, and living in a cold climate does not prevent occupational or leisure-time activities but are continued year-round. Despite this, different cold-related performance limitations, illnesses, and injuries are still common in northern societies, causing an economic burden in terms of lost productivity and costs to the health care systems.[39] However, relatively little attention has been given to the public health measures needed to prevent the adverse health impacts of cold climate. Adaptation to life in cold climates takes place at several levels and therefore the roles of individuals, communities, governments, and the private sector have to be considered in the planning of adaptation strategies.

Managing with cold includes awareness and assessment of its potential risks, as well as implementing different management strategies. Increasing the individual's awareness of the effect of cold on human performance and health is essential; as the modern lifestyle may have somewhat eroded the traditional skills for how to operate in cold climatic conditions. Increasing public awareness of the effects of cold can be achieved through targeted information campaigns, or by integrating this information into the education of health experts as well as the general population (comprehensive schools). Governments or local authorities should provide information about prevention and protection from cold during extreme cold periods to high-risk groups. Assessment of potential cold-related risks of both occupational and leisure-time activities is a prerequisite for planning. The different cold management strategies include organizational and technical measures, as well as the use of cold-protective clothing. In health care, the special needs of the susceptible population groups should be taken into account when planning and practising health care and when providing individual recommendations.

Global warming is likely to bring not only warmer average temperatures but also a greater frequency of extreme weather events, like cold spells, according to the Intergovernmental Panel on Climate Change. Health consequences related to cold climate in circumpolar areas, and in the northern parts of Europe, will remain common and represent the majority of climate-related adverse health effects. The aging population, urbanization, and the variable housing and socio-economic conditions in circumpolar countries may accelerate the emergence of health problems induced by cold climate and extreme weather events; hence, the need for public health responses is increasing. Many of the health effects of climate change will take place via numerous complex and unpredictable pathways and will require interdisciplinary analyses and integrated preventive planning.[40]

Box 14.2 A cold risk assessment tool for northern workplaces

The International Organization for Standardization has adopted a model and methods for risk assessment and management practices for cold workplaces and occupational health professionals. The document *Ergonomics of the Thermal Environment* (2005) contains informative guidelines on how to apply different international thermal standards and other validated scientific methods in the assessment of cold risks. The standard supports good occupational safety and health practices, which are reproduced here.

1. Cold risk assessment

Stage 1. Observation: identification of major cold related risks at workplaces (qualitative information, checklist).
Stage 2. Analysis: quantifying a specific problem at workplaces by occupational health and safety experts (quantitative information, measurements).
Stage 3. Expertise: quantifying a specific problem based on the lower stages of cold-risk assessment. This stage of analyses are performed by occupational health care units, occupational hygienists, or other similar expert institutes with adequate competence (quantitative information, measurements).

2. Assessment of health

Stage 1: Identification of major cold-related health risks (qualitative information, health checklist).
Stage 2: Individual health assessment (interview, clinical investigations).
Stage 3: Specialized analysis of health (clinical investigations, e.g., cold provocation tests).

3. Cold risk management

3.1. Organisational preventive measures: beforehand planning, scheduling of work, pauses, etc.

3.2. Technical preventive measures: tools, work areas, slippery surfaces, lighting, working at heights, climbing, etc.

3.3. Protective clothing: whole-body protection, hand and footwear, head protection, face and respiratory protection, use of personal protective equipment together with cold protective clothing.

3.4. Training and information: learning and guidance material.

3.5. Occupational health care actions for cold work.

4. Practices for cold risk assessment and management

4.1. Practices for cold risk assessment and workplaces.

4.2. Practices for cold risk management at workplaces.

Further details of the methods and practices are given in the annexes of the draft ISO standard (ISO DIS 15743).

NOTES

1 Holmér (1994).

2 Mäkinen, Raatikka et al. (2006). This is the FINRISK 2002 Study, the seventh national health survey which focused on cardiovascular risk factors in a representative sample of adults from several regions of Finland. A cold exposure substudy was conducted on a subsample (n=6,591) of the main survey.

3 Virokannas (1996).

4 Rintamäki, Pääkkönen, et al. (2004); Hassi, Mäkinen, and Rintamäki (2005).

5 Oksa, Ducharme, and Rintmäki (2002); Pienimäki (2002); Oksa, Sormunen, et al. (2006).

6 For a review of ethnic differences in thermoregulation, see Taylor (2006). Piazza, Menozzi, and Cavalli-Sforza (1981) plotted gene frequency maps showing the selective effect of climate.

7 This is now known as the Bergmann's and Allen's Rule. For their original papers, see Allen (1877) and Bergmann (1847).

8 Roberts (1953); Newman (1960); Katzmarzyk and Leonard (1998); Silva (2006).

9 Scholander, Hammel, Andersen, et al. (1958); Scholander, Hammel, Hart, et al. (1958); Andersen et al. (1960); Elsner, Andersen, and Hermansen (1960); Irving et al. (1960); Hammel et al. (1960).

10 See the reviews by Bittel (1992); Young and Blatteis (1996); Rintamäki (2001); Leppäluoto, Korhonen, and Hassi (2001); van Marken Lichtenbelt, Schrauwen, et al. (2002); and Stocks et al. (2004).

11 See notes 1 and 9.

12 See Elsner, Andersen, and Hermansen (1960), Elsner, Nelms, and Irving (1960), and Irving et al. (1960) for data on Canadian subarctic Indians; Hart et al. (1962) on the Inuit; Andersen et al. (1960) on the Sami; Galloway, Leonard, and Ivakine (2000) on Siberian Evenki; and Snodgrass et al. (2005) on the Yakuts. The meta-analysis by Leonard et al. (2002) included data on Inuit and subarctic Indians in Canada and Alaska, and Evenki and Buryat in Russia, as well as non-indigenous northern residents.

13 Hisdal and Reinertsen (1988); Mäkinen, Pääkönen, et al. (2004); van Ooijen et al. (2004).

14 Donaldson, Rintamäki, and Näyhä (2001); Eurowinter Group (1997).

15 van Marken Lichtenbelt, Westerterp-Platenga, and van Hoydonk (2001); Westerterp-Plantenga et al. (2002).

16 Enander (1984); Heus, Daanen, and Havenith (1995); Havenith (1995); Rissanen et al. (2001).

17 See Geurts, Sleivert, and Cheung (2005). Data on Arctic Indians were provided by Irving et al. (1960), Elsner, Andersen, and Hermansen (1960), and Elsner, Nelms, and Irving (1960); Inuit by Hart et al. (1962); Sami and northern Norwegian fishers by Krog et al. (1960); and French-Canadian fishers in the Gaspé region of Quebec by LeBlanc (1962).

18 Faulkner, Zerba, and Brooks (1990); Oksa (1998); Sargeant (1987).

19 Oksa, Rintamäki, et al. (1995, 2000), Rutkove (2001); Dewhurst et al. (2005).

20 Mäkinen, Rintamäki, et al. (2005); Gao and Abeysekera (2004); Demura et al. (2005); Piirtola and Era (2006).

21 See the reviews by Pilcher, Nadler, and Busch (2002), Palinkas (2001), and Hoffman (2001).

22 Coleshaw et al. (1983); Giesbrecht et al. (1993).

23 Teichner (1958); Bowen (1968); Davis, Baddeley, and Hancock (1975); Vaughan (1977).

24 Provins, Glencross, and Cooper (1973); Ellis (1982); Ellis, Wilcock, and Zaman (1985); Enander (1987); van Orden et al. (1990).

25 Palinkas, Mäkinen, et al. (2005); Mäkinen, Palinkas, et al. (2006).

26 Rosenthal et al. (1984); Mersch et al. (1999); Weingartner et al. (1981);

O'Brien, Sahakian, and Checkley (1993); Michalon, Eskes, and Mate-Kole (1997).

27   Pääkkönen (2002); Leppäluoto, Pääkkönen, et al. (2005); Reed (1995).

28   See the Antarctic studies by Reed et al. (1990, 2001), Reed (1995), and Palinkas, Reed, et al. (2001); and the occupational studies in the Arctic by Levine et al. (1995), Leppäluoto, Sikkilä, and Hassi (1998), and Hassi, Sikkilä, et al. (2001).

29   Mercer (2003); Hassi (2005); Eurowinter Group (1997); Donaldson, Ermakov, et al. (1998); Donaldson, Tchernjavskii, et al. (1998); Stocks et al. (2004).

30   Rytkönen, Raatikka, et al. (2005); Hassi, Remes, et al. (2000); Hassi (2005); Raatikka et al. (2007).

31   Spencer et al. (1998); Danet et al. (1999); Näyhä (2002); Hajat, Bird, and Haines (2004); Kloner, Poole, and Perritt (1999); Kloner (2006); Mercer (2003).

32   Kotaniemi et al. (2002, 2003); Larsson et al. (1998).

33   Kunst, Looman, and Mackenbach (1993); Eng and Mercer (1998); Kloner, Poole, and Perritt (1999); Healy (2003); Curriero et al. (2002).

34   Eurowinter Group (1997); Näyhä (2005).

35   Keatinge, Coleshaw, and Cotter (1984); Keatinge, Donaldson, and Bucher (2000); Woodhouse, Khaw, and Plummer (1993); Näyhä (2005).

36   Ramsey et al. (1983); Hassi, Gardner, et al. (2000); Hassi (2005).

37   Hassi and Mäkinen (2000); Hassi, Mäkinen, and Rintamäki (2005); Rintamäki (2000); Ervasti et al. (2004); Castellani and O'Brien (2005).

38   Long et al. (2005); Mallet (2002).

39   Hassi and Mäkinen (2000); Juopperi, Hassi, and Ervasti (2002); Ervasti et al. (2004); Rytkönen et al. (2005).

40   Intergovernmental Panel on Climate Change (2001); World Health Organization (2003a); Haines and Patz (2004); Patz et al. (2005); and Menne and Kristie (2006).

PART FOUR

Consequences

15 Infectious Diseases

ANDERS KOCH, MICHAEL BRUCE, AND PREBEN HOMØE

In the first part of the twentieth century and earlier, infectious diseases were major causes of death in Arctic communities, not only in terms of absolute numbers but also relative to other causes. Since then, infectious disease mortality rates have decreased markedly. In 1925 more than half of all deaths in Greenland were caused by acute infections and tuberculosis, compared with 5 per cent some seventy-five years later.[1]

In spite of this improvement, the overall burden of infectious diseases in the Arctic remains high, and higher than in southern populations. The present pattern of Arctic infectious diseases is characterized by a high incidence of infections common in developed countries (e.g., respiratory tract infections, otitis media) but also by less common infections such as hepatitis and trichinellosis. This chapter focuses on Alaska, Canada, and Greenland, particularly their Inuit populations, about which much information on infectious diseases is available.

Historic Menaces – Epidemics in the Past

Inuit settlements in the Arctic are characterized by their small sizes and scattered locations. In the past, many settlements were isolated for all or most of the year. This isolation provided some protection from infectious diseases, but when new pathogens were introduced, epidemics frequently occurred.

A missionary to Greenland, Hans Egede, wrote about respiratory tract infections in 1738, the speed with which they spread, and the more severe effects on the Inuit compared with the Danes. In the early twentieth century, the Danish physicians Gustav Meldorf and Alfred

Berthelsen described annual epidemics of respiratory tract infections which, in a matter of hours or days, infected most persons in a settlement and others nearby. Symptoms were of various grades of severity, ranging from the common cold to pneumonia. These epidemics likely occurred when weather changes made travelling possible.[2]

In Alaska, outbreaks of influenza and influenza-like illness were frequent in the nineteenth century, often arriving with European or American whalers and merchant ships during the summer. The 'Great Sickness' epidemic of 1900, a combined measles and influenza outbreak, hit western Alaska and caused the death of a quarter of Alaska's Eskimo population, but barely affected the non-Native population.[3]

Nor was the Arctic spared pandemics that affected much of the world. In October 1918, during the Spanish Flu pandemic, a ship left Seattle, Washington, for Nome, Alaska. Although precautions were taken to screen for sick passengers upon their arrival, the local people began to fall ill just days later. The death toll in affected areas was high: in nearby Brevig mission, 85 per cent of the adult population died in just five days. The spread of the pandemic to Alaska eventually helped elucidate the nature of the 1918 influenza virus and confirmed its avian origin. The viral genome was sequenced, using RNA fragments recovered from the lung tissues of a female Eskimo victim from Brevig, who had been buried in permafrost.[4] (Here is another example of research conducted in the Arctic with global implications.)

In Canada, 'virgin soil' epidemics occurred in the Arctic as late as the mid-twentieth century – for example, an outbreak occurred in the Yukon during the construction of the Alaska Highway by the U.S. Army during the Second World War. A major measles epidemic in 1952 reached Baffin Island and the Ungava peninsula in northern Quebec, which affected 99 per cent and killed between 2 per cent and 7 per cent of the population. The epidemic was traced to Inuit visitors to the Armed Forces base at Goose Bay, Labrador.[5]

Greenland was spared measles epidemics for a very long time due to the fact that the requisite long sea voyage exceeded the incubation time and the infectious period of the disease. The first case in Greenland did not appear until 1945. In the 1950s all but the most remote settlements had encountered one or more measles epidemics. Complications were frequent, mostly in the form of pneumonia, otitis media, and meningitis, but tuberculosis mortality also increased significantly during these outbreaks. The first measles vaccination campaign, using 'the Schwarz live further-attenuated measles vaccine,' was carried out in 1965 in those villages that had not yet experienced measles, and was incorporated into the general child vaccination program in 1976, preceding Denmark where the measles vaccination was not introduced until 1987.[6] Vaccinations substantially reduced the number of measles cases in the Arctic, although sporadic outbreaks have occurred, for example, in Greenland in 1990 and on Baffin Island in 1991.

In Greenland, the first polio epidemic was described in 1858 and the last major epidemic occurred in 1952–3, mostly as a result of outside contacts. Approximately 25 per cent of those infected died and another 25 per cent had persisting paralysis. Vaccinations began in 1955, and the last documented case was in 1962. In Canada, from 1948–9, 8 per cent of the Inuit population in Chesterfield Inlet in the Northwest Territories contracted polio from workers stationed in Churchill to the south, and 2 per cent of the population died. In 1956 in Alaska, an outbreak of polio was observed on St Paul Island.[7]

Tuberculosis

That tuberculosis was most likely present in the New World prior to European contact was supported by palaeopathological findings, including the identification of *Mycobacterium tuberculosis* DNA in mummified human remains.[8] However, its epidemic form was among the last major infectious disease to appear in the nineteenth century and did not come under control in the Arctic until well into the 1960s. Tuberculosis spreads through droplets from infected persons and is facilitated by crowded and poor living conditions, factors consistent with life in most Arctic indigenous communities.

In the Arctic, tuberculosis reached its peak by the middle of the twentieth century. In 1955, the incidence of tuberculosis was 2,300 per 100,000 in Greenland, a world record. Similar rates were reported in Alaska and Canada. It was during this era that large-scale population-based intervention programs were initiated to combat the disease, which also lay the foundation of the modern public health system in these regions.[9]

In the central and eastern Canadian Arctic, between 1950 and 1969, annual patrols by the coastguard ship *C.D. Howe* conducted X-ray surveys, administered BCG (Bacille Calmette-Guerin) vaccinations, and evacuated infected patients to hospitals in southern Canada. While undoubtedly this plan was effective in bringing the tuberculosis epidemic under control, it was achieved with great human costs.

Figure 15.1   Trends in the incidence of tuberculosis among Alaska Natives, Canadian Inuit, and Greenlanders

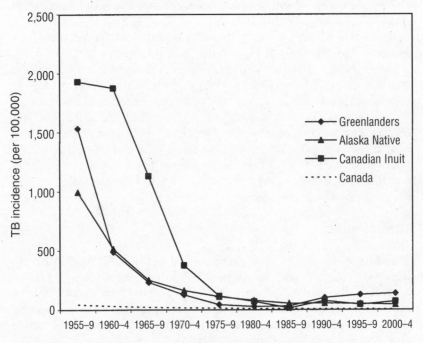

Sources: Updated from Bjerregaard and Young (1998: fig. 5.1); Alaska, Alaska Native and U.S. 1955–2002 data from Fortuine (2005: Appendix B); Greenland: 1995–2004 single year data from *Annual Reports* of the Chief Medical Officer (Embedslægeinstitutionen i Grønland); 5-year means for 1960-1994 period from the annual report for 2000; Canadian Inuit refer to Inuit in Northwest Territories (including Nunavut); after 1992 data refer to all Inuit in Canada; 1963–75 data from *Health Conditions of the NWT* (Health and Welfare Canada, various years); 1976–87 data from Health and Welfare Canada (1991) *Health Status of Canadian Indians and Inuit – 1990*; 1992–2004 data from Canadian Tuberculosis Reporting System (CTBRS).

Often, individuals who were identified as infected once they came on board were not allowed to go ashore to say goodbye or make arrange-ments for their families. The hospital stay in the south could last for many years and many persons lost contact with their families, their

Inuit language, and their way of life. Those who died were buried without their family's knowledge, and young children were sent from one hospital to the next without records. Today, many Inuit families remember the tuberculosis campaigns with sadness, horror, and anger.[10]

In Greenland in 1949, a BCG vaccination campaign was carried out on the west coast, with the aim of vaccinating all tuberculin-negative children. An increasing number of patients were sent to Denmark for treatment. In 1954, Queen Ingrid's Sanatorium in the capital Godhåb (now Nuuk) was built and, by 1959, all tuberculosis patients were receiving treatment in Greenland. A hospital ship, the *Misigssut*, sailed along the west coast every year from 1955 to 1971 to visit all settlements and summer camps to carry out tuberculosis examinations. By 1962, the situation was firmly under control and the sanatorium was converted into a general hospital. By the 1970s the incidence rate was approximately 10 per cent of that in the 1950s. Because of this reduction, Greenland abandoned routine BCG-vaccinations in 1990.[11]

Alaska adopted a different strategy. Following a survey in 1949–52, which showed that 25 per cent of susceptible Yupiks in the Yukon-Kuskokwin delta were infected each year, an intensive case finding, hospitalization, and out-patient treatment program was initiated. In 1954 home treatment with a combined regimen of para-amino-salicylic acid (PAS) and isoniazid (INH) was started as a trial and accepted for broad use two years later. In 1957, a field trial of INH prophylaxis was started in the Bethel area and, in 1963, it was offered to all residents in the region.[12]

While the incidence of tuberculosis has fallen quite dramatically since the 1950s, a substantial gap still exists between the Inuit and the national rates of Canada, Denmark, and United States. Tuberculosis remains a significant health threat in the Arctic. By the 1990s, the decline had begun to slow or even reverse (fig. 15.1).

In the Nunavik region in northern Quebec, 63 per cent of active TB cases in the period 1990–2000 were caused by ongoing transmission rather than reactivation of past epidemic strains. Previously unrecognized intervillage spread was found to be an important route of transmission. The resurgence of TB in Greenland was due to microepidemics in small, isolated settlements in the south. Molecular epidemiological studies showed the outbreaks to be locally confined. The increase made the authorities reintroduce BCG-vaccinations of newborns in 1997 and to strengthen TB monitoring and control. Drug resistance remains low in Greenland (only 0.5 per cent during 1998–2002), compared with Inuit patients in Denmark (13 per cent), offering hope for effective medical treatment.[13]

A particular problem in tuberculosis control is the identification of latently infected persons, who are then offered prophylactic treatment to prevent the development of clinical disease. In regions such as Greenland and northern Canada, the widespread use of BCG vaccinations makes the interpretation of the classic tuberculin test difficult. The availability of a new blood test (the gamma-interferon assay) for the detection of latent infection may become an important tool in the prevention of TB. Studies are underway in Greenland to evaluate its use.

Respiratory Tract Infections

Upper and lower respiratory tract infections (RTI) cover a wide spectrum of infections, from common colds to severe, life-threatening pneumonia. Otitis media and tuberculosis, also respiratory tract infections, are discussed separately in this chapter. Compared with the beginning of the twentieth century, mortality from RTI has declined substantially. However, it remains an important cause of childhood mortality, hospitalizations, and primary care visits today.[14]

Many Inuit children suffer from severe lower RTI early in life. A cohort of children from Nunavut on average experienced four episodes of lower RTI in their first year of life, which accounted for half of all hospitalizations of the cohort. In Nunavut and Alaska, rates of hospitalization for severe lower RTI in infants appear to be among the highest in the world, with rates exceeding 300 per 1,000 in the Baffin Region and 250 per 1,000 in the Yukon-Kuskowkwim delta. Twelve per cent of the hospitalized infants in Nunavut required mechanical ventilation, and readmissions were frequent. In addition, long-term consequences of lower RTI in the form of bronchiectases, bronchiolotis obliterans, and chronic atelectases appear to be unusually common in these populations.[15]

In a community-based prospective cohort study of RTI among children aged 0–2 years in Sisimiut, west Greenland, children reported having symptoms of RTI in 42 per cent of their time of observation. One-third of all episodes of RTI were lower respiratory tract infections. About 65 per cent of all episodes of RTI resulted in some kind of activity restriction and 40 per cent resulted in use of health care services.

The incidence and prevalence of childhood RTI in Greenland exceed the rates found in many developing countries.[16]

Little information is available on the microbiological causes of RTI in Arctic populations. Although a number of viral agents have been found in hospitalized Alaska and Canadian Inuit children with lower RTI (adenovirus, rhinovirus, influenza and parainfluenza), the respiratory syncytial virus (RSV) appears much more frequently in these children and is a leading cause of hospitalization and long-term sequelae.[17]

While factors such as crowding and poor housing quality, prevalent in many Inuit communities in the past, facilitated the spread of tuberculosis and other respiratory tract infections, living conditions have improved considerably in recent decades. The current risk-factor pattern appears to be much like that observed in developed countries. Among children in Sisimiut, major risk factors for RTI were attending childcare centres, domestic (night-time) crowding, and passive smoking. In Alaska, Native children experienced domestic crowding and their underlying medical conditions increased their risk of hospitalization for RSV bronchiolitis, while breastfeeding appeared to protect them against RSV. Indoor air quality was associated with severe lower RTI in Inuit children in Nunavut. Investigations in Greenland have suggested that genetically determined immune factors may also play a role.[18]

Otitis Media

The very early onset and frequent episodes of upper RTI among Inuit children start off a train of events that lead to recurrent episodes of acute otitis media (OM), secretory OM (also called otitis media with effusion, OME), chronic OM with tympanic membrane perforation and/or chronic suppuration, and finally to hearing loss and impaired learning and school performance. All forms are highly prevalent among the Inuit across the Arctic, which has been a known fact for decades. A medical report in 1839 from Greenland described that earaches were common problems among the inhabitants. A study of skeletal remains in Greenland showed evidence of the sequelae of chronic OM (in the temporal bones) in 5 per cent of pre-contact Inuit specimens and 18 per cent of those dated 100 to 200 years ago. Since the 1960s, systematic surveys have been conducted in Alaska, Nunavut, and Greenland to document the high prevalence of the various forms of OM.[19]

The prevalence of chronic OM varies among communities with rates between 3 per cent and 45 per cent. A cohort study in Greenland found that 40 per cent of Inuit children have had acute OM before one year of age. While the causative viral and bacterial agents involved are the same as in other parts of the world, there is heavy nasopharyngeal colonization by these microorganisms early on in life. The risk factors for OM include having a parental history of OM, domestic crowding, use of daycare, and passive cigarette smoking. Both long-term, exclusive breastfeeding and early bottle-feeding have been implicated in studies among the Inuit.[20]

Surgery is the treatment of choice for chronic OM when frequent irrigation and antibiotic eardrops fail. Results of surgery are generally worse than in the non-Native population. 'Fly-in' specialist surgical teams have been successfully deployed in Greenland and northern Canada. Clearly, the solution to the problem lies in postponing or preventing the first episodes of upper RTI and acute OM. Preventive strategies range from broad socio-economic improvement, longer maternal leaves, and higher hygienic standards to providing audiological assessments and upgrading local medical facilities (e.g., installing otomicroscopes) and surgical skills. The installation of sound field amplification systems in the schools may ameliorate the consequences of poor hearing.[21]

Hepatitis

Infectious hepatitis is a group of liver infections caused by five hepatitis viruses, labelled A to E, of which A, B, and C are the most important. These differ in their mode of transmission, clinical course, and long-term sequelae. Hepatitis A virus (HAV) is transmitted by the fecal-oral route, either through close personal contact with an infected person or through contaminated food and water. The disease is rarely fatal and usually self-limited, and it renders life-long immunity. Hepatitis B virus (HBV) is transmitted by sexual contact or via the blood stream. HBV infection may result in life-long immunity, but some cases progress into a chronic state with free virus in the blood. In a minority of chronic HBV-infected persons, long-term sequelae include liver cirrhosis and/or primary liver cancer. Hepatitis C virus (HBC) is transmitted via contaminated blood or direct needle inoculation and may result also in clinical hepatitis, cirrhosis, and liver cancer.

Hepatitis A and B virus occur at high and endemic rates in Arctic populations. HAV serosurveys have consistently shown that some 50–70 per cent of the adult population had previously been exposed, and that the prevalence increases with age. HAV tends to occur in epidemics. In Greenland, epidemics of jaundice were noted in the eighteenth and nineteenth centuries and about once per decade during the first half of the twentieth century. The last major epidemic occurred in 1970–4. From one imported case, 11 per cent of the population of Greenland contracted hepatitis, and 0.3 per cent died. In northern Canada, a major epidemic occurred in 1991–2, mostly in communities without running water or adequate sewage disposal, and resulted in 20 per cent of five- to twenty-year-olds becoming ill and 2 per cent developing fulminant hepatitis. In Alaska, prior to vaccine introduction, large epidemics occurred every seven to ten years with the highest attack rates among children aged five to fifteen years.[22]

In Alaska in 1992, an HAV vaccination program of more than 5,000 young persons in twenty-five villages was able to halt an epidemic within three weeks after administration in each community. Universal childhood HAV immunization was later initiated statewide to all Alaskan children age two and eighteen years in 1996, resulting in the rate of acute HAV falling from the highest in the country to the lowest within ten years. The use of immunoglobulin (passive immunization) proved to be unsuccessful during previous epidemics, as the pace of the epidemics were only slowed down temporarily while the public health system was disrupted. In Canada and Greenland, no such vaccination campaigns have been initiated, but the reduction in HAV epidemics may be caused by increased sanitary standards.[23]

In the 1970s, it became apparent that hepatitis B virus (HBV) infection was endemic in Arctic indigenous populations. In Greenland, a series of serosurveys between 1965 and 2004 showed the prevalence of HBV exposure between 42 per cent and 75 per cent and of chronic HBV infection between 7 per cent and 20 per cent. Seroprevalence was low in childhood but increased markedly in later ages, suggesting that transmission mainly took place in teenage years via sexual contact. In Canada and Alaska, somewhat lower prevalence figures have been found. Among Canadian Inuit, five serosurveys from 1980 to 1999 showed average rates of HBV exposure around 25 per cent and of chronic HBV infection of 5 per cent, about five and twenty-five times the rates among Canadians. For this population, the majority of HBV infections occurred in early childhood. In Alaska, rates of chronic infection of 6–14 per cent among Natives from south-west Alaska in the 1970s were reported. The proportion of those infected who developed clinical disease was highest among children, and 28 per cent of infected children under five years of age ultimately developed chronic infection.[24]

Rates of long-term sequelae of HBV infection, liver cirrhosis, and liver cancer are high among Alaska Natives but lower than expected in Canada and Greenland, given the high HBV prevalence. The extent to which under-reporting or other factors such as HBV subtypes, age at infection, or genetic factors may have contributed to this discrepancy is unknown. Eight different HBV genotypes exist, of which 5 (A, B, C, D, and F) have been found in Alaska, the largest number of genotypes observed in any region. The most prevalent was D. In Greenland, only genotypes B and D have been found. However, little is known about the clinical significance of these genotypes.[25]

Different preventive actions have been taken in the Arctic countries. In Alaska, a program of mass HBV screening and vaccination of seronegative persons was implemented in the 1980s. Furthermore, all infants were routinely vaccinated. This program had a profound impact, as the rate of acute HBV infection fell from 200/100,000 in 1981 to <5/100,000 in 2002 (fig. 15.2), and ten years after routine vaccination no children <10 years of age had developed chronic infection. In Canada, targeted and routine vaccination was introduced in 1985–9 and 1995–9, respectively. Target groups included communities with high HBV prevalence, health care workers, family contacts of chronically infected persons, and infants. This has led to a progressive decline in cases of acute HBV infections across northern Canada. In Greenland, HBV vaccinations are offered to health care workers and to newborns of chronically HBV-infected mothers, but the impact of this program has not been evaluated.[26]

There is much less information on hepatitis C virus (HCV) infection. However, seroprevalence in Greenland and Alaska is low (0.5 per cent and less), comparable with the rest of the U.S. and Denmark. In Canada, seroprevalence appears to be higher (between 1 and 18 per cent), although viremia is less frequent. The clinical impact of HCV infection in Arctic countries is essentially unknown.[27]

Sexually Transmitted Diseases

Sexually transmitted diseases as a group comprise gonorrhea, syphilis, infections caused by the human immunodeficiency virus (HIV),

Figure 15.2   Impact of statewide hepatitis B vaccination program on incidence of clinical infection in Alaska

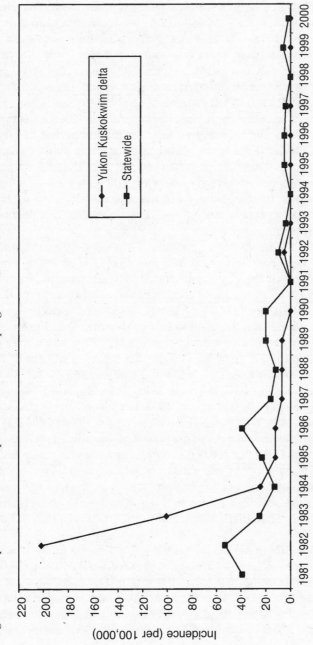

Source: B. McMahon, Arctic Investigations Program, Centers for Disease Control and Prevention, Anchorage, Alaska.

Chlamydia trachomatis, herpes simplex virus, human papilloma virus (HPV), *Trichomonas*, and several other less-common pathogens. Syphilis is generally a rare disease and occurs only sporadically, although in the recent past, there have been epidemics. For example, in Greenland in 1976–7 and in 1987, around 700 cases were noted per year. Gonorrhea and chlamydial infections are far more common, highly transmissible, and, if left untreated, can lead to significant morbidity, especially in women (pelvic inflammatory disease, ectopic pregnancy, and infertility). There is a long incubation period between infection with HIV and the onset of clinical symptoms that constitute the acquired immunodeficiency syndrome (AIDS). The use of anti-retroviral therapies also delays the onset of AIDS. Most jurisdictions report these two entities separately, but the extent of HIV testing that is done in the population varies, and cross-national comparisons should be done with caution.

In Greenland, the incidence of gonorrhea increased steadily during the 1950s and 1960s, reaching a peak in the late 1970s, at a staggering 20,700 per 100,000 of the population, or 31,000 per 100,000 of adults aged 15–59. (Such rates are more comprehensible when expressed as 207 per 1,000 and 310 per 1,000.) As figure 15.3 shows, the decline since then has been impressive, thanks to a systematic intervention strategy that includes partner tracing and treatment. The level has remained around 1,100 per 100,000 since the early 1990s, which is still about 100 times higher than in Denmark and is the highest among all Arctic regions. In Alaska, rates have been declining since the late 1980s, and averaged about 80 per 100,000 during 2000–4. Alaska Natives had substantially higher rates (160 per 100,000 in men and 390 per 100,000 in women). In the Nunavik region of northern Quebec the incidence rate of gonorrhea was 1,000 per 100,000 in 1990, approximately fifty times that of the rest of the province, with a decreasing trend through the 1990s. In the ethnically mixed Northwest Territories, the first few years of the twenty-first century saw the incidence of the disease reverting back to the levels of the late 1980s and early 1990s, around 360 per 100,000.[28]

In Greenland, chlamydia became a notifiable disease in 1995. Since then the incidence has almost doubled and exceeded 3,400 per 100,000 during 2000–4, more than ten times the rate in Denmark. In Alaska, rates have steadily climbed since the mid-1990s, and exceeded 660 per 100,000 in 2005. Rates for Alaska Natives were considerably higher (960 in men and 2,700 in women). In Nunavik, in 1990, the incidence

Figure 15.3   Trends in incidence of gonorrhea and chlamydia in Alaska, northern Canada, and Greenland

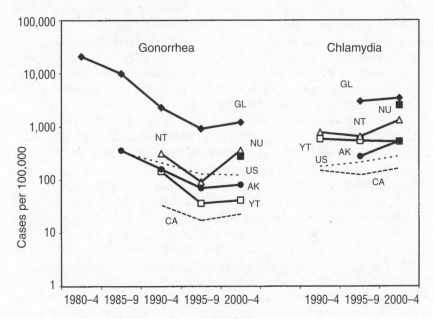

Notes: ······: US: United States;   ----CA: Canada
Δ NT: Northwest Territories; ■ NU: Nunavut; □ YT: Yukon; • AK: Alaska;
♦ GL – Greenland. Rates refer to notified cases per 100,000. Individuals with multiple infections were counted as separate cases; data are for all ethnic groups/races combined; y-axis in logarithmic scale.
Sources: Centers for Disease Control, Public Health Agency of Canada, Office of the Chief Medical Officer of Greenland – see note 28 for details.

was 3,400 per 100,000, which was twenty times higher than in the non-Native population of the province and showed no sign of decrease in the ensuing years.[29]

Given the high rates of STDs, there was much fear of HIV/AIDS spreading to the Arctic when the epidemic began in the 1980s. This has not happened, but HIV/AIDS nonetheless represents a major public health threat. Since the appearance of the first HIV case in 1985 in

Greenland, the number of cases has grown. By the end of 2004, the total number of HIV-positive individuals had reached 137, and the number of AIDS cases had reached forty-eight. Transmission was mainly (80 per cent) heterosexual and appeared mostly in a core group of persons from the two largest towns in Greenland, Nuuk, and Sisimiut. In Sisimiut in 1998, despite an extensive contact tracing program, a number of HIV-positive persons appeared without any known HIV-positive sexual contacts. After screening the total population of the town (5,500), no unknown HIV reservoir was detected.[30]

Elsewhere in the Arctic, eighty-seven cases of HIV and twenty-seven cases of AIDS had been reported from the three northern territories of Canada (all ethnic groups included) by the end of 2005. In Alaska, a total of 1,050 HIV cases (727 with AIDS and 323 without AIDS) had been reported by 2005. In terms of risk groups, men having sex with men accounted for almost half of the cases, with 15 per cent each for heterosexual contacts and injection-drug users. Almost a quarter of the cases (23 per cent) were Alaska Natives, slightly higher than their share of the state's total population (19 per cent). The incidence of AIDS in Alaska was lower than in the United States nationally.[31]

The prevention of HIV/AIDS and other STDs requires behavioural change related to sexual practices, such as condom use and limiting the number of sexual partners. Survey data on sexual behaviour, especially among youths, are presented in chapter 20.

Invasive Bacterial Diseases

An invasive bacterial disease is caused by bacteria invading a normally sterile body compartment, for example septicemia and meningitis. The Inuit are at particular risk for several invasive bacterial diseases.

Infection by *Streptococcus pneumoniae* (pneumococci) is one of the leading causes of pneumonia, bacteremia, septic shock, and meningitis. Incidence rates of invasive pneumococcal disease (IPD) in Inuit are approximately four times that of non-Inuit. Children under two and seniors aged sixty-five and above are at highest risk. Common serotypes reported in the Arctic during the period 1999–2004 were 1, 3, and 14. As all three are included in the 23-valent polysaccharide vaccine, and one serotype in the 7-valent conjugate vaccine, it has been estimated that 80 per cent of IPD occurring in Alaska, northern Canada, and Greenland are potentially preventable with use of these vaccines. In Alaska and select regions of northern Canada, routine use of the 7-valent vaccine began in 2001 and 2002, respectively. After its introduction in Alaska, a 90 per cent reduction in vaccine-type IPD rates among Alaska Native children < 2 years of age and an 80 per cent among non-Native children < 2 years of age were observed. In addition, there was a 40 per cent decline in vaccine-type IPD in adults and a reduction in antimicrobial resistant IPD for the entire population.[32]

Haemophilus influenzae can cause respiratory tract infections (otitis media, sinusitis, epiglotittis, pneumonia), meningitis, and septic arthritis. Among the six serotypes (a–f), *Haemophilus influenzae* type b (Hib) was the most common cause of childhood meningitis prior to the introduction of childhood conjugate vaccines in the early 1990s.

Prior to 1991, rates of invasive Hib disease among Alaska Natives were among the highest in the world, with rates >300 per 100,000 among those under five years of age, four times the non-Native rate in the state. Since the introduction of universal infant vaccinations, rates of disease have rapidly decreased. By 2001–4, the Native rates had decreased by 98 per cent to 5 per 100,000; however, the disparities persist because in the non-Native population and the rest of North America the disease has practically been eliminated. Continued surveillance for invasive diseases caused by all serotypes of *Haemophilus influenzae* is needed to monitor the impact of immunization programs and the emergence of other serotypes (i.e., a and f) that may replace Hib and cause severe illness.[33]

Another cause of bacterial meningitis is *Neisseria meningitides* (meningococci). While epidemics occur sporadically, the incidence of meningococcal disease in Alaska, northern Canada, and Greenland has remained relatively stable at 1–2 cases per 100,000 per year, with children under the age of two having the highest risk. The majority of the cases are caused by serogroups B and C. Group C is included in the quadrivalent conjugate vaccine in use in Alaska and the monovalent vaccine in use in Canada.[34]

Illnesses caused by group A streptococcus (*Streptococcus pyogenes*) or GAS range from mild sore throat and skin infections such as impetigo, to more severe and sometimes life-threatening diseases such as necrotizing fasciitis and toxic shock syndrome. A total of 186 GAS cases have been reported from Alaska and northern Canada since 2000. Over one-third of the cases presented with cellulitis. Only one case was reported from Greenland during this period. Indigenous children under two years of age were at the highest risk. There is no vaccine to prevent GAS infections. Control of these infections depends on case detection and giving antimicrobial prophylaxis to close contacts to prevent its spread.

Group B streptococcus (*Streptococcus agalactiae*) or GBS can cause a range of diseases, including sepsis, pneumonia, meningitis, and various infections associated with pregnancy. Fewer GBS than GAS cases have been reported in the three regions, and for this disease, non-Native children less than two years of age were at the highest risk.[35] No vaccine exists. Pregnant women in whom vaginal and rectal GBS colonization is detected are given antibiotics to reduce the risk of neonatal infection.

Helicobacter Infection

Helicobacter pylori infection causes stomach ulcers and increases the risk of chronic gastritis, mucosa-associated lymphoid tissue (MALT) lymphoma, and gastric adenocarcinoma. In developing countries, infection appears to take place early in life with chronic infection continuing during adult life, while in developed countries, the prevalence among children is low but increases with age. Low socio-economic status in childhood is a recognized risk factor. As the incidence of stomach cancer has increased in Greenland and Alaska in the latter part of the twentieth century, in contrast to global trends (see chapter 17), there is strong interest in studies on *H. pylori* in Arctic populations.[36]

A number of serosurveys have shown intermediate to high rates of *H. pylori* positivity among Inuit populations. In Greenland and Canada, the age-specific prevalence was intermediate between those of developing and developed countries with rates of 53–7 per cent among adults and 25–32 per cent among children under fifteen years of age. In contrast, a study of stored sera from Alaska Natives found 32 per cent positive among those aged 0–4 years, which increased to 67 per cent by age 5–9, and 78 per cent by age 10–14. A variety of risk factors have been proposed, including number of siblings, male gender, low weight for height in children, and sanitary conditions.[37]

As iron deficiency anemia is common among Alaska Natives, it has been suggested that blood loss from chronic gastritis due to *H. pylori* infection could be a contributing cause. A number of studies did find an association between *H. pylori* infection and anemia. An atypical type of hemorrhagic gastritis associated with *H. pylori* has also been observed among Yupik Eskimos. However, treatment of the infection with antibiotics has not been shown to improve the anemia.[38]

The consumption of antibiotics is high in many Arctic populations. Among Alaska Natives, a high proportion of *H. pylori* strains have been found to be resistant to antibiotics, both in urban and in rural settings. A person's previous use of antibiotics is significantly associated with subsequent isolation of antimicrobial resistant strains. Even after successful treatment and eradication of *H. pylori*, there is a high rate of reinfection. Similar studies have not been done in other Arctic regions, and the long-term impact on stomach cancer from *H. pylori* infection and its treatment remains to be explored.[39]

Zoonoses and Parasitic Infections

With their strong hunting traditions and subsistence based on wild game, Arctic indigenous peoples are at increased risk of zoonoses and parasitic infections acquired from infected meat. Zoonoses refer to a group of diseases caused by organisms that are usually present in animals but are transmitted to and cause disease in humans.

Trichinellosis is caused by ingestion of the nematode worm *Trichinella*. One of the nine subspecies, *T. nativa* is widespread in Arctic wildlife and is freeze-tolerant (which makes recommendations on freezing of meat irrelevant). The main animal sources of human trichinellosis include bear (polar, black and grizzly), walrus, and seals (ringed and hooded). First symptoms include diarrhea, nausea, and vomiting, followed by fever, edema, and muscle pains. In rare cases it may even be fatal. The disease occurs sporadically, but outbreaks in humans have been noted several times in Alaska, Canada, and Greenland, sometimes involving over a hundred cases. Despite the declining frequency of outbreaks, seroprevalence studies still show a high proportion of people with past exposure, especially in hunting districts and among older persons (10–70 per cent in persons >40 years in Greenland). The lower prevalence among younger persons reflects more recent changes away from the traditional diet. In Greenland, meat samples from hunted polar bear and walrus undergo mandatory microscopy, although test sensitivity is low. In the Nunavik region of Canada, a prevention program was implemented in the 1990s, based on pre-consumption testing of meat samples at a regional laboratory and rapid dissemination back to the communities. It was credited with successfully controlling an outbreak in 1997.[40]

A number of once common zoonoses has greatly decreased in significance with lifestyle changes. *Echinococcus granulosis* and *E. multilocularis* are common tapeworms in foxes and dogs and cause the highly lethal alveolar hydatid cyst disease in humans. The disease is less common as dog teams are being replaced by snowmobiles in many parts of the Arctic. *Diphyllobotrium* (fish tapeworm) has been found in 45 per cent of fecal samples from dogs in northern Quebec, and human infections have been reported in Alaska, Canada, and Finland. Anisakidae – 'Herring worm' (*Anisakis simplex*) and 'cod worm' (*Pseudoterranova decipiens*) – are highly prevalent in Arctic fish (approximately 70 per cent of cod from western Greenland), but antibodies are found in less than 1 per cent of Greenlandic children tested. Serological studies in northern Quebec have shown a high prevalence of toxoplasmosis (*Toxoplasma gondii*), affecting about 50 per cent of the population. There has also been evidence of women acquiring the infection during pregnancy. Seropositivity was associated with involvement with the skinning of animals (wolf, fox, and marten) and consumption of dried seal meat, seal liver, and raw caribou meat.[41]

Botulism is caused by ingestion of a neurotoxin produced by the anaerobic bacterium *Clostridium botulinum*, which grows in meat and fish stored under special conditions. Botulism results in muscle paralysis, eventually leading to respiratory arrest. In the Arctic, traditional processing of meat and fish involves fermentation by anaerobic storage at low temperatures (above freezing) without salting, which may lead to occasional outbreaks of botulism. In Canada, outbreaks occur almost exclusively among the Inuit in the North and the Natives in British Columbia. In Greenland, small outbreaks and single cases occur regularly. Although a decrease in the incidence of botulism should be expected because of the decline in the traditional diet, botulism is still a public health problem in the Arctic, especially in Alaska. Between 1990 and 2000, 103 cases and fifty-eight events of botulism occurred in Alaska, accounting for 39 per cent of all cases reported in the United States. Toxin type E caused 90 per cent of the cases in Alaska. In 2002, twelve Yupik Eskimos developed botulism after eating blubber and skin from a beached beluga whale. Although death rates from botulism have decreased in Alaska, incidence rates have increased. A contributing factor may be a shift away from traditional fermenting techniques towards the use of plastic bags and plastic containers, which facilitate growth of anaerobic bacteria.[42]

Parasitic and zoonotic infections are highly dependent on climate.

There is concern that present and future climate changes in the Arctic affecting temperature, humidity, flooding, and wildlife composition may increase the incidence of these infections in humans.[43]

Antimicrobial Resistance

The discovery of effective agents to prevent and treat infections caused by bacteria and other microorganisms is one of the most important developments of modern medicine. However, as antimicrobial agents are introduced into the environment, microorganisms respond to the selective pressures of these agents by becoming resistant – that is, able to survive and reproduce in the presence of the agent. The consequences are enormous: increased morbidity and mortality, use of more toxic and expensive drugs, and the use of greater resources to monitor the emergence of new patterns of resistance.

As discussed earlier in this chapter, invasive pneumococcal disease represents a significant public health threat in the Arctic. In Alaska, the percentage of invasive pneumococcal isolates demonstrating full resistance to penicillin increased from ~1 per cent in 1993 to almost 15 per cent in 2000. However, since the introduction of the heptavalent vaccine in routine childhood immunizations in the U.S. in 2001, this upward trend has been reversed. In other Arctic countries, the proportion of full resistance to penicillin among S. pneumoniae isolates is much lower – 3 per cent in northern Canada and < 1 per cent in Greenland, Iceland, Finland, and northern Sweden. In Greenland there has been considerable fear of introduction of penicillin resistant pneumococci, but despite the high consumption of antibiotics, penicillin-resistant pneumococci have not yet been isolated.[44]

Once considered to be an infection acquired only in health care institutions, methicillin-resistant Staphylococcus aureus (MRSA) infection, acquired in the community, is an emerging, though not yet widespread, public health challenge. In Alaska, outbreaks of community-acquired MRSA skin infections associated with antibiotic use have been reported. In Greenland, only a few imported cases of MRSA without secondary spread have been documented.[45]

Emerging Infections

Indigenous people in the North are at higher risk for many infections compared with other populations. The various diseases discussed in this chapter can all be considered as emerging. Some are more properly considered to be re-emerging, as they were once common and were thought to be under control. From time to time, completely new threats appear. For example, Alaskan waters were once thought to be too cold to support the growth of the bacteria *Vibrio parahaemolyticus*. However, in July 2004, an outbreak of *V. parahaemolyticus*–related gastroenteritis occurred among cruise-ship passengers who had consumed raw oysters in Alaska. The emergence of this infectious disease, associated with rising water temperatures in Alaska's Prince William Sound, may be a harbinger for the appearance of other novel pathogens in the North if temperatures continue to rise.

The emergence of highly pathogenic H5N1 avian influenza in the Arctic is also an area of concern. This virus has the potential to arrive via migratory birds travelling from endemic areas in Asia to Alaska and other regions of the circumpolar north. Surveillance for avian influenza viruses in migratory bird populations is yet another activity to be added to the long list of public health tasks in response to new infections.

Many interconnected factors are responsible for the continuing and growing importance of infectious diseases in the Arctic: changes in the size and composition of the population (overcrowding, migration from small rural communities to urban centres); changes in personal behaviours (increased travel, substance abuse, intravenous drug use, and risky sexual behaviour); health care practices (increasing use of antimicrobial agents); and changes in the physical environment (contamination of subsistence food supplies and greater human contact with altered wildlife habitats). Indeed, many of these factors not only contribute to the risk of infectious diseases but also are broad determinants of the population's overall health.[46]

Circumpolar Infectious Diseases Surveillance

A cornerstone in the control of infectious diseases is surveillance. While all Arctic countries and regions have public health agencies responsible for surveillance, the need for an international, circumpolar collaboration in data collection, analysis, and policy recommendations has long been recognized. Such a collaboration became a reality in 1999 when the International Circumpolar Surveillance (ICS) project was established, creating a network of hospital and public health laboratories throughout the Arctic.

The initial priority for ICS was invasive bacterial diseases caused by *Streptococcus pneumoniae, Haemophilus influenzae, Neisseria meningitidis,* and Group A and B streptococcus. These organisms were chosen because: (1) rates of diseases caused by many of these pathogens were elevated in the indigenous peoples of the Arctic; (2) strains of *S. pneumoniae* were rapidly acquiring resistance to antibiotics commonly used to treat these infections; (3) most clinical laboratories in Arctic countries routinely cultured these pathogens from clinical specimens; and (4) vaccines were available for clinically important serotypes of *S. pneumoniae, H. influenzae,* and *N. meningitidis.* While no vaccine is available for diseases caused by groups A and B streptococcus, surveillance is important in detecting outbreaks and assessing the effectiveness of control measures.

Canada and Alaska participated in ICS at the outset in 1999, covering only IPD. The program was expanded to include the other invasive bacterial diseases the following year. Greenland joined in 2000, followed by Iceland, Norway, and Finland in 2001, reporting national data on IPD. Northern Sweden (county of Norrbotten) joined in 2003, reporting invasive disease data on all five organisms.

When a case of invasive disease caused by an organism under surveillance occurs in an ICS member country, the identified case is reported to local public health personnel who perform a chart review to capture relevant clinical, demographic, and laboratory data. Local laboratories send the isolate to national reference laboratories for confirmation, serotyping, and antimicrobial susceptibility testing. These data are then forwarded to the ICS coordinator at the CDC's Arctic Investigations Program in Anchorage for analysis, report generation, and information dissemination. Data are reported in 'real time' from northern Canada and Alaska to ICS headquarters as cases occur, whereas cases from other countries are reported as end-of-year summary data.

The priorities and overall direction of ICS are governed by an international steering committee consisting of representatives from the participating countries, the WHO European regional office, and Arctic indigenous peoples' organizations. The steering committee has identified other infectious diseases of concern, such as tuberculosis, hepatitis B, respiratory syncytial virus, HIV/AIDS, and pertussis, for future inclusion in the surveillance program.

The collection of standardized laboratory and epidemiological data on infectious diseases among ICS member countries has led to the formulation of prevention and control strategies. In 2000, ICS assisted with the identification of an outbreak of invasive disease caused by *S. pneumoniae* serotype 1 occurring among young adults in two northern regions of Canada. The extent of the outbreak was determined using ICS data and resulted in vaccination of adults with 23-valent polysaccharide vaccine, and routine vaccination of children with 7-valent pneumococcal conjugate vaccine (PCV-7) starting in 2002. Norway began routine vaccination of children with PCV-7 in 2006, and this vaccine may come into routine use in other northern European countries in the future. ICS will continue to monitor how this vaccine affects the populations in all member countries.

In early 2004, an increase in the number of cases of invasive disease caused by non-type b encapsulated *H. influenzae* was detected in both Alaska and northern Canada. Non-type b *H. influenzae* (serotypes a, c, d, e, f) is an uncommon cause of invasive disease in children; however, with the decline in Hib disease in the post-vaccine era, the importance of infections caused by other non-vaccine serotypes has increased. ICS data, shared among Arctic countries, contributes to the detection of outbreaks occurring in the circumpolar north. The ICS is a valuable tool in evaluating vaccine effectiveness in northern countries whose dates of vaccine introduction are so varied.[47]

NOTES

1 Much of the historical information in this chapter is derived from Bjerregaard and Young (1998).
2 See the original reports in Danish by Meldorf (1907) and Berthelsen (1943). Egede's 1738 comment was quoted by Berthelsen.
3 Fortuine (1989) provided a comprehensive history of health and disease in Alaska. The 'Great Sickness' was described in further detail by Wolfe (1982).
4 The team of Reid et al. (1999) and Taubenberger et al. (2005) conducted the sequencing of the viral genome.
5 Marchand (1943) and Peart and Nagler (1954) described the epidemics in Yukon and Baffin Island, respectively.
6 Measles epidemics in Greenland were described by Christensen et al. (1954) and Fog-Poulsen (1957). The 1990 epidemic was reported in the annual report of the Chief Medical Officer for 1991 (Landslægeembdet 1992).
7 Adamson et al. (1949) reported the polio epidemic in the central Cana-

dian Arctic. The epidemics in Greenland in the 1950s were analysed by Fog-Poulsen (1955) and Eskesen and Glahn (1955).

8 The pre-Columbian origin of TB in the Americas was reviewed by Clark et al. (1987). Salo et al. (1994) identified mycobacterial DNA in a Peruvian mummy.

9 The TB situation at mid-twentieth century in Alaska was assessed by Fortuine (1989), in Canada by Wherret (1945), and in Greenland in the report of the Commission for Greenland to the Danish National Board of Health (Sundhedsstyrelsen 1950).

10 TB incidence trends for Canadian Inuit in different time periods were reported by Wherrett (1945), Grzybowski, Styblo, and Dorken (1976), and Hoeppner and Marciniuk (2000).

11 The early success of TB control in Greenland was discussed by Stein et al. (1968). Soborg et al. (2001) reported the alarming doubling of the incidence during 1990–7.

12 The Bethel trial showed the protective effect of INH to persist after nineteen years (Comstock, Baum, and Snider 1979). The TB field research of the U.S. Public Health Service in Alaska in the 1940s and 1950s was chronicled by Fortuine (2005).

13 The Nunavik outbreak was investigated by Nguyen et al. (2003). An overview of the re-emergence of TB in Greenland and the challenges it posed for the health service was provided by Thomsen, Lilleback, and Stenz (2004) and Skifte (2004).

14 The contribution of respiratory infections to infant mortality in Alaska was reviewed by Gessner and Wickizer (1997) and to hospitalizations in Nunavut by Banerji et al. (2001).

15 Jenkins et al. (2004) followed an Inuit infant cohort from Iqaluit. Severe complications were described by Karron et al. (1999), Singleton, Redding, et al. (2003), and Redding et al. (2004).

16 Koch, Sørensen, et al. (2002) described their Sisimiut child cohort study, conducted during 1996–8, which is the largest study of its kind to date in the Arctic.

17 Reports on RSV infections in Alaska include Singleton, Petersen, et al. (1995) and Bulkow et al. (2002).

18 Studies on risk factors include Koch, Mølbak, et al. (2003) in Greenland, Bulkow et al. (2002) in Alaska, and Orr et al. (2001) in Nunavut. Kovesi et al. (2006) conducted a pilot study on indoor air quality. See Koch, Melbye, et al. (2001) on the association of acute RTI with the gene for mannose-binding lectin insufficiency in Greenlandic children, which may play a role in the development of innate host immune system.

19 Homøe (1997) studied the pneumatization of the temporal bone in skele-

tal collections in Greenland. Baxter (1999) reviewed the three-decade experience of otological research and service by the McGill University medical project in Baffin Island. Several surveys on otitis media have also been conducted in Greenland (Pedersen and Zachau-Christiansen 1986; Homøe, Christensen, and Bretlau 1996).

20 Woods et al. (1994) conducted an audiological survey in the Kivalliq region of Nunavut. In a comprehensive series of studies in Greenland, Homøe, Prag, et al. (1996) and Homøe, Christensen, and Bretlau (1999a, 1999b) reported on the age of onset, frequency of recurrence, nasopharyngeal carriage of microorganisms and sociomedical risk factors. Schaefer (1971) conducted an earlier study on infant feeding habits and risk of otitis media.

21 Duval et al. (1994) reviewed the twenty-year surgical experience of the University of Manitoba Northern Medical Unit in the central Canadian Arctic. Eriks-Brophy and Ayukawa (2000) described the use of sound field amplification in classrooms in Nunavik.

22 McMahon (2004) provided a pan-Arctic overview of the various types of hepatitis. See Skinhøj, Mikkelsen, and Hollinger (1977), Minuk, Waggoner, et al. (1982), and Pekeles, McDonald, et al. (1994) for epidemiological data specific to HAV.

23 Alaska's successful HAV vaccination program was described in McMahon, Beller, et al. (1996).

24 There is a large literature on the epidemiology of HBV in the Arctic – see, for example, Skinkøj (1977), Olsen, Skinhøj, et al. (1989), and Krarup et al. (2005) in Greenland; Minuk, Ling, et al. (1985), Larke et al. (1987) and Minuk and Uhanova (2003) in Canada; and Barrett et al. (1977), Schreeder et al. (1983), and McMahon, Alward, et al. (1985) in Alaska.

25 HBV genotypes were identified in Alaska by Livingston et al. (2007) and in Greenland by Langer, Frosner, and von Brunn (1997).

26 For details of the HBV prevention program in Alaska, see McMahon, Rhoades, et al. (1987) and Harpaz et al. (2000). A Viral Hepatitis Workshop in the 13th International Congress on Circumpolar Health in Novosibirsk, Russia, reviewed the status of HBV control programs.

27 The limited data on HCV are presented in the reviews by McMahon (2004), Langer, Frosner, and von Brunn (1997), and Minuk and Uhanova (2003).

28 Data on gonorrhea for Greenland were obtained from the annual reports for years 2000–4 of the Chief Medical Officer (Embedslægeinstitutionen i Grønland); Alaska and U.S. data are retrieved from CDC Wonder, the online data access service at http://wonder.cdc.gov, and also Alaska

Department of Health and Social Services (2006c); data for Canada and the northern territories were obtained from the Public Health Agency of Canada's Notifiable Diseases Online at www.phac-aspc.gc.ca/surveil lance_e.html; and for Nunavik from Hodgins et al. (2002).

29 Data for chlamydia for Alaska are from Alaska Department of Health and Social Services (2006b); data for Greenland and Canada are from the same sources as indicated in note 28.

30 Data on HIV/AIDS in Greenland are from Embedslægeinstitutionen i Grønland (2004), and the studies by Lohse et al. (2004) and Olsen, Koch, et al. (2000).

31 Alaskan data are from the Alaska Department of Health and Social Services (2006a); Canadian data are from Public Health Agency of Canada (2006b).

32 Bruce et al. (2006) provided circumpolar data on IPD. See Christiansen, Poulsen, and Ladefoyed (2004) for studies in Greenland, and Davidson et al. (1994) in Alaska. Hennessy et al. (2005) evaluated the impact of the heptavalent conjugate vaccine in Alaska.

33 Singleton, Hammitt, et al. (2006) reviewed Hib surveillance data from 1980–2004 in Alaska and documented the disease's near elimination since the introduction of vaccination. There was a brief re-emergence during 1996–2000 when the vaccine was changed.

34 The epidemiology of meningococcal and other invasive bacterial diseases are reviewed by the International Circumpolar Surveillance team from the 13th International Congress on Circumpolar Health in Novosibirsk, Russia (Cottle, Bruce, and Deeks 2006).

35 Data on GAS and GBS are from the database of the International Circumpolar Surveillance project. See Castrodale et al. (2007) for an investigation of neonatal GBS cases in Alaska.

36 For a current overview of *Helicobacter pylori* infection, see Kusters, van Vliet, and Kuipers (2006).

37 Survey data from Greenland (Koch, Krause, et al. 2005), northern Canada (McKeown et al. 1999), and Alaska (Parkinson et al. 2000) are available.

38 The H. pylori–anemia association was investigated by Yip et al. (1997) and Baggett, Parkinson, et al. (2006). The randomized controlled trial of antibiotic treatment was reported by Gessner, Baggett, et al. (2006).

39 Antimicrobial resistance in *H. pylori* was investigated by McMahon, Hennessy, et al. (2003) and Bruce, Cottle, et al. (2006), and reinfections by McMahon, Bruce, et al. (2006).

40 See Dupouy-Camet (2000) for a global survey of the problem, and Moller et al. (2005) and Proulx, MacLean, et al. (2002) for the Greenland and

Nunavik experience. Results of human seroprevalence surveys are from the unpublished data of L. Moller, E. Petersen, A. Koch, and others.

41 Wilson, Rausch, and Wilson (1995) reviewed the surgical experience of treating alveolar hydatid cyst disease at the Alaska Native Medical Center in Anchorage. See Moller (2006) for a review of zoonoses in Greenland. Much research on zoonoses was conducted in northern Quebec: Tanner et al. (1987) tested five species in serosurveys, McDonald et al. (1990); and Pekeles, McDonald, et al. (1991) investigated a toxoplasmosis outbreak; and Desrochers and Curtis (1987) examined dog feces.

42 Sobel et al. (2004) reviewed surveillance data on botulism in the United States. McLaughlin (2004) and Chiou et al. (2002) investigated outbreaks in south-western Alaska.

43 Parkinson and Butler (2005) speculated on the potential impact of climate change on infectious diseases in the Arctic. Climate change is further discussed in chapter 10.

44 Prevalence data on antimicrobial resistance are provided by the International Circumpolar Surveillance project. Rudolph et al. (2000) reviewed the Alaskan experience in the 1990s. Hahn et al. (2005) examined prescription drug use among children in Greenland.

45 Community-acquired outbreaks of furunculosis (boils) caused by MRSA have been reported by Baggett, Hennessy, et al. (2004).

46 See Butler, Parkinson, et al. (1999) for an overview of emerging infectious diseases in the Arctic. McLaughlin et al. (2005) investigated the Alaskan cruise ship epidemic. See Check (2006) for a news story on Alaska as a frontline outpost in the detection of potentially infected migratory birds flying over the Bering Sea from Asia.

47 Parkinson, Bell, and Butler (1999) described the goals and objectives of ICS. The control of two northern Canadian outbreaks facilitated by ICS was described in Proulx, MacLean, et al. (2002) and Macey et al. (2002).

16 Cardiovascular Diseases, Diabetes, and Obesity

MARIT JØRGENSEN AND KUE YOUNG

In the circumpolar region, substantial lifestyle changes have occurred since the 1950s. Among indigenous peoples, the declining dependence on hunting and fishing, decrease in physical activity, and change from a traditional diet to a more Western diet have been observed. Such environmental factors, interacting with genetic susceptibility, have exerted a considerable influence on the prevalence and incidence of obesity, diabetes, cardiovascular diseases, and their risk factors.

Prevalence of Obesity and Overweight

Obesity is the excess of body fat or adipose tissue. While body fat serves a variety of essential metabolic functions, its excess can predispose an individual to significant health problems, including diabetes, coronary heart disease, hypertension, and certain cancers. In population surveys, excess body fat can only be indirectly measured. Body mass index (BMI) is a simple index of weight-for-height (weight in kg/ [height in metres]^2) that is commonly used to classify overweight and obese individuals. According to criteria adopted by the World Health Organization, 'overweight' is defined as a BMI of 25.0 to 29.9, and 'obese' is a BMI of 30 and above. However, it is now recognized that the distribution of fat, especially excess abdominal fat, is a more important risk factor for disease, which can be assessed by the waist circumference.[1]

In a pooled dataset from four studies conducted from 1990 to 2001 among Inuit in Alaska, Canada, and Greenland, it was found that 37 per cent of men were overweight and 16 per cent were obese, while 33 per cent of Inuit women were overweight and 16 per cent were obese. After age-standardization, the prevalence of obesity among the Inuit

Figure 16.1   Overweight and obesity among the Inuit in global perspective

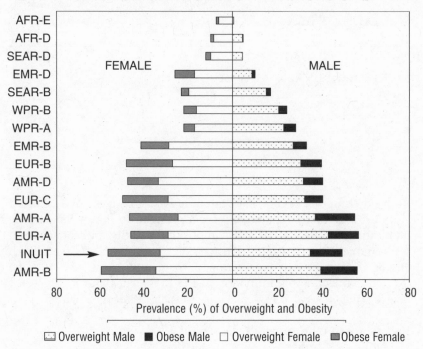

Notes: Bars represent WHO regions (AFR – Africa; AMR – Americas; EUR – Europe; EMR – Eastern Mediterranean; SEAR – Southeast Asia; WPR – Western Pacific); A, B, C, D, E refer to subregions; Inuit indicated by black arrow. Overweight: BMI 25-29.9; Obese: BMI 30+.
Source: Young et al. (2007), from American Journal of Public Health, reproduced with permission from American Public Health Association, Washington, DC.

ranked at the top among the highly developed countries of Europe and North America (fig. 16.1).[2]

Among women, the Inuit age-standardized mean waist circumference was higher than all reported populations, whereas Inuit men ranked quite low. A study of anthropometric measurements of body composition among Inuit in the Alaskan Siberia project confirms that the visceral fat content is high, and that measurements of abdominal fat are similar among men and women.

Secular trend data suggest that mean BMI has increased since the 1970s among both men and women. In Greenland, the prevalence of obesity increased among women from 12 per cent to 26 per cent between two population surveys in 1993 and 1999. The prevalence of overweight increased from 27 per cent to 35 per cent. Among men, the prevalence of obesity and overweight remained unchanged. Also, body composition has changed; judged by measurements of waist circumference and skin folds, body fat and central fat patterns have increased, whereas lean body mass has decreased.[3]

Self-reported data on obesity among Alaska Natives are available from the Alaska Behavioral Risk Factor Surveillance System (BRFSS). Figure 4.4 shows the trend in BMI in Alaska, while figure 16.2 compares BMI categories in various demographic groups. It can be seen that the combined prevalence of overweight and obesity is higher in males than females, and higher in Natives than non-Natives. It increases with age, education, and income but declines again among those belonging to the highest category. Among the Inuit (predominantly Yupik) in the Yukon-Kuskokwim region of Alaska in the early 2000s, 65 per cent of adults were overweight or obese. The mean BMI and waist circumference were higher among women than men.[4]

Body weight and obesity were analysed in a population-based cohort study in Finnmark county in Norway. Sami men had mean BMI comparable to other ethnic groups in Finnmark, whereas Sami women were more obese but they did not suffer more from diabetes. It was suggested that higher levels of physical activity compensated for the increased diabetes risk attributed to obesity. Among Swedish Sami, the mean BMI was not significantly different from a comparison group of non-Sami matched by age, gender, and area of residence.[5]

Data on obesity among children in the Arctic are less readily available. In a survey of Dene children in five communities in the Yukon and Northwest Territories, 32 per cent of children were overweight or at risk of overweight (>85th percentile of reference standard), compared with only 14 per cent of Canadian children. The prevalence was similar between boys and girls. In Nuuk, Greenland, school entry records of six- to seven-year-old children showed a 6 per cent increase in mean BMI between 1980 and 2000, and an increase in prevalence of overweight/obesity from 8 per cent to 22 per cent. Since different criteria were used, these populations could not be directly compared.[6]

Figure 16.2   Prevalence of overweight and obesity in Alaska by selected sociodemographic groups

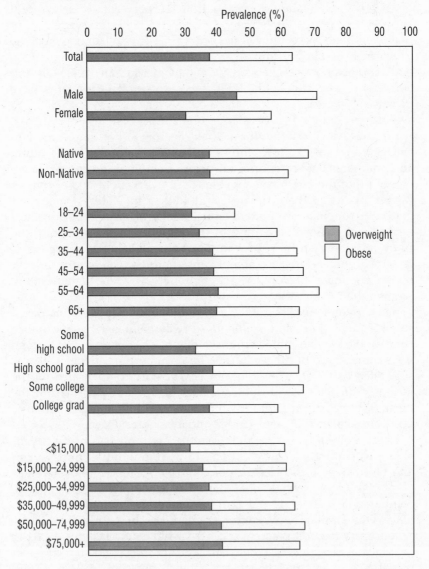

Source: Alaska Department of Health and Social Services, *Annual Report of the Behavioral Risk Factor Surveillance System*, for 2002–3 and 2004–5.

Metabolic, Behavioural, and Sociocultural Aspects of Obesity

The association between obesity and health problems such as diabetes and cardiovascular disease is well documented among circumpolar peoples. However, among the Inuit the metabolic impact of increasing levels of obesity, at least cross-sectionally, appears to be much less compared with Europeans, especially for indicators such as HDL-cholesterol, triglycerides, and blood pressure. These data indicate that universal criteria for obesity may not indicate the same degree of metabolic risk for populations such as the Inuit. On the other hand, Inuit migrants in Denmark seem to follow the same pattern in the association between obesity and metabolic risk factors as a Danish comparison population, thus indicating that lifestyle rather than genetic factors are likely responsible for the observed ethnic-specific differences in cardiovascular risk associated with obesity.[7]

Among the Inuit in Canada, some obesity indices were associated with high income, mixed ethnicity, fluency in the Inuit language, and less time spent on the land. In Alaska, obesity was associated with certain food items (butter, fried foods, Eskimo potatoes, cereal). In Greenland, the consumption of seal meat was found to be weakly associated with a high waist/hip ratio. The results from the 1999 Greenland survey indicated that the modernization process among the Greenland Inuit was accompanied by a decrease in BMI and central fat patterning, especially among women.

Health promotion efforts to exhort individuals to reduce weight need to take into account any given population's cultural understanding of what is unhealthy and what is not ideal in regards to 'looking-good.' Hence, in some cultures where scarcity of food has been common and excess fat becomes a symbol of wealth, overweight and obesity is considered attractive and desirable. It seems reasonable that this is the case also in Arctic populations – a perspective that should be taken into consideration when planning interventions to decrease obesity and improve physical activity behaviour. According to the Santé Québec survey in the early 1990s 55 per cent Inuit, compared with 94 per cent in Quebec, believed that obesity was associated with an increased risk of health problems. However, 37 per cent Inuit also believed that fat layers increase protection from cold, although this proportion declined with years of education. In terms of attempts to lose weight, the Inuit were the least interested compared with the rest of the province or with the Cree Indians, even among those who were overweight or obese.[8]

Diabetes and Glucose Intolerance

Estimates of diabetes incidence and prevalence are dependent on the data sources used. Data on diabetes in the Arctic region are available from registries of diagnosed diabetes and from population surveys involving the oral glucose tolerance test (OGTT). International criteria exist that define diabetes on the basis of plasma glucose levels in the fasting and two-hour values of the OGTT. As well, there are categories of 'impaired glucose tolerance' (IGT) and 'impaired fasting glucose' (IFG) that have been described informally as representing the pre-diabetic state, as individuals in these groups are at substantially increased risk to become diabetic in the future.[9]

A circumpolar comparative study of registry-based prevalence of diagnosed diabetes during the late 1980s showed that Alaskan Aleuts had the highest age-standardized prevalence, followed by Alaskan Indians. Inuit in Alaska and Inuit and Dene in northern Canada all had low prevalence, while the indigenous population of Chukotka had the lowest. The Aleut's rate approached that of the United States all-race rate of that period, and all Arctic indigenous groups had diabetes prevalence that was substantially below the epidemic levels reported among Native Americans in southern Canada and the United States. Within Canada, there was a clear north–south gradient.[10]

The Alaska Area of the U.S. Indian Health Service established a diabetes registry in the mid-1980s based on its patient care information system. (It is now managed by the Alaska Native Tribal Health Consortium.) It provides trend data for different groups of indigenous peoples. In 1985, the age-adjusted prevalence (standardized to the 1980 U.S. population) was 0.9 per cent for Inuit, 2.2 per cent for Indians (all tribes), and 2.7 per cent for Aleuts. By 1998, they had all increased, to 1.9 per cent among Inuit, 3.5 per cent among Indians, and 4.9 per cent among Aleuts. The highest prevalence was reported from the Tsimshian Indians of Annette Island in southeastern Alaska (7.6 per cent). While data exclusive to Dene are not available, the population of the Interior Unit is predominantly Dene, and the prevalence there was 2.9 per cent. While the Inuit rate was still the lowest, and remained lower than the United States national rate for that period, its rate of increase (110 per cent) was the greatest of the three ethnic groups. The registry can also generate incidence rates: for the period 1986–93, they were 22.2/10,000 for Aleuts, 18.5/10,000 for Indians, and 10.0/10,000 for Inuit, compared with a U.S. rate of 24.2/10,000.[11]

Data based on patient care registries may underestimate prevalence because of undiagnosed cases, typically accounting for 50–70 per cent in most epidemiological studies. The most accurate assessment of the burden of diabetes is one based on OGTT. Until recently it has been a widely accepted opinion that the prevalence of diabetes among Inuit in Greenland was low. The Greenland Population Study in 1999 was the first population-based study in Greenland where all participants received an oral glucose tolerance test. A high prevalence of diabetes and impaired glucose tolerance (IGT) was found (table 16.1). Surprisingly, diabetes was more common in the villages compared with the towns. Family history of diabetes, overweight, sedentary lifestyle, and alcohol consumption increased the risk for glucose intolerance whereas frequent intake of fresh fruit and seal meat were inversely associated with diabetic status. The proportion of individuals with previously unknown diabetes among the diabetic individuals was remarkably high, 70 per cent, highest in the least Westernized areas compared with the capital Nuuk. The proportion of unknown cases may be influenced by several factors, including the prevalence of symptoms in untreated cases, unawareness of diabetes in the health care system, and regional differences in access to diabetes health care.

Alaskan Inuit in the GOCODAN study appear to have a lower prevalence of diabetes compared with the Greenland Inuit, especially among men, despite a higher prevalence of abdominal obesity; a difference which is only partly explained by age-differences and a more restrictive definition of diabetes in Alaska where self-report diabetes was not included as a part of the diagnosis. Among men, 3.9 per cent had diabetes according to the WHO criteria; the prevalence among women was 9.1 per cent. The Alaska-Siberia study from 1994 also indicated a lower prevalence of diabetes than that in Greenland. However, when correcting for the change in diagnostic WHO criteria for diabetes from 1985 to 1998, there is no significant difference.[12]

The high prevalence of impaired glucose tolerance among Inuit indicates that diabetes prevalence may increase further in the future. A recent modelling of future diabetes in Greenland illustrates that if the development in BMI continues, the prevalence of type 2 diabetes will increase from 10 per cent to 23 per cent in women from 1999 to 2014. The increase in prevalence for men is estimated to be 10 per cent to 11 per cent. Type 2 diabetes is predicted to be responsible for approximately half of the cases of hypertension, dyslipidemia, IHD, and stroke. Alaskan Inuit with diabetes had a higher incidence of stroke

Table 16.1 Prevalence of diabetes and impaired glucose tolerance in selected Arctic populations based on OGTT screening

Ethnic group	Survey year	Sample size	Age	% with IGT	% with diabetes
Central Yupik, Alaska	1962[a]	535	20+	–	1.1
		296	40+	–	1.7
	1972[b]	320	40+	–	7.5
	1987[c]	766	40+	2.3	4.7
	1994[d]	106	25+	14.2	2.8
		47	45+	23.4	4.3
Siberian Yupik, Alaska	1994[d]	239	25+	6.7	9.6
		126	45+	12.7	15.1
Inupiat, Alaska	1994[d]	109	25+	6.4	3.7
		57	45+	10.5	7.0
	2000[e]	787	18+	15.6	6.9
Inuit, Greenland	1999[f]	917	35+	12.2	9.7
Dene, Alaska	1965[g]	306	20+	–	1.0
		163	40+	–	1.8
	1987[h]	110	40+	4.5	10.0
Aleut, Alaska	1973[i]	335	10+	–	6.0
		156	35+	–	11.5
Chukchi, Chukotka	1983[j]	493	30–59	49	0

[a]Mouratoff et al. (1967): 10 villages, Yukon-Kuskokwim region, 100 gm OGTT.
[b]Mouratoff and Scott (1973): 6 villages, Yukon-Kuskokwim region 100 gm OGTT.
[c]Murphy et al. (1992): 10 villages, Yukon-Kuskokwim region, OGTT in case of random glucose >6.7mmol/l.
[d]Ebbesson et al. (1998): 4 villages, Bering Straits region; 75g OGTT.
[e]Carter et al. (2006): Norton Sound region; 75g OGTT; figure in IGT column actually refers to IFG only (impaired fasting glucose).
[f]Jørgensen, Bjerregaard, and Borch-Johnsen (2002): Nuuk, Qasigianguit, and 4 villages in Uummannaq district; 75g OGTT.
[g]Mouratoff et al. (1969): 7 villages, Yukon-Kuskokwim region; 100 gm OGTT.
[h]Murphy et al. (1992): 4 villages, Yukon-Kuskokwim region; OGTT in case of random glucose >6.7mmol/l.
[i]Dippe et al. (1975): Pribilof Island; 75 gm OGTT.
[j]Stepanova and Shubnikov (1991): only men; coastal villages; 75 g OGTT.

compared with other Alaska Natives and U.S. whites; whereas the incidence of myocardial infarction, end-stage renal disease, and amputations were lower.[13]

Little data exist on the prevalence of diabetes among the Sami, but among Sami in Finnmark in Norway, the incidence of diabetes in a population-based cohort study was 6.1 per 1,000 person-years, not different from that in the other ethnic groups in the same area but somewhat lower than in the general Norwegian population.[14]

Genetic Susceptibility

The high and increasing prevalence of diabetes among peoples in the Arctic region raises the question whether diabetes develops due to genetic defects or whether the disease is caused by a specific constellation of 'normal genes.' Chapter 13 discusses in detail various genetic investigations that have been conducted among Arctic indigenous peoples. Genes favouring fat deposition intra-abdominally and in skeletal muscles could have been selected during evolution. This hypothesis is called the 'thrifty genotype' hypothesis. In accordance with this theory, hunter-gatherers would have had a better chance of survival if they were able to store energy as fat, especially in the fast turnover depots in the abdomen, instead of glycogen in the transient depots in muscle and liver. In that respect, it is more cost-effective to store energy as fat than as glycogen. It means that subjects with a low capacity for insulin-mediated glycogen synthesis have a better chance of surviving. These subjects suffer from reduced insulin-mediated glucose uptake in skeletal muscles, and it is therefore suggested that insulin resistance may have been a protective mechanism during evolution. In our time, where overfeeding and physical inactivity is a bigger problem than starvation, this tendency to store fat may result in obesity and diabetes.

In contrast to the 'thrifty genotype' hypothesis, there is an alternative explanation called the 'thrifty phenotype' hypothesis, which focuses on the association between the early development of disease and chronic disease in later life. In this hypothesis, the organism adapts to poor nutrition in early life by programming its insulin metabolism to expect a similarly depleted environment in later years. This adaptation appears to operate through insulin resistance as well as insulin secretion. It can be hypothesized that living conditions among the Inuit generations ago increased the risk for inadequate nutrition during fetal or early life. What has become broadly known as the 'life course' perspective recognizes the early life (fetal, infant, and childhood) influences on a whole spectrum of health outcomes, including chronic diseases such as diabetes and cardiovascular diseases, throughout life.[15]

Prevalence and Correlates of Hypertension

Hypertension is an important risk factor for cardiovascular diseases, and is itself considered a disease with its own determinants. Several studies of blood pressure have been conducted among the Inuit since the 1950s, but they are difficult to compare because of methodological differences. Their conclusions have ranged from significantly lower, to similar, or even slightly higher blood pressures among the Inuit compared with the general European or North American populations.[16]

In Alaska, diastolic blood pressure was found to be positively associated with fasting insulin levels among Siberian Yupiks on the St Lawrence Island. Among Yupiks and Athabascan Indians blood pressure increased with an increase in the consumption of store-bought food relative to traditional food, body mass index, mechanized activity, and glucose intolerance. In Greenland, however, there was no association of systolic or diastolic blood pressure with the consumption of traditional marine food.

The datasets of four surveys among the Inuit in Canada, Alaska, and Greenland (previously discussed under obesity) conducted during the 1990s were merged. Mean systolic blood pressure among the Inuit ranked intermediate on a global scale, and lower than most European populations. Systolic blood pressure increased with age. Male gender, obesity, and being a non-smoker were associated with high systolic and diastolic blood pressure. When adjusted for age, body mass index, smoking, and anti-hypertensive treatment, blood pressure differed significantly among the four Inuit populations – it was lowest in Nunavik, intermediate in Alaska and Greenland, and highest in Kivalliq.

Plasma Lipid Profiles

Since at least the 1930s there has been considerable interest in lipid metabolism among the Inuit. Surveys in northern Canada, Alaska, and Greenland have generally demonstrated a favourable lipid profile of low levels of triglycerides (TG) and high levels of high-density lipoprotein cholesterol (HDL), although for total cholesterol (TC) and low-density lipoprotein-cholesterol (LDL) the data are inconsistent. As more subfractions of plasma lipids were discovered, they too were tested on the Inuit, who continued to show higher levels of protective factors such as apolipoprotein A-I and lower or similar levels of apolipoprotein B and lipoprotein (a), factors associated with higher risk of ischemic heart disease.[17]

Studies from Nunavik and Greenland showed a direct association between a marine diet, estimated by n-3 fatty acids in serum or reported consumption of seal and the favourable lipid profile. Further studies among Greenlanders with different degrees of Inuit ancestry and exposure to Westernization (who lived in Nuuk, a medium-sized town, or in four villages in Uummannaq district, or in Denmark) found that those with three or more Inuit grandparents ('full heritage') had higher HDL than those of mixed heritage in both sexes, independent of other factors such as diet, alcohol, smoking, and residence. For full-heritage Inuit men, TG was also significantly lower than those of mixed heritage. For full-heritage Inuit women, however, TG and LDL were also higher, countering the benefits of the high HDL. As expected, Westernization was associated with a shift to a more unfavourable lipid profile, but this was observed only within Greenland. When Inuit had migrated to Denmark, their lipid profile improved. This could be the result of complex dietary changes, belying the simplistic view that 'Westernization' is always associated with poor health outcomes. Inuit from the villages in Greenland likely consumed less seal and other traditional n-3 fatty acid-rich meats than those from larger towns. However, those who migrated to Denmark likely consumed more fruits, vegetables, and plant oils.[18]

The Metabolic Syndrome

It has been recognized since the 1970s that various cardiovascular risk factors, such as obesity, glucose intolerance, dyslipidemia, and hypertension, tend to cluster in the same individuals. Since the 1980s, the concept that these metabolic abnormalities constitute a distinct clinical-pathological syndrome, perhaps unified under insulin resistance as the primary defect, has gained ground. Various names have been applied over the years, but the term 'metabolic syndrome' (MetS) is now the generally accepted one. Individuals with MetS have also been shown to be at increased risk of developing diabetes and cardiovascular diseases. There are two widely used definitions and sets of diagnostic criteria, generally referred to as the National Cholesterol Education Program (NCEP) and World Health Organization (WHO) definitions. Under NCEP, MetS is present when three of five criteria are satisfied: (1) abdominal obesity based on waist circumference; (2) high TG; (3) low HDL; (4) high blood pressure; and (5) high fasting glucose. The WHO definition has additional criteria and slightly different numerical cut-off points, and includes some measure of insulin resistance and also microalbuminuria. Studies in various populations have shown that the different definitions result in different prevalence rates composed of sets of individuals that do not completely overlap.[19]

The prevalence of MetS has also been determined among various regional groups of circumpolar Inuit. Using the NCEP definition, the prevalence was 16 per cent among the Yupik of the Yukon-Kuskokwim region, 14 per cent in the Kivalliq region of Canada, and 18 per cent in Greenland. In all regions, the prevalence was higher among women than men. These rates are lower than among North American Natives or white Americans/Canadians. Among Inuit in Greenland the effects of Westernization on metabolic risk was different for men and women. For men there was an increase in prevalence of MetS with Westernization within Greenland, while among women, westernization was accompanied by a decrease in MetS prevalence. For men, physical inactivity associated with Westernization seemed to increase the metabolic risk; for women, higher education was associated with a more favourable risk profile.[20] The significance of MetS in predicting future disease among the Inuit can only be clarified through prospective cohort studies.

Trends in Cardiovascular Disease

Table 16.2 compares the mortality rates of ischemic heart disease and cerebrovascular disease (stroke) in various circumpolar regions, all age-standardized to a common standard population to facilitate comparison, obtained from the Circumpolar Mortality Database created for this book (described in chapter 1). Finland has much higher rates than other countries in Scandinavia and North America. Within Scandinavia, northern regions have higher rates than the national averages. Northern Canadian regions have lower ischemic heart disease rates but comparable stroke mortality rates than the Canadian national rate.

Among Alaska Natives, mortality from ischemic heart diseases increased during the 1980s, and began to decline during the mid-1990s. At the same time, rates have declined dramatically among

Table 16.2   Age-standardized mortality rates for cardiovascular diseases in selected circumpolar regions

Country/region[a]	Ischemic heart disease[b]	Cerebrovascular disease[c]
Denmark	115.0	59.9
Greenland	135.5	119.5
Finland	162.2	62.2
Finnish Lapland	172.4	59.8
Sweden	117.2	54.9
Norbotten and Västerbotten counties	129.7	60.6
Norway	105.5	53.3
Finnmark, Troms, and Nordland counties	125.5	58.0
Canada	103.7	37.2
Yukon	98.6	49.5
Northwest Territories	117.2	49.6
Nunavut	66.3	47.6
United States	135.7	42.1
Alaska	95.3	43.2
Alaska Natives	90.5	48.0

[a]Denmark and Greenland data cover the period 1999–2001; all other regions cover the period 2001–3.
[b]Ischemic heart disease ICD-10 codes I20-I25.
[c]Cerebrovascular diseases or stroke ICD-10 codes I60-I69.
Source: Circumpolar Mortality Database.

American whites. As table 16.2 shows, the Alaska Native rate is still lower than that of the state or national all-race rates. For stroke, the mortality rates have consistently been higher among Alaska Natives during the 1980s and 1990s, and remained elevated while that of white Americans have decreased.[21] In the multi-ethnic population of the Northwest Territories in Canada the age-standardized mortality rate for both ischemic heart disease and stroke are higher than in Canada, whereas for the predominantly Inuit Nunavut, only stroke mortality is higher (table 3.2).

It is a long-held belief that ischemic heart disease is rare among the Inuit, who have benefited from the protective effects of the traditional arctic diet with its high content of monounsaturated and polyunsaturated fatty acids of marine origin. However, poor mortality statistics, and the lack of incidence data, put doubts to this assertion. Mortality rates from ischemic heart disease in the various Inuit populations are similar to, whereas mortality from stroke tend to be higher than, European populations. In terms of a history and electrocardiographic evidence of past ischemic heart disease, data from Greenland and Alaska showed that the prevalence of ischemic heart disease among Inuit is high and similar to that in American populations and approaches that observed in the middle range of European populations. The studies challenge the traditional hypothesis that the Inuit are protected against ischemic heart disease from a high consumption of marine n-3 fatty acids, and there is a need for critical rethinking of cardiovascular epidemiology in this population.[22]

Cardiovascular risk factors in circumpolar populations since the 1950s may have affected trends in cardiovascular disease incidence. The prevalence of type 2 diabetes and obesity has increased dramatically. Furthermore, physical activity has most likely declined and dietary changes have moved towards a more Western diet, although the consumption of marine mammals and fish is still high compared with western European countries (see chapter 11). These changes in risk factors are likely to have contributed to an increased incidence of cardiovascular diseases. However, prevalence rates of smoking have declined at least in some regions, which could have reduced the rates. Against such background, it is intriguing that mortality from ischemic heart disease has decreased in Greenland since the 1960s and in Alaska since the 1990s. Cardiovascular diseases among Sami are discussed in greater detail in chapter 9.

NOTES

1 For a general review of obesity and health and the criteria of obesity, see World Health Organization (2000). International comparative data on the prevalence of obesity are available from the online database of the International Obesity Task Force, www.iotf.org/database, and from the WHO document on global health risks (Ezzati et al. 2004, vol. 1: 497–596).
2 Details on the pooled dataset can be found in Young, Bjerregaard, et al. (2007). The original surveys were conducted in 4 communities in the Bering Strait region of Alaska (n=454); 8 communities in the Kivalliq region of Nunavut territory, Canada (n=380); 14 communities in the Nunavik region of northern Quebec, Canada (n=400); and in 2 towns and 4 villages on the west coast of Greenland (1,311). See Young (1996b),

Risica et al. (2000), Dewailly, Blanchet, et al. (2001), and Jørgensen, Glumer, et al. (2003) for descriptions of the original four surveys.

3 Martinsen et al. (2006) compared data from the 1993 and 1999 Greenland surveys.

4 Preliminary data from the CANHR Study was reported by Mohatt et al. (2007).

5 The Finnmark study was reported by Njølstad, Arnesen, and Lund-Larsen (1998). Swedish Sami data are presented in Edin-Liljegren et al (2004). Box 9.1 describes the methodology involved in creating the Swedish Sami cohort.

6 Nakano, Fediuk, Kassi, Egeland, et al. (2005), in their directly-measured BMI study in northern Canada, used the 2000 U.S. Centers for Disease Control growth charts as reference standard, which defined BMI-for-age >95th percentile as 'overweight' and between the 85th and 95th percentile as 'at risk for overweight.' The Greenland study by Schnohr, Sørensen, and Niclasen (2005) used the International Obesity Task Force reference standard and definitions of 'overweight' and 'obesity.' For a brief review of the use of BMI in children and adolescents, see Must and Anderson (2006).

7 More detailed analyses from the four-survey pooled data set are available in Young, Bjerregaard, et al. (2007); for Greenland specific data, see Jørgensen, Glumer, et al. (2003); and Jørgensen, Borch-Johnsen, and Bjerregaard (2006) on Greenlandic migrants in Denmark.

8 See Young (1996b) for Canadian Inuit data; Murphy, Schraer, et al. (1995) on Alaska; and Bjerregaard, Pedersen, and Mulvad (2000) and Bjerregaard, Jørgensen, et al. (2002) on Greenland. Furnham and Baguma (1994) discussed cross-cultural differences in perception of male and female body shapes. Data from the Santé Québec survey was reported in Jetté (1994).

9 See World Health Organization (1999) for international criteria for the definition and classification of diabetes. Diabetes is defined as either a fasting plasma glucose (FPG) value of 7.0 mmol/L or a 2-hour value of 11.1 mmol/L; impaired glucose tolerance (IGT) is defined as FPG <7.0 mmol/L and 2-hr value 7.8 and <11.1 mmol/L. The American Diabetes Association (Expert Committee 2003) defined impaired fasting glucose (IFG) as fasting glucose 5.6-6.9 mmol/L. Diabetes can be further divided into type-1 and type-2, formerly referred to as 'juvenile-onset' and 'adult-onset.' Type-2 accounts for over 90 per cent of all cases of diabetes. In this chapter, 'diabetes' refers to type-2. Discussion of type-1 diabetes can be found in chapter 20.

10 The circumpolar indigenous poulations were standardized to the 'world' population (Young, Schraer, et al. 1992). Reports from different countries tend to use their national populations as standard – age-standardized rates using different standard populations cannot be directly compared. Young, Szathmary, et al. (1990) mapped diabetes prevalence among the Aboriginal population by tribes, language families, culture areas, longitude and latitude, and geographical remoteness.

11 Trend data from Alaska are available from Schraer, Mayer, et al. (2001) and Naylor et al. (2003).

12 Compare Alaskan data from Carter et al. (2006) and Ebbesson, Schraer, et al. (1998) with Greenlandic data in Jørgensen, Bjerregaard, and Borch-Johnsen (2002). GOCADAN refers to Genetics of Coronary Heart Disease in Alaska Natives Study.

13 Martinsen et al. (2006) performed the projections in Greenland. Naylor et al. (2003) compared complications rates in different Alaskan ethnic groups.

14 See Njølstad, Arnesen, and Lund-Larsen (1998) for Sami data from Finnmark. No other studies have investigated diabetes in different ethnic groups in northern Scandinavia.

15 The thrifty genotype hypothesis was advanced by James Neel originally in 1962. For an update see Neel, Weder, and Julius (1998). The thrifty phenotype hypothesis originated with Barker – for a recent overview, see Barker et al. (2002). Kuh and Ben-Shlomo (2004) provided a comprehensive text on the life course approach to chronic disease epidemiology.

16 For a review of the earlier studies on blood pressure and the analysis of the merged dataset from the four surveys, see Bjerregaard, Dewailly, et al. (2003b). Alaskan Native data were reported by Schraer, Ebbeson, et al. (1996) and Murphy, Schraer, Thiele, et al. (1997); and Greenland data in Bjerregaard, Pedersen, and Mulvad (2000) and Bjerregaard, Jørgensen, et al. (2002). The combined Inuit dataset was compared to published results of the INTERSALT study. While lower than most European samples, the Inuit were higher than several Asian populations and the Amazonian Indians.

17 Bjerregaard and Young (1998:130–2) reviewed the earlier literature on blood pressure. For details on regional data, see Dewailly, Blanchet, et al. (2001) for Nunavik; Young, Nikitin, et al. (1995) and Young, Gerrard, and O'Neil (1999) for Kivalliq; Gerasimova et al. (1991) for Chukotka; and de Knijff et al. (1992) and Bjerregaard, Pedersen, and Mulvad (2000) for Greenland.

18 Lipid and lipoprotein data on Inuit from the Greenland Population Study of 1998–2002 conducted in Greenland and Denmark were reported in Bjerregaard, Jørgensen, and Borch-Johnsen (2004).

19 The NCEP definition was provided in the 2001 report of its Adult Treatment Panel III (ATP III). It is promoted, especially in the U.S., for clinical use as it involves laboratory measurements that are commonly performed. The WHO definition of MetS was included in its 1999 consultation document revising the classification and diagnosis of diabetes. The International Diabetes Federation (2005) modified the ATP III, making abdominal obesity an essential requirement for diagnosis, and also providing ethnic-specific criteria (at least for Europeans, and South and East Asians). The criteria are available from IOTF at www.iotf.org.

20 Jørgensen, Bjerregaard, et al. (2004) compared the prevalence of the metabolic syndrome as determined by the two definitions. Young, Chateau, and Zhang (2002) and Liu et al. (2006) compared Inuit with subarctic Indians and Euro-Canadians. From Alaska, Mohatt et al. (2007) provided preliminary Yupik data from the Yukon-Kuskokwim region. Gender differences in the association between Westernization and the metabolic syndrome were reported by Jørgensen, Moustgaard, et al. (2006).

21 Day and Lanier (2003) reviewed Alaska Native mortality. Schumacher, Davidseon, and Ehrsam (2003) reviewed cardiovascular incidence and mortality trends.

22 Dyerberg and Bang have done pioneering research on the role of plasma lipids in ischemic heart disease in Greenland – see, for example, the review in Dyerberg (1989). Bjerregaard, Young, and Hegele (2003) argued against the rarity of IHD among the Inuit. Jørgensen, Bjerreaard, et al. (2007) and Ebbesson, Risica, et al. (2005) provide evidence from EKG studies.

17 Cancer

JEPPE FRIBORG AND SVEN HASSLER

Cancer is a collective term for a group of diseases with different etiologies, clinical presentations, and pathological features, all sharing the uncontrolled growth and spread of abnormal (malignant) cells. Because it affects different body organs and tissues, cancer is generally classified according to anatomic site (i.e., where the 'primary' cancer originates, to be distinguished from 'secondary' sites where it may have spread or metastasized). However, within each site, there may well be several different histological types (such as squamous cell carcinoma, adenocarcinoma, etc). Cancer may be detected at different stages in its natural history, often a reflection on the quality of preventive and diagnostic health services. Cancer can also be categorized according to various known or suspected risk factors (such as tobacco, radiation, viruses), which is a scheme that is more useful in terms of potential interventions.

The burden of cancer in a population can be assessed in terms of its mortality, incidence, health care utilization, and economic costs. The most accurate way to measure cancer incidence is through a cancer registry, especially if it is population-based. Cancer is one of the few chronic diseases for which registries exist, at least in most developed countries, including those in the circumpolar region. Because of its high lethality, cancer mortality rates are often used where incidence data are not available. However, it should be recognized that mortality rates also reflect the availability and effectiveness of treatment services. Figure 17.1 provides a comparative view of cancer mortality in the circumpolar countries and their northern regions. It is evident that the highest rates are reported in Greenland and Nunavut, two regions where the Inuit form the overwhelming majority (>85 per cent) of the population. Since the incidence of cancer from all sites combined for

Figure 17.1   Age-standardized mortality rates of cancer in the circumpolar region

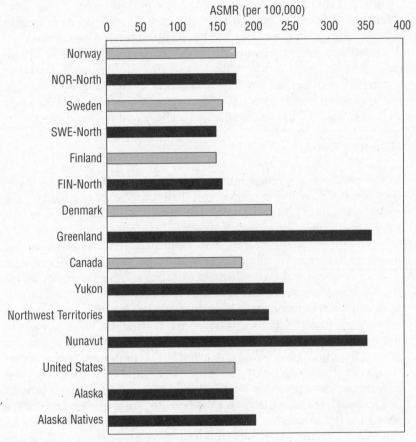

Notes: All rates (per 100,000) are standardized to the European Standard Population; all cancer sites combined; NOR-North: Nordland, Troms, and Finnmark combined; SWE-North: Norbotten and Västerbotten combined; FIN-North: Lapland.

Sources: Circumpolar Mortality Database, with data compiled from EUROSTAT (for national data for Denmark, Sweden, Norway and Finland and regional data for Norway and Sweden), Statistics Greenland, Statistics Finland (for Lapland data), Statistics Canada, and the National Center for Health Statistics (for U.S., Alaska, and Alaska Natives data); all rates are mean for 2001–3, except Denmark and Greenland, which are based on 1999–2001 data.

the Inuit is similar to that of non-Inuit in these regions, the excess mortality is indicative of poorer survival (discussed towards the end of this chapter). It should also be noted that cause of death information from death certificates are particularly subject to inaccurate recording in remote regions, so these data need to be interpreted with caution.

This chapter focuses primarily on cancer among the Inuit in Greenland, Alaska, and Canada, with special case studies on the Sami in northern Scandinavia (box 17.1) and cancer in Arkhangelsk Oblast in north-western Russia (box 17.2). Discussion of cancer among the Dene in Alaska and Northwest Territories can be found in chapter 8.

Historical Trends

In the middle of the nineteenth century, the first reports of malignant diseases in Greenland appeared, but the reports were few, and by the end of the century, cancer among the Inuit was thought to be practically non-existent. However, in 1904 the first microscopically verified case of cancer (of the breast) was published. A subsequent careful investigation covering all of Greenland in the years 1913–20 revealed that not only did malignant diseases exist but also the frequency, when the age distribution of the inhabitants was accounted for, was comparable with that in Denmark.[1] Already in the 1920s a high proportion of salivary gland carcinomas was observed. During the 1970s, studies in the Arctic areas revealed the existence of a distinctive cancer pattern among the Inuit, which were characterized by high frequencies of carcinomas of the nasopharynx, salivary glands, and esophagus, and low frequencies of tumors common in Western countries, such as cancers of the breast, skin, prostate, and the hematological system (fig. 17.2).[2] As a result of increasing survival of the Inuit population into cancer-prone ages, better detection, and changing risk factors during the twentieth century, malignant disease has moved from being a medical curiosity to a major health problem in the Arctic today.

In the period 1924–33, cancer was stated as the cause of death in less than 2 per cent of all deaths in Greenland. Although this proportion might have been underestimated, the high mortality rate due to infectious diseases and the consequent modest life expectancy made cancer a rare disease. However, during the twentieth century, the frequency of malignant diseases increased steadily in parallel with the reduction in the burden of infectious diseases, and by the beginning of the twenty-first century, cancer constituted 27 per cent of all deaths in Greenland.[3]

Figure 17.2   Standardized incidence ratio of selected cancers in Greenland
compared with Denmark

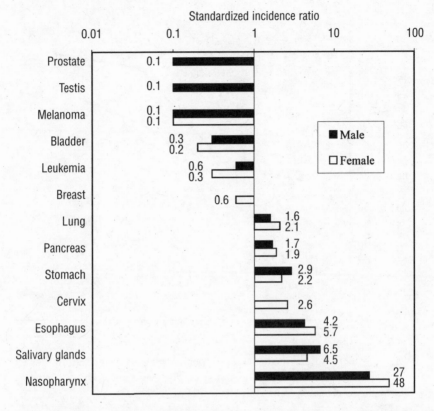

Note: Data refer to 1988–97 period; age-standardized to the IARC World Standard Population
Source: Adapted from Friborg et al. (2003).

Since the early 1970s, when reliable cancer registries in the Arctic
were developed, age-standardized incidence rates among the Inuit
have increased simultaneously in Greenland, Canada, and Alaska by
approximately 50 per cent. While overall rates among the Inuit in the
1950s and 1960s seemed to be below their respective national rates,
they appeared to have caught up. This increase, however, has not been
evenly distributed among different cancer sites. While the incidence of
more traditional Inuit cancers such as nasopharyngeal, salivary, and

Figure 17.3   Divergent trends in incidence of traditional and non-traditional Inuit cancers in Canada, Alaska, and Greenland

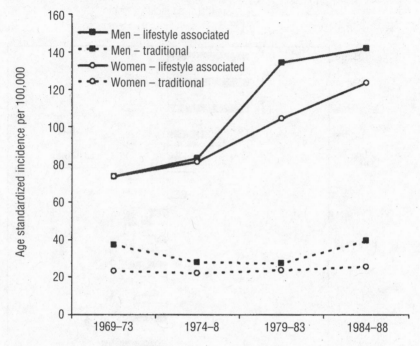

Note: Age-standardized incidence rates (per 100,000), standardized to the IARC World Standard Population; data refer to 1969–88 period.
Source: Based on data reported in Nielsen et al. (1996).

esophageal cancers has remained constant, the 'modern' cancers, primarily lifestyle-associated ones such as lung, colon, breast, and prostate cancer, have increased (fig. 17.3), likely the result of changes in smoking, reproductive, and dietary patterns. Only cancer of the uterine cervix has shown a consistent decline since the 1980s. The commonest cancers among Greenlandic men during the period 1988–97 were lung (27 per cent), colorectal (9 per cent), and esophageal (8 per cent); among women, they were lung (18 per cent), breast (16 per cent), uterine cervix (15 per cent), and colorectal (8 per cent).

While men generally are at greater risk of cancer than women, the opposite is observed in Greenland where the risk of cancer among females is approximately 10 per cent higher than among males. This is primarily because of the very low rates of prostate cancer in Greenlandic men and the high rates of cancer of the uterine cervix in Greenlandic women. In Nunavut, there appears to have been a steady increase of cancer among women during the 1990s, such that by the end of the decade, the female rate exceeded the male one.[4]

Sources of Data

While cancer registries exist in all Inuit areas, there are operational differences. In Greenland, reporting of cancer cases to the Danish Cancer Registry is mandatory. In Alaska, cases among Inuit are collected by the Alaska Native Tumour Registry, which is a full participant of the U.S. National Cancer Institute's Surveillance, Epidemiology, and End Results (SEER) program and adheres to its standards on data collection and coding. It includes Alaska Native patients living in Alaska at the time of diagnosis who are eligible for Indian Health Service benefits. In Canada, each province and territory maintains its own registry of cancer cases, information on which is then forwarded to and collated by the Canadian Cancer Registry maintained by Statistics Canada.

In Canada, Inuit status among cancer cases can be identified for those who are residents of the Northwest Territories and Nunavut, but not those residing in the provinces (the Nunavik region in Quebec, Labrador, and southern urban centres). While Alaskan Inuit (as distinct from the other Native groups, Indians, and Aleuts) are identifiable at the individual record level based on self-reports, such information is not consistently available. Routine cancer statistical reports tend to cover all Alaska Natives as a group. Information on ethnic affiliation is not available in Greenland, and cancer and other health statistics from Greenland have traditionally used individuals born in Greenland as a proxy.

About 4 per cent of cancer cases were coded as 'unspecified' in both Greenland and Alaska, comparable to that in Denmark. Histological verification is available for 78 per cent of cases in Greenland, which is lower than in Denmark, and reflects the lack of facilities for biopsy in remote areas.

Lung Cancer

Lung cancer has become a pandemic during the twentieth century, and rates of lung cancer have increased markedly in all Inuit populations since the 1960s. Compared with rates worldwide, Inuit men and women rank at the top, and the rates among women are probably the highest reported. While lung cancer rates in other populations began to decline by the end of the twentieth century, this development seems to be delayed in the Arctic. Although rates of lung cancer among Inuit men seem to have reached a plateau in the 1990s, rates among women continue to rise. The single most important risk factor for lung cancer is smoking, and the overall trend in lung cancer among the Inuit most likely reflects changes in the smoking prevalence. The per capita consumption of cigarettes in Greenland based on import statistics more than doubled between 1950 and 1980, although a decline was noted in the 1990s. Between 1993 and 2000, the smoking prevalence among adult Greenlanders actually decreased from 80 per cent to 70 per cent, which is still extremely high. With a latency period of several decades between smoking and cancer development, the lung cancer epidemic, especially among Inuit women, may not have reached its peak.[5]

Other factors are known to influence the risk of lung cancer. The observation of high lung cancer rates among Canadian Inuit in the 1950s prior to the smoking epidemic gave rise to speculations that open-flame lamps could have been the source of potential exposure to hydrocarbons and other volatile substances.[6] Moreover, as a diet rich in vegetables and fruits has been shown to be associated with a decreased risk of lung cancer, the low intake of these foods in the traditional Inuit diet may contribute to an increased risk. These are unlikely to be significant factors, as lung cancer rates continue to rise while housing standards and dietary quality have improved.

Attention has also been focused on the possible influence of long-term exposure to radon gas, formed from the decay products of radium and uranium that may infiltrate the house from underlying rocks and soil. A survey in Greenland found the proportion of houses exceeding the recommended radon levels to be slightly higher than in Denmark. However, substantial geographic variation was present as none of the houses in Nuuk but 28 per cent of houses in Narsaq, in the southern part of Greenland, exceeded recommendations.[7] Thus, while radon exposure may add to the high lung cancer rates in some areas of the Arctic, the overall contribution is probably small.

In conclusion, cigarette smoking remains the predominant cause of lung cancer among the Inuit, and given the avoidable nature of this exposure, may be the main area of intervention.

Smoking is a risk factor that is shared with bladder cancer. However, bladder cancer is uncommon among Inuit, whose risk is only 20–40 per cent that of Europeans. Unlike lung cancer, bladder cancer rates have remained· stable since the 1970s. Inuit communities are not exposed to chemical industries known to be associated with bladder cancer (rubber, dyestuff, leather, and paints), but Inuit do smoke, so it is puzzling why there is an increase in lung cancer and not bladder cancer. A possible explanation could be the traditional Inuit diet, which is rich in vitamin A, believed to protect against bladder cancer. In that case, rates of bladder cancer may increase in the future, as the intake of traditional foods decreases.

Breast Cancer

The incidence of breast cancer has traditionally been low among the Inuit, but a considerable increase since the 1970s has been observed, with rates now approaching those observed in their respective national populations. Nunavut appears to remain a low-risk region, with rates at about 40 per cent that of Canada.

In Greenland, the increase is particularly noted among women older than fifty years of age. There is a shift from the pattern seen typically in low-risk countries with stagnating or falling rates after menopause to the pattern commonly seen in Western countries with increasing rates after menopause (fig. 17.4). While improved diagnosis could have contributed to the increase, one would expect to see the increase across all age groups, and not only among post-menopausal women.

Most of the ethnic and international differences in the risk of breast cancer can be explained by differences in environmental exposures and lifestyle, particularly reproductive and hormonal factors. The birth rate among the Inuit has been steadily falling, and the maternal mean age at first birth has increased. Both factors are known to increase the risk of breast cancer. Increased risk of breast cancer has also been associated with obesity after menopause and large weight gains after the age of eighteen years. The increase in breast cancer rates is therefore consistent with the increasing prevalence of obesity and type 2 diabetes in the Inuit populations (see chapter 16). A contributing factor could be changes in the pattern of breastfeeding, as prolonged breastfeeding is associated with a decreased risk of breast cancer in both pre-and post-menopausal women. Prolonged breastfeeding, practically continued through the childbearing years, was common in the Inuit populations at the beginning of the twentieth

Figure 17.4   Change in age-specific incidence of breast cancer among Greenlandic Inuit

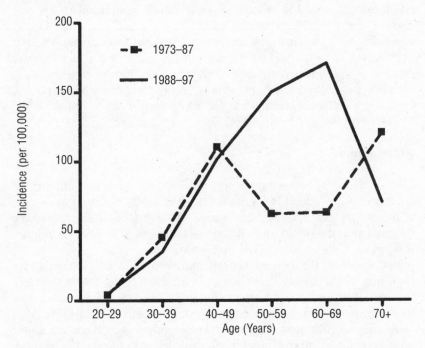

Note: Age-standardized incidence rates (per 100,000), standardized to the IARC World Standard Population
Source: Adapted from Friborg et al. (2003).

century, but decreased throughout the century, and the pattern of breastfeeding is now similar to what is seen in Western populations. The traditional Inuit diet may also offer protection against breast cancer as fatty acids originating in fish is suggested to have a protective effect.[8]

Low parity, late age at first birth, and obesity are risk factors that are shared with two other hormone-associated cancers: uterine and ovarian cancer. Compared with Western populations, cancers of the uterus and ovary are rarer among the Inuit. The fact that incidence rates of these two cancers have not increased in parallel with breast cancer rates indicates that factors other than those associated with reproductive history may also be important for the increasing incidence in breast cancer.

·Colorectal Cancer

The global variation in colorectal cancer rates is substantial, with high rates observed in Western populations and low rates in Asian populations. During the past decades rates have generally increased worldwide, although the trend towards increased incidence now seems to be reversed in North America. The Inuit populations have also experienced a significant increase in rates since the 1970s, and colorectal cancer is now one of the most common malignancies. Geographical differences are present among the Inuit, and rates among Alaskan Inuit, especially women, have consistently been higher than among Inuit in Canada and Greenland. While rates of colorectal cancer among Inuit in Northern Canada and Greenland approach the levels in Canada and Denmark, rates in Alaskan Inuit exceed those of U.S. whites (fig. 17.5). Whether this reflects an earlier introduction of risk factors in Alaska or differences in registration is not entirely clear. Better diagnostic services, especially access to endoscopies, might contribute to the increase, but diagnostic development alone cannot explain the differences in colorectal cancer rates observed among different ethnic groups in the same region.[9]

More likely, the rapid increase in colorectal cancer rates among Inuit indicates the influence of environmental risk factors, with diet being the most important. Both an energy-dense diet rich in fat, refined carbohydrates, and animal protein and a sedentary lifestyle increase the risk of colorectal cancer significantly. These factors probably influence colorectal carcinogenesis via insulin pathways, and a higher risk of disease has been found in diabetes patients.[10] The main component of the diet today consists of imported food, and obesity and diabetes are increasing (see chapters 11 and 16). Thus, it seems likely that the dietary transition among the Inuit, together with a less physically active lifestyle, has had a considerable impact on colorectal cancer rates.

Prostate Cancer

A high caloric diet, obesity, and low physical activity are risk factors that are shared by colorectal and prostate cancer. Thus, rates of prostate cancer among the Inuit would have been expected to increase

Figure 17.5   Trends in Alaska Native incidence of colorectal cancer

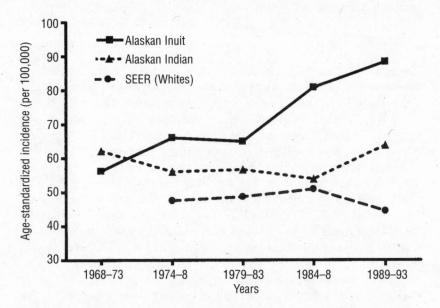

Note: Age-standardized incidence rates (per 100,000), standardized to the
1970 United States all-races population; Alaskan data refer to 1969–93 period;
Whites refer to SEER data from Western Washington state during 1974–93.
Source: Based on data reported in Brown et al. (1998).

in parallel with colorectal cancer rates. However, prostate cancer is traditionally rare and, unlike the increase in rates seen in other low-risk
areas, rates have remained very low among the Inuit in Greenland
compared with European populations. Rates of prostate cancer among
Inuit men in Alaska are increasing, although they are still lower than
among U.S. whites and Alaskan Indians and Aleuts. In Nunavut, rates
are only 10 per cent that of Canada as a whole.

Transurethral resection of the prostate and the test for prostate-
specific antigen (PSA) are not widely used in the Arctic and underesti-
mation of the frequency is possible. However, the low prevalence of
prostate cancer has been confirmed by an autopsy study among Inuit
men. Reasons for the lower risk of prostate cancer are unknown. It has
been suggested that the Inuit are protected against prostate cancer by
their traditional marine-based diet, which contains high intake of

omega-3 polyunsaturated fatty acid and selenium. Although no studies have addressed this in Inuit populations specifically, a high familial risk of prostate cancer is found in other populations.[11]

Nasopharyngeal Cancer

Globally, the occurrence of nasopharyngeal carcinoma (NPC) shows remarkable geographic and ethnic variation. NPC constitutes less than 1 per cent of all cancers in most populations, but a high incidence is found in areas of southern China, South-East Asia, North Africa, and among Inuit in the Arctic. NPC is twenty-five to forty times more common among Inuit compared with Caucasians.[12]

The undifferentiated carcinomas constitute the majority of NPCs in high-incidence areas, and more than 85 per cent of NPCs among Inuit belong to this group. Undifferentiated NPC has been causally linked to Epstein-Barr virus (EBV) infection. The evidence for causality is based on (a) the detection of viral genomes and proteins in the vast majority of tumors from high-incidence areas, including the Arctic; (b) the detection of clonal EBV in all tumour cells, indicating that EBV infection of the epithelium precedes tumour growth; and (c) the presence of EBV-specific antibodies and antibody titers in NPC patients years before diagnosis.[13]

Other environmental factors than EBV are also known to be involved in NPC development, although these have not been investigated in detail among Inuit. In Chinese populations, studies have demonstrated an association between high intake of preserved foods, especially salted fish, and subsequent NPC risk. Whether comparable high-risk foods are present in the Arctic is not clear, but in a small study from Alaska, NPC patients reported the use of salted fish during childhood more often than controls. A high content of nitrosamines has also been found in Greenlandic dried fish, equivalent to the high levels found in Chinese salted fish. Among risk factors implicated in other types of pharyngeal cancers, smoking only exerts a minor influence on NPC risk, while alcohol has no association at all.[14]

The familial risk of NPC is among the highest of any malignancy, and in Greenland first-degree relatives of an NPC patient had an eightfold increased risk of the disease. Familial aggregation of disease can be the result of genetic susceptibility, common environmental exposure, or both. The possible genes remain elusive, but certain HLA haplotypes and polymorphisms of metabolic enzyme genes have been reported to be associated with an increased risk of NPC in Chinese populations.[15]

Since the 1980s, the rates of NPC have decreased considerably in other high-incidence areas parallel to changes in lifestyle. The relatively modest decrease among the Inuit could indicate that genetic risk factors may play a larger role, or that environmental risk factors have not changed for a sufficiently long time period to clearly influence the incidence. However, it seems likely that the incidence of NPC will decrease further in the future.

Salivary Gland Cancer

Carcinoma of the salivary glands among the Inuit shares many similarities with NPC. Histopathologically, salivary gland cancer resembles NPC, and the tumour is also associated with Epstein-Barr virus. While rare in most populations, salivary gland cancer occurs among the Inuit with rates among the highest in the world, and the tumor is five to ten times more frequent among the Inuit compared with Europeans. Little is known about risk factors for salivary gland cancer in the Arctic, but the observation of an increased risk in families with prior cases of NPC indicates that the two cancers share risk factors. This unity with NPC has not been described in other high NPC-incidence populations and could indicate that genetic or environmental factors different from those present in Chinese populations influence the risk of Inuit EBV-associated cancers. The rates of salivary gland cancer seem stable in the Inuit populations, although the relatively low numbers limit the interpretation.[16]

Esophageal Cancer

The incidence of esophagus cancer is high and the cancer continues to be of considerable public health importance. Migration studies in other populations have indicated that environmental factors are important and smoking and alcohol are confirmed risk factors. However, rates of esophageal cancer among the Inuit have not followed the increasing trend of lung cancer, and other risk factors may be relevant in the Arctic. Human papilloma virus (HPV) has been found in a high proportion of esophageal cancers among Alaska Natives. Another suggested risk factor is the traditional Inuit diet, as a high content of nitrosamines (a group of known carcinogens) has been found in certain foods.[17]

One histological subtype, adenocarcinoma of the esophagus (and also of the upper part of the stomach), is associated with obesity, and in Western populations this cancer type has increased with a rate of 5–10 per cent per year and now accounts for more than 50 per cent of all esophagus cancers. An increase among the Inuit has not yet been observed. But as Inuit cancer surveys are not routinely stratified by histological subtypes, an obesity-driven increase in adenocarcinomas of the esophagus could be obscured by a simultaneous decrease in rates of squamous cell carcinomas.

Stomach Cancer

Contrary to the stable rates of esophageal cancer, increasing rates of stomach cancer have been reported in both Greenland and Alaska. The increase is especially clear among males, in contrast to global trends for this malignancy. Reasons for the increase are unknown, as improved diagnosis would probably have affected the rate of esophageal cancer also. While smoking is known to increase the risk of stomach cancer, the large increase in male stomach cancer rates is not accompanied by similar increases in male lung cancer rates, just as the large increase in female lung cancer rates is not accompanied by an increase in female stomach cancer rates. Stomach cancer has also been associated with *Helicobacter pylori* infection, and the high seropreva-lence of *H. pylori* (50–60 per cent) is higher than in Western popula-tions. As no time series of *H. pylori* occurrence is available for any Inuit population, the role of *H. pylori* in the stomach cancer rate increase cannot be estimated, although a large increase in *H. pylori* seropreva-lence appears unlikely in the light of the sociocultural changes in Inuit communities. Thus, the increase in stomach cancer rates remains largely unexplained.[18]

Cervical Cancer

It is now established that the sexually transmitted human papillo-mavirus (HPV) is a necessary cause of cancer of the uterine cervix. There are over 100 types of HPV, of which types 16 and 18 are the most oncogenic. Non-sexual factors such as smoking, diet, and parity may influence the acquisition and persistence of the infection and the pro-gression from infection to invasive cancer. A significant decreasing trend for cancer of the cervix has been observed among the Inuit, although rates are still higher than among the general rates in the U.S.

and Denmark. While increased screening activity may account for some of the decrease, a reduced prevalence of HPV infection may also contribute. Although time trends of HPV infection rates among the Inuit are not available, it could have paralleled the steadily falling incidence of other sexually transmitted diseases such as gonorrhoea documented in some jurisdictions. Increased use of condoms, advocated for family planning and HIV prevention, also decreases the risk of HPV infection.[19]

The viral etiology of cervical cancer offers opportunity in terms of screening, diagnosis, and prevention. Detection of HPV in cervical samples increases the sensitivity of cervical cancer screening, and may be a useful substitute for Pap smears. A recombinant vaccine directed at four HPV subtypes was licensed by the United States Foods and Drugs Administration in 2006 for use in girls and women between the ages of nine and twenty-six. The vaccine reduces the risk of both HPV infection and HPV-related cervical intraepithelial neoplasia (the preinvasive lesion). The implementation of the vaccine in Arctic communities could have an extensive impact on the burden of cervical cancer.

Liver Cancer

Chronic hepatitis B virus (HBV) infection is associated with an increased risk of hepatocellular carcinoma (HCC). Hepatitis B is prevalent among the Inuit (see chapter 15), and rates of HCC are proportionally high compared with their respective national populations. However, there is regional variation – the incidence of HCC among Inuit in Greenland is lower than in Alaska, despite higher rates of hepatitis B infection.

Prevention of hepatitis B through vaccination in Alaska has clearly shown to reduce the risk of chronic hepatitis B, and studies in other hepatitis B-endemic populations report an equivalent protective effect of vaccination against development of HCC. As a consequence, newborns in Alaska and in the Northwest Territories are routinely vaccinated, while newborns in Greenland are offered vaccination if the mother is HBV-infected. The detection of hepatitis B-specific antigens in blood can also be used for large-scale diagnostic and screening purposes, as demonstrated in Alaska. Another hepatitis virus, hepatitis C, is an important risk factor for HCC in other populations, but due to a generally low prevalence in the Arctic, the significance of this virus as a risk factor for HCC among the Inuit is still small.[20]

Box 17.1 Cancer among the Sami of northern Scandinavia

Chapter 9 provides an overview of the patterns of health and disease among the Sami. While there is a general lack of information on health issues specific to the Sami population, cancer is one area that has attracted some attention. That cancer has been relatively well studied is probably due to the fact that the greater part of Sápmi suffered heavily from nuclear fallout from the bomb tests on the Kola Peninsula during the 1950s and 1960s and the Chernobyl accident in Ukraine in 1986. Studies on cancer incidence and mortality among the Sami has so far only been done separately in the Sami populations of Norway, Sweden, and Finland.[21] These studies cover both reindeer herders and non-herders. Generally, they show great concordance regarding the risk of cancer relative to the non-Sami population (table 17.1). Except for Swedish Sami women, the cancer risk among the Sami tends to be lower. Particularly low risks are observed for colon (both sexes in Norway and male in Sweden) and prostate (all three countries). Lower risk for breast cancer is observed among Finnish Sami women, and lung cancer among Norwegian Sami men.

The overall low risk of cancer has been attributed to dietary factors, such as the high intake of selenium from reindeer meat and the high consumption of n-3 fatty acids from fish and freely grazing reindeers. High levels of physical activity may contribute to a lower risk, while genetic factors may have been protective. A higher risk for stomach cancer among the Sami in Sweden may reflect a historical high incidence of stomach cancer among rural-living Sami with a high intake of smoked and salted meat and fish and a lower intake of fruit and vegetables. Although the incidence of stomach cancer is decreasing in the general population, a similar trend is not observed among the Sami. (Lifestyle factors such as diet, smoking, and physical activity are discussed in greater details in chapter 9.)

The importance of lifestyle factors for the development of cancer among the Sami were indicated in a Finnish study where it was reported that a subpopulation, the Skolts, showed a non-reduced overall risk for cancer in contrast to the general Sami population for which the cancer incidence was significantly reduced. The Skolt Sami live in a specific region in north-east of Finland and they have a different language and partly different habits and lifestyle. However, among the Sami in Sweden, an equally low mortality from cancer was found among reindeer-herding and non-herding Sami men. As it was assumed that the non-herding Sami had adopted a lifestyle similar to the non-Sami population, the low mortality from cancer suggested genetic rather than lifestyle-related explanations.

Table 17.1   Age-standardized incidence ratios of selected cancers among Sami in Norway, Sweden, and Finland

Site	Finland Both sexes	Norway		Sweden	
		Male	Female	Male	Female
Stomach	1.20	0.91	1.06	1.23*	1.53*
Colon	0.72	0.50*	0.62*	0.74*	1.19
Rectum	0.58	1.06	0.72	0.89	1.24
Lung	0.94	0.63*	0.60	0.81	0.84
Breast	0.36*	–	0.85	–	1.01
Ovary	1.50	–	0.88	–	1.51*
Prostate	0.25*	0.57*	–	0.76*	–
All sites	0.64*	0.78*	0.84*	0.90*	1.04

*95% confidence interval excluding unity.
Note: Different comparison groups of non-Sami were used in different countries – the Finnish national population, the rural population of the three northernmost counties of Norway, and a demographically matched non-Sami cohort in Sweden.
Sources: Norway: Haldoren and Tynes (2005); Sweden: Wiklund, Holm, and Eklund (1990); Hassler et al. (2001); Finland: Soininen, Järvinen, and Pukkala (2002).

In Sweden, prostate cancer was studied among different Sami groups, which were differentiated according to the extent of presumed adherence to a Sami lifestyle and the degree of Sami heritage. Both the incidence and mortality from prostate cancer were significantly lower among herding Sami living in the mountain areas, where the traditional Sami lifestyle is strongest, compared with those herders living in other regions of the country. No differences in cancer risks were observed when the herders were subdivided according to degree of Sami heritage, lending support to the view that the low risk for prostate cancer is related to traditional Sami lifestyle rather than to genetic factors.

The only Nordic collaborative initiative regarding Sami health was aimed at studying cancer incidence among reindeer-herding Sami in Norway, Sweden, and Finland in relation to the radioactive fallout from the atomic bomb testing on the Kola Peninsula and the fallout from Chernobyl. Although enhanced quantities of the isotope Cesium 137 in lichen, reindeer meat, as well as in whole-body content among reindeer herders have been found, there had been no detectable excess of either leukemia or thyroid cancer. On the contrary, slightly smaller than expected number of cases were found. Similarly, the incidence of prostate, lung, breast, and colorectal cancer was lower than in the rest of the population. These results suggest that radiation doses received by the reindeer-herding Sami were too small to have substantially affected cancer incidence.[22]

Cancer Control and Prevention

The control of cancer requires multiple strategies directed at different stages in the natural history of the disease: (a) primary prevention, by reducing the prevalence of risk factors before the occurrence of disease; (b) early detection or screening, sometimes referred to as secondary prevention, to abort the progression to invasive cancer; and (c) treatment for those diagnosed with cancer, to improve survival and quality of life.

In the discussion of individual cancers above, several risk factors emerge as particularly important for the Inuit, and their elimination or reduction in the population holds promise for primary prevention. As in most populations worldwide, tobacco is by far the most important cause of cancer, responsible for the very high rates of lung cancer, and a contributing factor in the development of cancers of the esophagus, stomach, and kidneys. Even if smoking prevalence is dramatically reduced today, one would expect a time lag of some thirty years before any impact on lung cancer rates can be observed. (Chapter 12 discusses further the smoking trends in the Arctic and strategies for tobacco control.)

Heavy alcohol consumption is associated with the development of a number of cancers, including those of the oral cavity, pharynx (but not nasopharyngeal cancer), esophagus, and liver.[23] The frequency of alcohol consumption in different populations is difficult to compare due to methodological differences (discussed further in chapter 12). The drinking pattern among the Inuit tends to be episodic ('binge' drinking), as opposed to the increasing daily consumption over many years observed in other populations. The control of heavy alcohol drinking should be part of a cancer-control strategy, with the added benefit of reducing other health problems such as injuries (see chapter 18).

The dietary transition that Inuit have undergone has had both positive and negative effects on the risk of cancer. The traditional Inuit diet, while low in fresh vegetables and fruits, contains high contents of vitamin A and fatty acids of marine origin, which are protective of some cancers. However, the high content of nitrosamines identified in several traditional food items probably contribute to the high risks of nasopharyngeal and esophageal cancer. The modern diet, while containing more vegetables and fruits, is also energy-dense with high levels of saturated fat, which together with reduced physical activity has led to an increase in obesity and diabetes. Obesity and diabetes increase the risk of several cancers, while regular physical exercise appears to lower the risk. The public health recommendations for a diet rich in fruits and vegetables, the maintenance of a healthy weight and a physically active lifestyle would have benefits in the prevention of cancer as well as other chronic diseases.

While most cancer risk factors involve individual behaviours or lifestyles, the physical environment also plays a role. The accumulation of organic pollutants and heavy metals in the Arctic food chain has attracted a lot of attention (see chapter 10). Their importance in cancer development, however, is difficult to assess. Although some have shown mutagenic and carcinogenic potential in animal studies, the evidence from human observational studies is inconclusive. Their effect is likely small or the induction period for these contaminants too long for the influence to be detectable in cancer trends.

The viral etiology of HPV in cervical cancer and HBV in hepatocellular carcinoma discussed above opens up the exciting possibility that some types of cancer can now be prevented by vaccination. The population-wide effectiveness of HBV vaccine is now well established, whereas the use of HPV vaccine was only licensed in 2006, and its long-term impact remains to be determined. Although vaccination against EBV is not yet available, the association between EBV and nasopharyngeal cancer has been utilized for diagnostic purposes in other high-incidence populations. Probably more relevant for the Inuit is the detection of EBV in blood or pharyngeal scrapings from individuals with suspected NPC. Such techniques can be applied to select high-risk individuals to undergo a more thorough clinical examination. Among Inuit, close family members of NPC patients have an increased risk of NPC, and in this group, EBV-based screening methods could become an important tool.[24]

Early detection of cancer either through organized screening or medical vigilance is dependent upon a well-organized health care system. The Arctic generally lags behind in terms of such efforts. In Greenland, a centralized population-based program for cervical cancer screening was not implemented until 1999, decades after its implementation in Denmark. In Nunavut, only about 50 per cent of eligible women received a Pap smear during the period 1998–2000, making it the jurisdiction with the lowest screening participation rate in Canada. However, by 2005, the proportion of women aged eighteen to sixty-nine who had at least one Pap test in the preceding three years had risen to 79 per cent in Nunavut, exceeding the Canadian national average of 73 per cent. The other two northern territories also had higher than national rates (Yukon 79 per cent, Northwest Territories 84 per cent). Clearly, intensive promotion of participation in preventive services in the target population can be achieved. The use of innovative technology is particularly suitable for the Arctic with its scattered and sparse population. In the central Canadian Arctic, a colposcopy suite was established in the 1990s in the regional hospital for the diagnosis and management of cervical intraepithelial neoplasia, eliminating the need to transfer patients another 1,000 kilometres further to the south to Winnipeg.[25]

Definitive diagnosis of most cancers requires sophisticated and complex tools (such as computed tomography, magnetic resonance impedance scans, endoscopy, surgical pathology, and biomarkers), and by necessity such tools are concentrated in regional centres. The unique challenges of health care delivery in the Arctic is the need to strengthen primary health care at the community level to ensure that patients with possible cancer are identified and referred promptly for further investigations.

The treatment of cancer is also highly specialized and includes surgery, chemotherapy, and radiotherapy. Thus, Inuit patients are often required to travel long distances and to be away from home during treatment. Some of the more basic chemotherapy treatments, that is, the treatment of lung and breast cancers, have been moved from Denmark to Greenland. While such decentralization of treatment will likely increase in the future, given the small size of the Inuit populations, it will only be restricted to the most common types of cancer.

There is some evidence that the management of cancer in the Arctic is less than optimal. Data from Alaska suggest that Alaska Natives tend to be diagnosed at later stages of their disease than U.S. whites. Their survival rates were lower, in both men and women, for all sites combined. However, there is ground for optimism as the survival rate had increased between the periods 1969–83 and 1984–94, particularly for colorectal and live cancer.[26]

Finally, comprehensive cancer control requires ongoing surveillance and monitoring. The international collaborative project that collected consistent and comparable incidence data for the circumpolar Inuit covered the period 1969–88, and a monograph was published in 1996. Since then, only regional studies have been performed, and only questions concerning the most frequent cancer types have been reasonably addressed. Given the characteristic cancer pattern, the challenging infrastructure and the rapid change in living conditions in the Arctic, a renewed effort in circumpolar surveillance is long overdue.

Box 17.2 Cancer in the Arkangelsk Oblast in northwestern Russia

Comparison of cancer statistics from Russia (and the former Soviet Union) with other countries and regions has been difficult due to methodological differences in diagnosis, reporting, and registration. In the late 1990s, an international collaborative project between the University of Tromsø in Norway and the Oncological Hospital in Arkangelsk developed a population-based cancer registry for the Arkangelsk Oblast, a region of over 1.3 million people in north-western Russia (see map 8). Each year between 3,500 and 4,000 new cancer cases were reported to the registry. About 80 per cent of cases were verified histologically and/or cytologically. About 2–3 per cent of cases were derived from death certificates only, comparable to the Norwegian Cancer Registry.[27]

The project included site visits to two district hospitals to cross-validate the files of active living patients against registry records in terms of the accuracy and completeness of different types of information. About 6 per cent of cases randomly selected from the district hospitals were not registered. A pathologist from Tromsø also reviewed the histological slides. Several groups of residents were likely to be under-enumerated: the indigenous Nenets from the Nenets Autonomous Okrug, many of whom live in the tundra as herders and hunters and

Figure 17.6   Age-standardized incidence rates of selected cancer sites, Arkangelsk Oblast and Norway

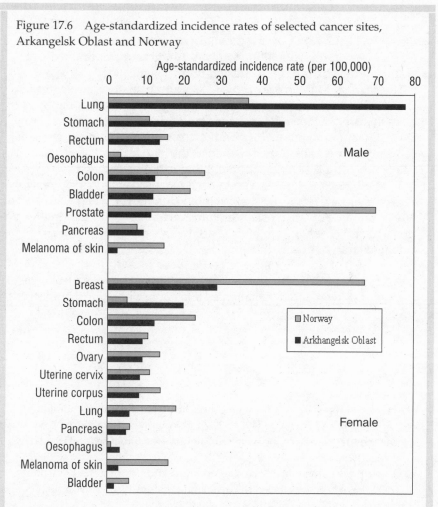

Age-standardized incidence rate (per 100,000)

Note: Age-standardized incidence rates (per 100,000) standardized to the IARC World Standard Population.
Sources: Arkangelsk Oblast data from Vaktskjold et al. (2005); Norwegian data (mean of 1993–2001) obtained from *Cancer in Norway 2001* (www.kreftregis teret.no).

have little contact with the health care system, and the rural elderly poor who may not be have been able to access district-level specialist facilities due to transportation costs. Military and shipyard personnel (engaged in the construction of nuclear vessels) and their families had their own health care system and might not have been captured by the registry. Population mobility (mainly out-migration) since the disintegration of the USSR has also created problems for the registry.

The registry was able to provide a portrait of the cancer burden in the oblast. During the period 1993–2001, there were some 35,000 cases registered. Overall, the age-standardized incidence rate was 281/100,000 for men and 164/100,000 for women. The male rate was comparable to that of Norway, whereas the female rate was only about 60 per cent of the Norwegian rate. Lung cancer accounted for 16 per cent of all cases, followed by stomach (15 per cent). As figure 17.6 shows, there are some very substantial differences when compared with Norway. Elevated risks (three to four times) were reported for stomach and esophagus in both sexes. Lung cancer was twice as high among men in Arkangelsk than in Norway, whereas among women it was only 0.3 of the Norwegian rate. Reduced risks were also reported in Arkangelsk, relative to Norway, for prostate (0.2) among men, breast (0.4) among women, and malignant melanoma of skin (0.2) in both sexes.

NOTES

1 Historical reports (in Danish) on cancer in Greenland can be found in Rink (1857) and Bertelsen (1904). The first comprehensive review covering the first decade of the twentieth century was published in German by Fibiger (1923).

2 Descriptive epidemiologic studies on Inuit cancer during the 1960s and 1970s have been conducted in Greenland (Nielsen 1986), Alaska (Blot et al. 1975), and Canada (Schaefer et al. 1975).

3 Causes of death data in Greenland from 1924–33 were reported by Bertelsen (1937). Contemporary data are available from Statistics Greenland.

4 Data for the period 1969–88 are available for the circumpolar Inuit from the international collaborative project, and are published a special issue of *Acta Oncologica* 35 (1996). For a summary, see Nielsen et al. (1996). Updates on incidence up to 1997 for Greenland (Friborg, Koch, et al. 2003) and up to 1998 for Alaska (Lanier et al. 2001b) have been published. A comprehensive report on cancer among Alaska Natives from

1969–2003 (Lanier, Kelly, et al. 2006) is available from the Alaska Native Tribal Health Consortium, www.anthc.org/cs/chs/epi/pubs.cfm. For Canada, Inuit-specific data are available for Nunavut for the period 1992–2001 (Healey, Plaza, and Osborne 2003) and the Northwest Territories from 1990–2000 (Northwest Territories Department of Health and Social Service 2003). These sources will be used extensively in the rest of the chapter.

5 For an epidemiologic overview of lung cancer, see Alberg, Brock, and Samet (2005). Greenland's cigarette consumption data can be found in Bjerregaard and Young (1998:198), updated in Statistics Greenland, *Greenland in Figures 2005*. Smoking prevalence data are cited from Bjerregaard (2004).

6 Hildes and Schaefer (1984) pointed out that lung cancer affected elderly women predominantly, who had the domestic task of tending to open seal-oil lamps almost around-the-clock. There is some palaeopathological evidence to support this as black pigmentation (anthracosis) has been found in the lungs of female Eskimo mummies from several centuries ago in Alaska and Greenland, long before the advent of tobacco and environmental pollution (see Zimmerman and Aufderheiden 1984; Hansen, Meldgaard, and Nordquist 1985).

7 Data are from the Asiaq Survey report by Petersen, Boe, and Persson (2005).

8 See chapter 7 for further discussion of Inuit fertility. Lipworth, Bailey, and Trichopoulos (2000) reviewed the evidence of the protective effect of breastfeeding in breast cancer. Maillard et al. (2002) conducted a case-control study of breast cancer and n-3 and n-6 fatty acids in breast adipose tissue.

9 Global patterns are described in the *World Cancer Report* (IARC 2003). See Brown, Lanier, and Becker (1998) for the Alaskan situation between 1969 and 1993, updated to 2003 by Lanier, Kelly, et al. (2006). See Storm and Nielsen (1996) for circumpolar comparisons.

10 For a review of the evidence linking diabetes and colorectal, see Chang and Ulrich (2003).

11 Snyder, Kelly, and Lanier (2006) tracked prostate cancer among Alaska Natives from 1969–2003 and contrasted Inuit with Aleuts and Indians. The autopsy study in Greenland was reported by Dewailly, Mulvad, et al. (2003). For a review of the association between fish consumption and reduced prostate cancer, see Terry et al. (2001). Hansen, Deutch, and Pedersen (2004) assessed dietary intake and blood levels of selenium among Greenland Inuit.

12 See Lanier and Alberts (1996) for circumpolar comparisons. More recent data are available for Greenland from Friborg et al. (2003); for Alaska from Lanier, Kelly, et al. (2006); and for Nunavut from Healey, Plaza, and Osborne (2003).

13 Studies on the association between EBV and NPC were conducted in Alaska in the 1970s by Lanier, Bender, et al. (1980) and Lanier, Bornkamm, et al. (1981). For a review of the current status see Raab-Traub (2002).

14 See studies on dietary risk factors for NPC in Alaska by Lanier, Bender, et al. (1980) and Poirier et al. (1987). Yu and Yuan (2002) reviewed the epidemiology of NPC.

15 The familial clustering of NPC cases in Greenland has been studied by Albeck et al. (1993) and Friborg, Wohlfahrt, et al. (2005). For genetic studies of NPC among Chinese in Taiwan, see Hildesheim et al. (1997, 2002).

16 Saemundsen et al. (1982) and Raab-Traub et al. (1991) investigated EBV infection in salivary gland carcinoma in Greenland and Alaska respectively. Albeck et al. (1993) reported on salivary gland carcinoma in Greenlandic families.

17 Miller et al. (1997) found HPV-type 16 DNA in cancer specimens. For the global pattern in esophageal cancer, see the *World Cancer Report*.

18 The association between H. pylori and stomach cancer was reviewed by Prinz, Schwendy, and Voland (2006). Seroprevalence surveys were conducted by Koch, Krause, et al. (2005) in Greenland and McKeown et al. (1999) in Canada, the latter also detected *H. pylori* in community water supplies.

19 For a review of the epidemiology of HPV and its association with cervical cancer, see Trottier and Franco (2006). Roden and Wu (2006) examined the ramifications and outstanding issues surrounding the vaccine.

20 The epidemiology of viral hepatitis and HCC in the Arctic has been reviewed by McMahon (2004) and McMahon, Lanier, and Wainwright (1998). The screening and vaccination programs in Alaska were described in McMahon, Rhoades, et al. (1987) and McMahon, Bulkow, et al. (2000).

21 These studies include Haldoren and Tynes (2005) for Norway 1970–97; Wiklund, Holm, and Eklund (1990); Hassler, Sjölander, et al. (2001) for Sweden 1961–97; and Soininen, Järvinen, and Pukkala (2002) for Finland 1979–98.

22 Impact of the Chernobyl fallout was investigated by Strand et al. (1992) and Mehli et al. (2000), and fallout of the earlier Kola nuclear tests by Westerlund, Berthelsen, and Berteig (1987). The pan-Nordic study on

cancer among Sami reindeer herders was reported by Auvinen et al. (2002).

23 See Boffetta and Hashibe (2006) for a review of alcohol and cancer.

24 Chan and Lo (2002) and Tune et al. (1999) evaluated these diagnostic techniques involving EBV.

25 Data on Pap smear screening in Nunavut was obtained from Healey, Plaza, and Osborne (2003) and the 2005 Canadian Community Health Survey from Statistics Canada (CANSIM Table 105-4042). The colposcopy program was described by Martin et al. (1998).

26 Lanier, Holck, et al. (2001a) is the first study ever that looked at cancer survival in Alaska Natives. While for all cancer sites combined, the Native rate is 80 per cent that of the white rate, for cancer of the liver, Alaska Natives actually reported a higher survival rate.

27 Information presented in this box is obtained from Vaktskjold et al. (2005).

18 Injuries and Violence

KUE YOUNG AND SVEN HASSLER

In the decades since the 1940s, among the most serious health problems affecting northern peoples, particularly the indigenous population, are injuries sustained as a result of accidents and violence. This trend is reflected in excessive mortality, morbidity, health care utilization, residual disability, and social and economic costs. This chapter will not discuss suicide in detail, which is covered in the next chapter on mental health. However, data on suicide are included in some statistical tables covering all injuries. The main geographical focus is on northern Canada, supplemented by data and case studies from other circumpolar jurisdictions.

Basic Concepts of Injury Control

The study of injury epidemiology and control has undergone a conceptual shift since the 1970s, due especially to the pioneering work of William Haddon. The term 'accidents' is no longer considered adequate or appropriate by some schools of thought, as it suggests something that is unpredictable and unavoidable, a random event, or an 'act of God.' From a preoccupation with individual behaviour or susceptibility, the larger role played by the physical and social environments are also recognized. Injury can be defined as any damage sustained by the human body, which occurs rapidly and usually is immediately apparent. The causative agent is energy or an agent that interferes with energy exchange in the body. The forms of energy include mechanical (e.g., car crash, fall, suffocation), thermal (e.g., burn, cold exposure), chemical (e.g., drug overdose), electrical (e.g., electrocution) and ionizing radiation. Tissue damage is caused by rapid transfer of excessive amounts of energy or by interference with normal exchange patterns of energy that overwhelms the body's ability to withstand the transfer.[1]

Among the major contributions made by Haddon is his conceptualization of injury control in the form of a matrix, which has since become known as Haddon's matrix. The matrix is a 3x3 table, where one axis divides the injury into three time phases: pre-event, event, and post-event; and the other axis refers to factors contributing to the injury in terms of personal, equipment, and environmental factors. The matrix is useful both for understanding causation and implementing control measures.

Classification of Injuries

In the tenth edition of the *International Classification of Diseases* (ICD-10), injuries are grouped under chapter xix, entitled 'Injury, Poisoning, and Certain Other Consequences of External Causes,' with codes S00-T98, which are based on the nature of the injury (e.g., fracture, burns, poisoning, etc). Injuries are also listed in chapter xx, 'External Causes of Morbidity and Mortality,' with codes V01-Y98, which correspond to the 'E codes' of the previous edition, ICD-9. Individual jurisdictions may configure the grouping differently, making comparisons of categories of injuries difficult. From a public health perspective, the external causes are more useful and informative because of their relevance to prevention. Thus, it is important to code an injury as a fall and identify its causes, regardless of the type of fracture that results.

Injuries can be broadly classified according to whether they are intentional, unintentional (or 'accidents'), or undetermined intent. Within the 'intentional' category, injuries may be self-inflicted (i.e., suicide if resulting in death), or inflicted by others (i.e., assault if the victim lives, and homicide if otherwise).

Note that ICD-10 continues to use the term 'accidents' in referring to unintentional injuries. The ICD is uni-dimensional and its codes mutually exclusive. As part of an international collaborative effort on injury surveillance, the Centers for Disease Control published a matrix approach in analysing and reporting injuries by cross-tabulating mechanism against intent. This highlights the importance of mechanism in injury prevention – often modification of consumer products and environments can be effective regardless of intent (see table 18.1).[2]

Table 18.1   An example of injury classification based on mechanism and intent

	Intent or manner				
Mechanism	Unintentional	Self-Inflicted	Assault	Undetermined	Other*
Firearm	W32–34	X72–74	X93–95	Y22–24	Y35.0, 35.1, 36.4
Poisoning	X40–49	X60–69	X85–90	Y10–19	Y35.2, 36.7

*The 'other' column covers legal intervention (Y35), such as being shot by the police or operations of war (Y36).

Extent of the Problem

The importance of injuries can be gauged from the per cent distribution of all deaths. In Canada during 2001–3, injuries accounted for 14 per cent of all deaths in the Yukon, 19 per cent in the Northwest Territories, and 34 per cent in Nunavut, compared with only 6 per cent of all Canadians. A similar excess is also observed in Greenland (21 per cent) when compared with Denmark (6 per cent). In Alaska, 17 per cent of all deaths in the state resulted from injuries (and 22 per cent among Alaska Natives), compared with 7 per cent in the United States nationally. However, in the northern regions of Sweden and Norway, the proportionate mortality due to injuries was similar to the national figures – around 5 per cent. Finland had a slightly higher proportion – 8 per cent nationally and 10 per cent in Lapland.

Figure 18.1 compares the age-standardized mortality rates from all injuries (or external causes) in the circumpolar countries and their northern regions. It is evident that injuries are a particularly serious problem in those regions with a high proportion of indigenous peoples.

In Alaska and Northern Canada, the age-standardized mortality rates (ASMR) for injury were about twice their respective national rates. Greenland's injury ASMR was four times that of Denmark. In northern Fennoscandia, the rates were a little different from the respective national rates. In all jurisdictions, injury mortality was higher among men than women.

Within the North, there is also a substantial difference between indigenous and non-indigenous people. In Alaska, the ASMR for all injuries among Alaska Natives was three times that of the U.S. all-races

Figure 18.1   Age-standardized mortality rate for all injuries in the
circumpolar region

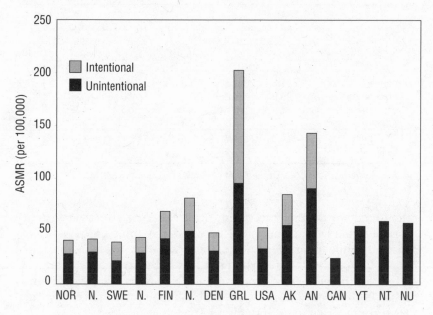

Notes: All rates (per 100,000) are standardized to the European Standard
Population.
N: North
NOR: Norway; North: Nordland, Troms and Finnmark combined
SWE: Sweden; North: Norbotten and Västerbotten combined
FIN: Finland; North: Lapii
DEN: Denmark
GRL: Greenland
USA: United States (all races); AK: Alaska (all races); AN: Alaska Natives in
Alaska
CAN: Canada; YT: Yukon; NT: Northwest Territories; NU: Nunavut
Source: Circumpolar Mortality Database, with data compiled from EURO-
STAT (for national data for Denmark, Sweden, Norway and Finland and
regional data for Norway and Sweden), Statistics Greenland, Statistics
Finland (for Lapland data), Statistics Canada, and the National Center for
Health Statistics (for U.S., Alaska, and Alaska Natives data); all rates are
mean for 2001–3, except Denmark and Greenland, which are based on
1999–2001 data.

Table 18.2   Unintentional injury mortality and hospitalizations in the Northwest
Territories by ethnicity, 1990–9

	Mortality (per 100,000)			Hospitalization (per 100,000)		
	Dene	Inuit	Others	Dene	Inuit	Others
All injury	121.3	162.3	50.6	2,383	2,460	1,031
All unintentional	95.9	99.2	30.1	1,601	1,523	833
Motor vehicle traffic	22.9	19.4	8.4	157	138	96
Other transport	5.3	14.5	2.8	95	136	56
Drowning	19.3	16.9	3.2	–	–	–
Falls	–	–	–	710	523	298

Source: Northwest Territories Department of Health and Social Services (2004b).

rate. In the Northwest Territories during the 1980s, the overall injury
mortality rate was comparable between the Inuit and Dene First
Nations, while their rates were twice as high as non-Aboriginal
people.[3] In the 1990s, while the Inuit had higher mortality overall for
all injuries than the Dene, in some specific injuries, the Dene rate was
higher. Both indigenous groups reported higher rates than non-indigenous people for all injuries (table 18.2).

The burden of injury has changed over time. There has been a
general decline in injury mortality rate in northern Canada since the
1980s, although the gap from the rest of Canada remains substantial
(fig. 18.2). In health planning, a useful index of premature mortality
that gives more weight to deaths among younger people (and hence
more 'valued' by society on the whole) is the 'potential years of life
lost' or PYLL. Conditions that kill mostly younger people, such as
injuries, contribute more to PYLLs than chronic diseases, which affect
primarily older people. From such a perspective, the impact of injuries
is heightened. In the Northwest Territories during the 1990s, injuries
accounted for 23 per cent of all deaths but 43 per cent of all PYLLs.[4]

Not all injuries are fatal. The extent of non-fatal injuries can be
gauged by health interview surveys. In Canada, the Canadian Community Health Survey (CCHS) posed the question: 'In the past 12
months, were you injured seriously enough to limit your normal activities?' Additional questions covered the type of injury (e.g., fracture,
burn), body site (e.g., head, legs), place of occurrence (e.g., home,
street), activity when injured (e.g., sports, work), cause of injury (e.g.,

Figure 18.2 Trend in injury mortality rate: Canada compared with the three northern territories

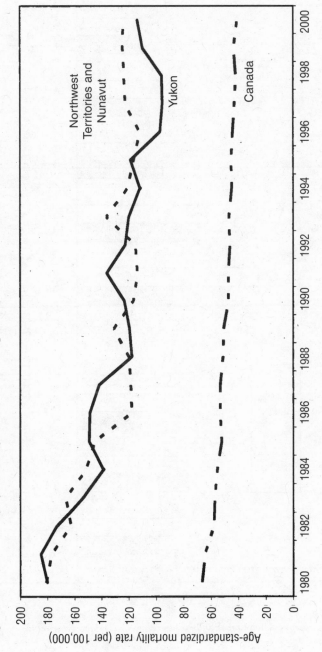

Notes: Age-standardized rates (per 100,000), standardized to the 1991 Canadian population; rates for Yukon and Northwest Territories/Nunavut smoothed by 3-year averaging.

Source: Public Health Agency of Canada. *Injury Surveillance On-Line* (http://dsol-smed.hc-sc.gc.ca/dsol-smed/is-sb/index_e.html).

Figure 18.3 Age- and sex-specific prevalence of serious injury in past year: Aboriginal and non-Aboriginal people in the northern territories of Canada

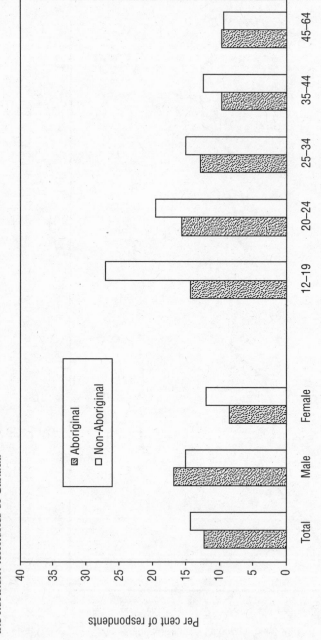

Source: Canadian Community Health Survey, 2000–1 and 2003 combined; based on data in Tjepkema (2005).

Table 18.3 Age-standardized mortality rates for selected injuries in the circumpolar region: Alaska and the Canadian North

Cause of death (ICD-10 codes)	USA	Alaska	Alaska Native	CAN	Yukon	NWT	Nunavut
All injuries (V01-Y89)	53.5	85.2	143.0	39.1	73.3	87.3	144.6
Accidents (V01-X59)	33.7	55.8	90.8	24.9	55.2	59.9	58.2
Transport accidents (V01-V99)	16.2	24.8	38.7	9.6	16.8	14.8	20.5
Accidental falls (W00-W19)	4.4	3.2	2.8	4.6	1.9	9.6	2.6
Accidental drowning/ submersion (W65-74)	1.2	3.5	8.8	0.9	4.1	3.2	11.0
Accidental poisoning (X40-X49)	5.7	11.7	17.7	2.8	8.3	8.0	7.4
Suicide (X60-X84)	10.6	18.9	30.4	11.3	16.4	20.2	81.3
Homicide, assault (X85-Y09)	6.0	6.3	13.3	1.4	1.7	5.1	5.1

Note: Circumpolar Mortality Database, all rates (per 100,000) standardized to Standard European Population.
Sources: Circumpolar Mortality Database, Statistics Canada, and the National Center for Health Statistics (for U.S., Alaska, and Alaska Natives data); all rates are mean for 2001–3.

transportation, assault), and injury-caused activity limitation. The CCHS shows that in the three northern territories, the prevalence of injuries was 12 per cent among Aboriginal people, not significantly different from non-Aboriginal residents (fig. 18.3). It would appear that the risk of sustaining a serious injury (that did not result in death) as reported to a health survey is comparable between Aboriginal and non-Aboriginal people in the North, but the risk of dying from an injury is much higher for Aboriginal people.[5]

Unintentional Injuries

The most important contributions to injuries are accidents, or unintentional injuries. The age-standardized mortality rate for various types of accidents in the circumpolar countries and their northern regions are shown in tables 18.3 and 18.4. Canada, the United States, and the Nordic countries (with the exception of Finland) all have similar rates. The northern regions in the Nordic countries reported only marginally higher rates than the national rates, whereas Greenland was three times Denmark's. In North America, the northern jurisdictions of Alaska, Yukon, Northwest Territories, and Nunavut had similar rates,

Table 18.4   Age-standardized mortality rates for selected injuries in the circumpolar region: Northern Fennoscandia and Greenland

Cause of death (ICD-10 codes)	*NOR*	North	*SWE*	North	*FIN*	North	*DEN*	GRL
All injuries (V01-Y89)	*41.5*	*42.6*	*39.8*	*44.2*	*81.6*	*58.5*	*48.7*	*202.4*
Accidents (V01-X59)	*28.7*	30.3	*22.2*	29.6	*50.2*	31.0	*31.5*	95.6
Transport accidents (V01-V99)	*7.6*	10.6	*6.2*	9.9	*13.2*	10.7	*9.1*	19.4
Accidental falls (W00-W19)	*10.9*	9.5	*3.9*	5.8	*18.7*	6.6	*9.0*	30.0
Accidental poisoning (X40-X49)	*3.9*	2.6	*3*	3.7	*7.5*	5.9	*3.3*	5.8
Suicide (X60-X84)	*11.2*	11.4	*11.9*	9.9	*25.2*	21.8	*12.5*	89.5
Homicide (X85-Y09)	*0.9*	0.8	*1*	0.9	*4.0*	3.6	*1.1*	11.7

Notes: Circumpolar Mortality Database, all rates (per 100,000) standardized to Standard European Population; NOR: Norway; North: Nordland, Troms, and Finnmark combined; SWE: Sweden; North: Norbotten and Västerbotten combined; FIN: Finland; North: Lapii; DEN: Denmark; GRL: Greenland.
Sources: Circumpolar Mortality Database, with data compiled from EUROSTAT (for national data for Denmark, Sweden, Norway and Finland and regional data for Norway and Sweden), Statistics Greenland, Statistics Finland (for Lapland data); all rates are mean for 2001–3, except Denmark and Greenland, which are based on 1999–2001 data.

and ranged from 1.7 to 2.5 times their respective national rates. The rate for Alaska Natives was similar to that of Greenlanders, and was almost three times the U.S. all-races rate (fig. 18.4).

Transport Injuries

Given the importance of transportation in our everyday life, it is not surprising that the means of transportation are an important, and often the most important, cause of injuries. In discussing transport injuries, distinction is made in terms of the type of vehicle involved: train, motor vehicle (e.g., automobiles), trucks, motorcycles, snowmobiles, all-terrain vehicles, other road vehicles (e.g., bicycles), watercraft, or aircraft; and also the type of persons injured: pedestrian, driver, passenger, motorcyclist, or pedal cyclist. Among motor vehicle collisions, a distinction is made between 'traffic' that occurs on public roads and 'non-traffic'that includes off-road recreational or sporting activities. Note that 'motor vehicle collisions' may involve the collision of a motor vehicle with a person, another vehicle, or a stationary object.

Figure 18.4 Age-standardized mortality rate for unintentional injuries in the circumpolar region

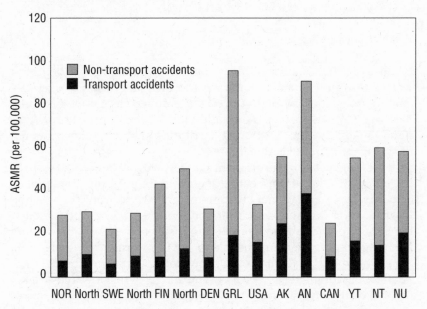

Note: Circumpolar Mortality Database, all rates (per 100,000) standardized to Standard European Population; for abbreviations and sources, see note to fig. 18.1.

Figure 18.4 provides a circumpolar perspective on mortality resulting from transport accidents. Although accident mortality rates are only marginally higher in the northern regions of Scandinavia than the rest of the country, the differential is highest for transport accidents. Greenland, Alaska (all races and Alaska Natives) and northern Canada all have rates that are between 1.5 and 2.5 times higher than their respective national rates.

In the Northwest Territories the death rate from land transport injuries during 1993–2002 was highest in the smaller communities, compared with the regional centres and Yellowknife, the capital city.[6] Table 18.2 shows that the Dene experienced higher motor vehicle traffic injury rate (both mortality and hospitalization) than the Inuit, perhaps due to the fact that Dene communities are generally road-accessible. Inuit communities, however, are far more dependent on off-road vehicles, which may explain their higher mortality (and hospitalization) from 'other transport' injuries.

Water-Related Injuries

Because of the proximity of many northern communities to bodies of water, drowning is an important cause of injury deaths, especially among indigenous peoples. According to data collected by the Canadian Red Cross Society, the drowning rate during the 1990s for Aboriginal people in the Northwest Territories and the Yukon was ten times higher than the national rate.[7]

In the Northwest Territories, during the 1990s, 42 per cent of drowning deaths resulted from boating incidents, 14 per cent from aquatic activities (e.g., recreational swimming), and 22 per cent from falling into the water through ice or from the shore. The Dene rate exceeded the Inuit rate, and both indigenous groups were five to six times more likely than non-indigenous people to die from drowning (table 18.2). Some transport accidents (e.g., snowmobile breaking through ice, automobiles plunging into water, and aircraft crashing into a lake) involve deaths in water, although they are not coded as 'drowning.' Inclusion of such deaths would increase the drowning rate in the Northwest Territories by 10 per cent.[8]

In Alaska, drowning is a particularly serious problem, with the mortality rate among Alaska Natives some seven times higher than the national rate. Among the northern territories of Canada, Nunavut reported the highest rate, which was some twelve times the Canadian national rate (table 18.3).

Intentional Injuries and Violence

The relative importance of intentional versus unintentional injuries in the circumpolar countries can be gauged from figure 18.1. Suicide, or intentional self-harm, is discussed in more detail in chapter 19. For homicide, the northern regions of Fennoscandia generally do not show excessive rates when compared with their respective countries as a whole (table 18.4). The greatest disparity in homicide rates was shown by Lapland, even then it was only 1.7 times the Finnish rate. The highest rates were found among Alaska Natives and Greenlanders. Greenland's homicide rate was eleven times that of Denmark. The rate for Alaska Natives was only twice that of the U.S. all-races rate, which

Table 18.5 Intentional injury mortality and hospitalizations in the Northwest Territories by ethnicity, 1990–9

	Mortality (per 100,000)			Hospitalization (per 100,000)		
	Dene	Inuit	Others	Dene	Inuit	Others
All intentional	24.6	62.9	19.3	611	878	184
Suicide/Self-inflicted	14.1	53.3	16.1	272	523	110
Homicide/Interpersonal	10.6	9.6	3.2	339	355	74

Source: Northwest Territories Department of Health and Social Services (2004b).

was because the United States nationally had high homicide rates, even exceeding those of the northern territories of Canada (table 18.3). Table 18.5 compares intentional injury rates in the Northwest Territories according to ethnicity.

When classified according to mechanism rather than intent, a review of firearm deaths in the Northwest Territories during 1990–8 revealed that the rate was almost four times that of the whole of Canada. The Northwest Territories is tied with the Yukon in having the highest rate of firearm ownership, with 67 per cent of households reporting their presence in the home, compared with the national average of 26 per cent. Firearm deaths in the North are exclusively committed by rifles and not handguns, and in 2001–3, ten out of sixteen firearm deaths were committed with unsecured weapons, that is, they were used by someone other than the registered owner.[9]

To assess the extent of violence in the community, one needs to go beyond the health care sector to the social service and justice systems. After falling for much of the 1990s, the crime rate in the Northwest Territories began rising again towards the end of the decade. However, the increase was largely due to less serious offences, particularly property damage and disturbing the peace. The rate of assaults remained relatively steady during the period 1993–2002. The smaller communities reported the highest crime rate overall and the highest assault rate compared with the regional centres and territorial capital city.[10]

Of increasing importance to the health and well-being of circumpolar peoples is family violence, including child abuse and neglect. Data are generally lacking, especially those with specific reference to the North. Chapter 20 discusses child abuse and neglect in further detail.

Box 18.1 Occupational hazards of reindeer herding

Unlike other indigenous populations, fatal accidents among the reindeer-herding Sami are mostly work-related. Male Swedish Sami reindeer herders are at a significantly increased risk of death from all injuries (1.7 times), vehicle accidents (1.7 times), snowmobile or all-terrain vehicles (7.3 times), and drowning (1.8 times) compared with a demographically matched non-Sami cohort, whereas no such excess is observed among non-herders or among Sami women.[11]

Reindeer herding is associated with many hazardous tasks and environments, especially during the gathering of the reindeer for migration or slaughter. During these periods, the herders use a variety of vehicles (motorcycles, snowmobiles, helicopters, airplanes, and boats) to gather the reindeers, and the work is often executed during long hours in a harsh climate and terrain. It has been shown that most reindeer-herding men spend more than 800 hours per year on the snowmobile.

The everyday use of motor vehicles in the reindeer-herding industry has intensified exposure to static work in seated positions (often in combination with head rotation) and to vibrations and heavy liftings. These working conditions have resulted in a high prevalence of musculoskeletal symptoms and hearing loss among reindeer herders in Finland and Sweden. Increasing mechanization is probably related to increasing pressure from Swedish society to develop profitable reindeer-herding companies, forcing many to make expensive investments in vehicles to save time and personnel costs.

According to self-reported data on the division of working time among reindeer herders in Finland, the slaughtering, gathering, and reindeer separation in late autumn are the most labour-intensive periods. More than half of the annual work-related accidents occur during those periods. Among Swedish reindeer herders, fatal accidents are fairly evenly distributed throughout the year and do not peak during the holiday months as commonly observed in the non-Sami population. More than 90 per cent of the fatalities were observed among the men who are most exposed to the hazardous herding operations.

The high number of work-related accidents among reindeer herders puts reindeer herding at the top of the most hazardous occupations in Sweden. Work-related fatal accidents are two to six times more common among reindeer herders than other workers in the agricultural (including farming, forestry, fishing, hunting, and reindeer herding) and building-construction sectors.

It should be quite possible to reduce the number of both fatal and non-fatal work-related accidents by suitably adjusted preventive measures, for example, education, modified work organization, technical improvement on vehicles, better clothing, and improved communication equipment. Promising attempts to bring down the number of accidents and musculoskeletal pain conditions among reindeer herders have been reported previously. An obstacle for implementation of such measures, however, is the poor financial situation within the reindeer-herding sector, which comes at a time when the need for investments in activities that promote occupational health is very high.

Risk Factors

The causes of injuries can be analysed in terms of the person, agent, and environment. Under 'person' are individual factors relating to personality, inborn characteristics, health and fitness, behaviours and practices, level of knowledge, hazardous exposures, and so on. Under 'agent,' which includes equipment, are the inherent design and mechanical fitness of vehicles, engineering products and other equipment, as well as safety devices installed or available for protection. The 'environment' refers to both the physical (e.g., terrain, season, weather, time of day) and social (e.g., community infrastructure, laws and regulations). Multiple risk factors are usually involved and interact among themselves. There are also direct/indirect and proximate/ remote determinants in the causal pathway of injuries. Some, especially those that operate in the event and post-event phases, determine the extent and severity of the injury once it has occurred.

There are certain determinants that are common to most injuries, such as basic demographic characteristics of age and sex. Figure 18.5 shows the age-specific hospitalization rates of injuries in the Northwest Territories. It can be seen that there are major differences in the pattern for intentional and unintentional injuries. The former affect young adults the most, while with the latter category, the incidence increases with age. Similar patterns are observed elsewhere.

Figure 18.5   Age-specific hospitalization rate for injuries in the Northwest Territories

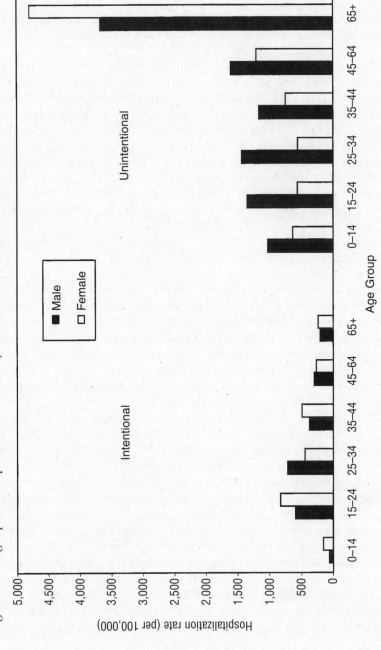

Source: Northwest Territories Health and Social Services (2004b).

Table 18.6   Risk factors for transport injuries

Person	Agent/Equipment	Environment
• Low rate of use of occupant restraints, protective devices • Wearing dark clothing (cyclists/pedestrians) • Walking on roads • Driver fatigue • Driving at high speed • Use of alcohol • Inadequate driving skill (especially ATV)	• Poor mechanical fitness of vehicles, lack of maintenance facilities • Unstable ATVs (especially 3-wheelers)	• Remote location of communities – long road distances, dependent on small aircraft • Poor road conditions; icy in winter; wildlife on country roads; no road/path • Bad weather • Lack of enforcement of traffic regulations, driver licensure

A study in the Northwest Territories found that male sex, increasing age, residence in remote communities, and location above 66° N were independent predictors of injury death on multivariate modelling, whereas ethnicity was not. However, when analysed separately by community remoteness and latitude, Inuit and Dene did have increased risk of 2.3 to 3.4 times in excess of non-Aboriginal residents.[12]

The use of alcohol at the time or shortly prior to the injury is often a factor contributing to the occurrence of the injury, both intentional and unintentional. In a review of data from 1999 to 2003 collected by the Chief Coroner's Office of the Northwest Territories, alcohol was found to be involved in 35 per cent of injury deaths, with men five times being more likely than women to have used alcohol. Overall, alcohol was judged to have been involved in 41 per cent of unintentional injury deaths, 29 per cent of homicides, and 35 per cent of suicides.[13]

While personal factors are clearly important determinants of injury, individual safety practices are also sensitive to socio-economic factors such as household income, education, employment, family structure and size, and community infrastructure. Such social determinants operate in most health conditions, including injuries. Substantial evidence exists to indicate that many northern communities are severely disadvantaged in these regards (see chapter 10).

Table 18.6 lists risk factors that are known to promote the occurrence of motor vehicle and other transport injuries. In the Northwest Territories, the 1999 Labour Force Survey included a safety and injury

Table 18.7   Use of safety devices in transport vehicles in the Northwest Territories:
Per cent of respondents reporting 'always' or 'most of the time'

	Helmet on all-terrain vehicle	Helmet on snowmobile	Lifejacket in boat	Seatbelt in car or truck
Sex				
Male	62	71	76	76
Female	66	65	82	83
Age Group				
15–24	58	72	71	76
25–39	63	69	80	80
40–54	74	70	81	82
55 +	54	43	81	73
Ethnicity				
Dene	27	48	71	71
Inuit	60	26	57	47
Other	85	86	84	86
Community				
Yellowknife	88	90	83	85
Regional centres	72	77	83	85
Small communities	37	42	69	66

Source: Northwest Territories Labour Force Survey, reported in Northwest Territories
Department of Health and Social Services (2004b).

module. In terms of the wearing of helmets in ATVs and snowmobiles,
lifejackets in boats, and seatbelts in cars and trucks, usage is generally
lower in the smaller communities and among indigenous people, particularly for helmets (table 18.7).

An alternative source of information on use of protective devices is
a survey that is based on direct observation of use rather than on
respondent recall. Transport Canada conducts periodic surveys, usually over a one-week period in September, lasting two hours during
daylight hours. The Yukon and Northwest Territories were found to
have the lowest rates of occupants using seat belts (66 per cent and 65
per cent, respectively), far below that of the national average (87 per
cent).[14]

Among non-traffic unintentional injuries, risk factors can also be
categorized as relating primarily to the person, the agent, and/or the
environment (table 18.8).

Table 18.8 Risk factors for non-traffic injuries

Person	Agent/Equipment	Environment
Fires/flame injuries		
• Careless smoking • Use of alcohol • Leaving stove unattended • Lack of supervision of children – playing with matches, lighters • Children and elderly more at risk because of larger body surface	• Unsafe woodstoves and electric heaters • Faulty electrical wiring • Lack of hot water temperature control	• Non-adherence to building codes • Non-use of flame-retardant materials • Absence of fire brigade with functional equipment • Absence of functioning smoke/CO detector, fire extinguisher • Blocked exits
Drowning		
• Lack of supervision of children near/on water • Use of alcohol • Misjudgment of ice thickness in winter	• Lack of personal flotation devices on boats	• Proximity of communities to lakes and rivers • Cold water temperature – hypothermia • Access to emergency response
Falls		
• Advanced age, frailty, poor vision, coordination, mobility, balance • Use of alcohol • Social isolation • Use of medications	• Unsafe furniture, beds, cribs, walkers • Slippery baths for elderly	• Unsafe playground • Unsafe home or streets – inadequate lighting, clutter, and obstacles • Icy walkways in winter • Lack of handrails, support

Social and Economic Impact

In the immediate aftermath of an injury, if it is of sufficient severity but not fatal, the injured person comes into contact with the health care system. Such contacts are likely to be long term and involve not only the acute care sector but also rehabilitation services. Institutionally based trauma registries are usually able to provide clinical information regarding severity, length of stay, and discharge disposition. There is, however, very little published on the health care experience of injury patients in the North. It is likely that many Aboriginal patients requiring prolonged rehabilitation will have to leave their communities and stay for long periods in large urban centres and be faced with considerable social, economic, and cultural challenges in their new environment.

The Canadian Community Health Survey (CCHS) provided some information on the impact of injury. In the northern territories, 59 per cent of Aboriginal people with a serious injury in the past year received treatment within forty-eight hours, not significantly different from the experience of non-Aboriginal people. Aboriginal people, however, were more likely to be admitted overnight to hospital for treatment – 15 per cent in the territories, significantly higher than the experience of non-Aboriginal people (8 per cent). In the territories, there is no significant differences between Aboriginal and non-Aboriginal people regarding the prevalence of injury-caused activity limitation.[15]

Estimating the costs to the health care system of a specific health condition is technically complex, limited by data availability and the need for assumptions and extrapolations. Costs include both direct costs (hospitals, drugs, physicians, other institutions, etc.) and indirect costs (i.e., costs to society in terms of lost productivity due to premature mortality and disability).

Prevention and Control

Haddon, the pioneer in injury prevention, developed a systematic approach consisting of ten strategies that are basic to and theoretically available in all situations. These are still relevant today. As a guide to policy they ensure that consideration is given to all possible control measures, regardless of the extent of current knowledge of causation.[16] These ten strategies are:

1 To prevent the creation of the hazard in the first place.
2 To reduce the amount of hazard brought into being.
3 To prevent the release of the hazard that already exists.
4 To modify the rate or spatial distribution of release of the hazard from its source.
5 To separate, in time or space, the hazard and that which is to be protected.
6 To separate the hazard and that which is to be protected by interposition of a material barrier.
7 To modify relevant basic qualities of the hazard.

8 To make what is to be protected more resistant to damage from the hazard.
9 To begin to counter the damage already done by the environmental hazard.
10 To stabilize, repair, and rehabilitate the object of the damage.

These are only potential strategies. They need to be priorized according to the prevalence of the problem and the effectiveness of the intervention. Generally, emphasis on individual education to change behaviour alone is not adequate ('active' measures); it must also be combined with 'passive' measures relating to product modification, environmental redesign, and legislative action. Taken collectively, injury prevention requires the three E's of Education, Engineering, and Enforcement.

A variety of government and non-governmental organizations in Canada have targeted injury prevention and control as a priority and are engaged in various consultative processes in developing strategies.[17] The Federal/Provincial/Territorial Sub-Committee on Injury Prevention and Control identified three key elements of an injury prevention model:

1 Injury causes – understanding how injury occur.
2 Priority populations – targeting groups that experience a disproportionately high injury burden.
3 Points of intervention – identifying a continuum of points where injuries can be prevented or their impact modified.

The Canadian Collaborating Centres for Injury Prevention and Control, an alliance of national and provincial injury prevention and control organizations, defined injury prevention as 'making positive choices about minimizing risk at all levels of society while maintaining healthy, active and safe communities and lifestyles. These choices are strongly influenced by the social, economic and physical environments where one lives, works, learns and plays.' It also developed an 'Integrated Canadian Injury Prevention Strategy,' consisting of four components:

1 Leadership and public policy development – developing healthy public policy to create supportive environments that enable

people to lead healthy and safe lives through the cooperation of all sectors and levels of government.

2 Knowledge development and translation – collecting information on effective injury interventions and making it available to people who can use it in a form that is most useful to them.

3 Community development and infrastructure – supporting community-based initiatives, involving community stakeholders, and integrating injury programs into community life.

4 Public information – developing a communication strategy aimed at changing public perceptions about the preventability of injury.

Any successful strategy requires the identification and implementation of specific interventions that have been shown to be effective in rigorous research studies and evaluations. Since the 1970s and 1980s various expert groups have taken on the task of preparing critical literature reviews and publishing guidelines for health professionals. Notable examples include the Canadian Task Force on the Periodic Health Examinations and the U.S. Preventive Services Task Force in 1984. Both were directed mainly at personal health services, especially those under the supervision of physicians and/or the primary care system. In 1996 a Task Force on Community Preventive Services, under the leadership of the U.S. Centers for Disease Control and Prevention, was convened to conduct and publish systematic reviews on community-based interventions to prevent disease and promote health. These reviews are posted on the Guide to Community Preventive Services website.[18] Each review provides the following:

- intervention location – e.g., school, day-care centre, city/provincial/national
- intervention strategy – e.g., behaviour modification, environmental change, safety training
- population characteristics – e.g., adolescents, preschool children
- review type – e.g., systematic review, meta-analysis
- methodological quality rating – rating scale from 0–10, based on votes submitted by readers

There are also examples of successful interventions in other circumpolar countries. The experience of the Harstad Injury Prevention Study is summarized in box 18.2.

Box 18.2 Case Study:
Community-Based Injury Prevention Study in Harstad, Norway

An example of community-based intervention directed at reducing traffic injury is the Harstad Injury Prevention Study (HIPS), which was initiated in the northern Norwegian city of Harstad (population 23,000) in 1988.[19] The project utilized multiple interventions, both active (i.e., requiring individual action) and passive measures.

Active
• Dissemination of local injury statistics and narratives in a quarterly newsletter.
• Promotion of traffic safety in local media.
• Counselling to increase parental vigilance in traffic safety for children.
• Speeches to community organizations, clubs, service agencies, and schools.
• Participation in health fairs.

Passive
• Local restrictions on beer sale in grocery stores and curfews for serving alcohol in bars and restaurants.
• Building of separate pedestrian and cyclist roads, lowering of speed limits, installing speed bumps, and road modification in black spots.
• Checks on vehicle for mechanical fitness and speed limit enforcement by police.
• Installation of additional high-mounted stop lights.
• National law making local health authorities responsible for injury prevention.

Of particular interest was the use of injury statistics as a tool of health promotion. HIPS responded to requests for local data from school districts, city planners, and private and public agencies. Based on local injury data, media campaigns were launched to lobby for road improvements. Data were also provided to clubs and schools to promote behavioural change.

Figure 18.6   Comparison of traffic injury rates between Harstad and Trondheim, Norway

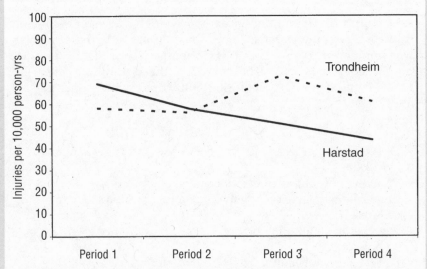

Source: Based on Ytterstad and Wasmuth (1995) and Ytterstad (2003).

To evaluate the effectiveness of the interventions, traffic injury rates over ten years were compared between Harstad and Trondheim, the non-intervention city (population 140,000) in the central part of the country (fig. 18.6). Between periods one and four, traffic injury rates declined 37 per cent in Harstad, compared with only 5 per cent in Trondheim. Sample surveys were also conducted post-intervention among 1,500 adults in each city to evaluate changes in knowledge, attitude, and behaviours. The surveys showed that a higher proportion of Harstad residents reported 'often' and 'quite often' having discussions among friends and family on traffic safety issues. A higher proportion of Harstad residents also reported that traffic injuries were preventable. More than half of Harstad respondents reported having acquired useful information or advice from the traffic injury newsletter, the majority of whom cited it as providing the stimulus for initiating discussions on traffic issues.

NOTES

1 For a definition of injury, see Barss et al. (1998:12), an international text-book on injury epidemiology and prevention. For an overview of Haddon's pioneering work, see his 1980 review paper and the reap-praisal by Runyan (2003).
2 Centers for Disease Control and Prevention (1997).
3 Northwest Territories data from the 1980s are reviewed in Young et al. (1992).
4 Northwest Territories Department of Health and Social Services (NTDHSS) (2004b).
5 The analysis of CCHS injury data was reported by Tjepkema (2005).
6 See Leamon (2005).
7 Health Canada (2001).
8 NTDHSS (2004b).
9 See Kinney (2005).
10 Northwest Territories Department of Health and Social Services (2005).
11 Data on fatal injuries among Swedish Sami reindeer herders are from Hassler, Sjølander, Johansson, et al. (2004) and Hassler, Johansson, et al. (2005). Pekkarinen, Anttonen, and Hassi (1992) provided Finnish data. The musculoskeletal complications are discussed in Daerga, Edin-Liljegren, and Sjölander (2004) and Rehn et al. (2002), and hearing loss in Anttonen, Virkonnas, and Sorri (1994).
12 Cited in Mo (2001), one of the few multivariate studies of a northern health problem.
13 See Santos (2005).
14 Transport Canada (2005). Available online from www.tc.gc.ca/road safety/tp2436/rs200501/menu.htm.
15 See Tjepkema (2005).
16 Haddon's strategies can be found in Runyan (2003). For a review of the role of environmental interventions, see Peek-Asa and Zwerling (2003). Gielen and Sleet (2003) reviewed the application of behaviour-change theories and methods to injury prevention.
17 The various Canadian government documents are cited in Northwest Territories Health and Social Services (2004b:82–4).
18 The guide has reviewed interventions for motor vehicle occupant injuries (e.g., use of child safety seats, safety belts, and reduction of alcohol-impaired driving), and violence (e.g., behavioural, health educa-

tion, and public policy interventions). For further information, visit www.thecommunityguide.org.

19 Further details about the Harstad study can be found in Ytterstad and Wasmuth (1995) and Ytterstad (2003).

19 Mental Health and Suicide

ANNE SILVIKEN AND SIV KVERNMO

Circumpolar peoples are subject to immense mental stress as their communities undergo profound social and cultural changes. Particularly for indigenous peoples, the second half of the twentieth century has been a period when the traditional life irrevocably gave way to Western lifestyles. Among the mental health/psychosocial health problems experienced by indigenous peoples, suicide is clearly the most significant, more so in some populations and regions than in others. This chapter will first discuss general mental health and well-being and then focus on suicide among the Sami and Inuit.

Mental Well-Being

Mental well-being can be evaluated by the presence or absence of common mental symptoms such as gloom, unhappiness, anxiety, and distress, or by asking questions to determine one's mental health status such as is found in the General Health Questionnaire.[1] In addition to straightforward mental symptoms, a number of other symptoms (headache, sleeplessness, fatigue, palpitations) may be indicators of both mental and physical disease. The presence of these symptoms usually does not make its way into statistics of mortality or hospital admissions, and in primary health care, mental symptoms are often disguised or misinterpreted as signs of physical illness. Furthermore, uniform registration of minor mental health problems is difficult and comparisons over time or place probably next to impossible.

A study of adolescents' well-being in Greenland showed that 67 per cent of boys and 90 per cent of girls had at least one of eight symptoms of anxiety and depression, including sleep disturbances, nightmares, feeling gloomy every day, and anxiety attacks. On average the boys reported 2.9 symptoms and the girls 4.6 symptoms. This prevalence was not significantly different from adolescents in Denmark. The mental well-being score was significantly related to suicidal behaviour. Among adult Greenlanders, 19 per cent of Inuit men and 34 per cent of women interviewed for the 1993–4 Health Interview Survey reported having had mental symptoms during the past two weeks. Twenty-three per cent of the population (16 per cent of men and 29 per cent of women) had been gloomy, depressed, or unhappy while 12 per cent (8 per cent of men and 15 per cent of women) had been nervous, distressed, or anxious. Approximately half reported both types of symptoms. That depressive symptoms occur twice as often as anxiety has also been found in a number of studies from other populations. It is especially older women who report mental symptoms; among those sixty years and above, 38 per cent have reported depressive symptoms and 19 per cent have reported anxiety as compared with men who reported 22 per cent and 11 per cent, respectively. Depression and anxiety were associated with several social variables in univariate analyses: not being in the labour force, experience of suicides among relatives or friends, sexual violence, and other types of violence. Alcohol abuse was not related to either type of symptoms.[2]

The North Norwegian Youth Study provides comprehensive information about adolescents' mental health. The study involved 3,200 high school students aged fifteen to twenty-one during the 1990s. The overall prevalence of behavioural/emotional problems was 10 per cent among Sami adolescents, not significantly different from their Norwegian or Kven (a Finnish-speaking minority) counterparts. The prevalence tends to be higher among girls than boys, while those living in marginal Sami areas had higher rates of problems than those living in the Sami core area.[3]

With regard to body attitudes and eating problems, Sami girls were more satisfied with their body than non-Sami girls, reflecting the different norms, values, and ideals about the body in Sami culture. Sami girls also had fewer eating disorders (1.5 per cent bulimic or anorexic) compared with Sami boys (4.8 per cent bulimic, 2.6 per cent anorexic) or Norwegian girls.

Psychiatric Illnesses

The reasons for seeking psychiatric consultations offer some insight into common psychiatric illnesses. The main reasons for psychiatric referral in the eastern Canadian Arctic are depression (28 per cent), suicidal thoughts or attempts (24 per cent), familial relationship problems (15 per cent), and grief reaction (11 per cent). Depression is significantly more common in women than in men while suicidal behaviour is more common in men. In a study from Nunavik, the single most common diagnosis in patients referred for psychiatric consultation was major depression with melancholia. The loss of significant relationships, the presence of great burdens of care due to illness of dependents, and persistent family violence are the main stresses associated with depression in women. In men the most common stressors are lack of meaningful work and the break-up of partnerships. Among Inuit women there appears to be a correlation between depression and marital disconcord, conflict related to the new role of women in the culture at large, alcohol use within the family, and economic difficulties. The women often present with problems related to their difficult life circumstances with issues relating to cultural change, economic deprivation, bereavement, and a variety of physical and sexual abuse.[4]

The classical psychoses, schizophrenia, manic-depressive illness, and organic brain syndromes are encountered in Greenland as frequently as they are in Denmark. The lifelong risk in developing schizophrenia requiring hospitalization is not greatly different, although the first admission to a hospital occurs earlier in Greenland.

Three so-called culture-bound psychiatric syndromes unique to the Arctic have been described. Arctic hysteria (*pibloktoq*), a transitory state of disturbed consciousness, motor disturbances, shouting, screaming, and so on. It has been interpreted as a defence mechanism against external pressure and at the same time a warning to other people that something is wrong. Another phenomenon known in traditional Inuit culture is the mountain wanderer or *qivittoq*. Someone who becomes angry and turns his/her back on society wanders into the wilderness where he/she is believed to become a monster. Qivittut are possibly only known in West Greenland and not in other Inuit communities. Finally, kayak anxiety or kayak dizziness (*nangiarneq*) is a phobic condition. The same expression is also used for the fear of walking on thin ice or the fear of heights.[5]

Suicide in Historical and Cultural Perspective

Since 1950 global suicide rates have continued to rise, and today suicide is an important public health problem all over the world. There are substantial variations in suicide rates among countries and, within the same country, among different ethnic groups and geographical regions. Suicide has become the leading cause of death for young indigenous people, especially among males, and is a significant contributor to potential years of life lost.[6]

In the *International Classification of Diseases* (ICD-10), suicide is classified under intentional injuries (see chapter 18 of this volume). Suicidal behaviour can be considered as a continuum ranging from merely thinking about ending one's life, through developing a plan and obtaining the means to do so, to attempting suicide and, finally, to completed suicide. Suicide can be regarded as a conscious and intended act, which the person does to harm himself/herself and where the harm has resulted in death. Although the intent to die is a central aspect in suicide, such intent is not always obvious in suicidal behaviour. For many suicidal people, the most pronounced intent is to escape intense pain or an unbearable situation. Non-fatal suicidal behaviour, most commonly called suicide attempt or deliberate self-harm, includes any intentional act of self-injury or self-poisoning (overdose), irrespective of the apparent motivation or intention. Suicidal ideation refers to the thought of killing oneself, being tired of life, or believing that life is not worth living.[7]

Although suicide among young indigenous people is often characterized as a modern phenomenon, suicide did exist in the distant past. However, such suicide has been described as 'voluntary death,' which occurred rarely and took place mainly among the elderly and infirm or members of the family and community who were no longer economically productive. Among older Chukchi in Siberia, death by suicide/violence is thought to be preferable to death from disease or old age. Subsequently, they have a particular term for voluntary death in their language, 'single fight.' There is no documented description of suicide in traditional Sami culture in Norway, but it is reasonable to assume that suicide is not unknown.[8]

In traditional Inuit society, suicides were carefully considered acts, and undertaken after extensive consultation with the family. In the 1880s, the noted anthropologist Franz Boas observed among the Central Eskimo that suicide was not rare, 'as according to the religious ideas of the Eskimo the souls of those who die by violence go to Qudlivun, the happy land. For the same reason it is considered lawful for a man to kill his aged parents.' Hanging was the most common method. Working among the Netsilik Eskimo in the 1950s and 1960s, Balikci reported that over the preceding fifty years, suicide occurred on the average of once every year and a half, in a population of around 300 people. Suicide of the 'traditional' sort among the elderly by then accounted for only a small proportion; most cases were committed by younger adults, including a ten-year-old boy. While hanging was still the predominant method, guns were also being used. Misfortune, either personal or affecting a close relative, was cited as the main reason. Balikci attributed the rise of non-traditional suicide to the socio-economic changes already evident then: the splitting up of extended families, migration to trading posts, disruption of preferred marriage patterns and weakening of kinship bonds. The availability of superior firearms also reduced cooperation among hunters and encouraged individual achievements.[9]

The suicide found in traditional indigenous culture can be characterized as social or institutionalized suicide, in contrast to the suicide observed today, which is an individual act and primarily a problem among young people. Suicide rates among elderly indigenous people are actually low compared with the majority populations where suicide risk increases as a function of age.

Suicide Trends and Patterns in Arctic Populations

Norway had relatively low suicide rates compared with its neighbouring Nordic countries, but from the end of the 1960s there has been a general increase in the suicide rates, reaching a peak in 1988 (17 per 100,000). Since then the rates have steadily decreased (to 11 per 100,000 in 2003). There was a marked increase in suicide among young males aged fifteen to twenty-four years from the 1970s to the beginning of 1990s. The northernmost counties of Norway have generally reported higher rates than the rest of the country. For the period 1991–5, the suicide rate for adolescents and young adults aged fifteen to twenty-four years was 21/100,000, compared with the national rate of 15/100,000.[10]

As there is no ethnicity information in the national population register in Norway, there are neither official statistics of health and living conditions nor suicide rates for the Sami. The most compre-

Table 19.1   Standardized mortality ratios (SMR) for suicide by selected characteristics among Sami in northern Norway compared with regional rural population

	Men	Women
Total cohort	1.27	1.27
County of residence		
Finnmark	1.50*	1.55
Troms	0.74	no Sami cases
Nordland	0.42	3.17
Sami density in population		
Sami core area	1.54*	1.31
Coastal area	1.24	1.21
Southern area	0.41	1.51
Reindeer herding		
No	1.30*	1.34
Yes	1.06	0.66
Age		
0–14	no Sami cases	no Sami cases
15–24	1.82*	3.17*
25–34	1.35	1.83
35–44	1.40	1.13
45–54	1.45	0.72
55–64	0.81	1.36
65+	0.29	0.00
Time period		
1970–80	1.17	1.14
1981–90	1.36	1.92
1991–98	1.20	0.81

*95% confidence intervals not enclosing unity indicated in italics.
Note: SMR = observed number of suicides among Sami/expected number of suicides according to a regional reference population.
Source: Silviken, Haldorsen, and Kvernmo (2006).

hensive study on suicide to date tracked a cohort of 19,801 Norwegian Sami between 1970 and 1998. In the national census of 1970, a survey on Sami ancestry was conducted in selected census tracts in the three northern counties, from which the Sami cohort was defined. The Sami population was divided into three groups based on the proportion of Sami in the population of the municipality of residence: (1) southern area, low density (< 25 per cent), (2) coastal area, medium density (25–60 per cent), and (3) Sami core area, high density (>60 per cent).[11]

Figure 19.1   Trend in suicide mortality among Norwegian Sami

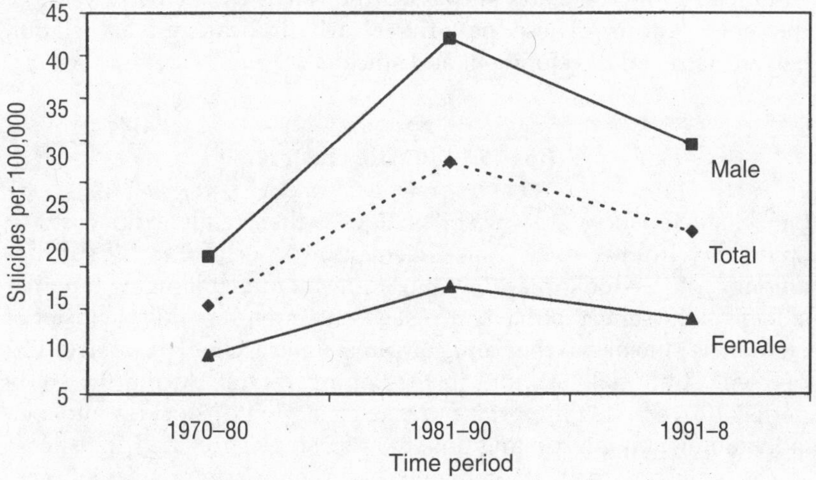

Source: Silviken, Haldorsen, and Kvernmo (2006).

This study showed that the Sami had about 30 per cent higher risk of suicide (both sexes and all ages combined) compared with the northern Norwegian reference population (SMR 1.27, 95 per cent confidence interval 1.02–1.56). As table 19.1 indicates, significantly higher risks were present among those aged fifteen to twenty-four in both sexes, among men living in Finnmark or the Sami core area, and among non-reindeer herders. In the study period, suicide mortality among Sami followed the same time trend as in the non-Sami population and also the national rates. In the time period 1981–90, there was an increase in suicide mortality among both Sami males and females (fig. 19.1). This peak corresponds with the clusters of suicide in the Sami core area.

Elsewhere in the Arctic, among Alaska Natives, Greenlanders, and Canadian Inuit, the increase in suicide rates did not occur at the same time (fig. 19.2). It happened first among Alaska Natives, later in Greenland, and still later in the Nunavik and Baffin regions in the eastern Canadian Arctic, with each later 'epidemic' more severe than the preceding one. In Greenland, a distinct regional pattern in the epidemic curve of suicides shows that suicide mortality rates first increased in the capital Nuuk, with a peak in the 1980s. In other central towns, suicide mortality peaked in the 1990s, while in the villages, suicide continued to increase and surpassed the towns by the early years of the new century. These patterns clearly indicate an association between societal development and suicide.

Box 19.1 Suicide clusters

One characteristic of adolescent suicides is their tendency to occur in epidemics. In one study from Greenland, 60 per cent of all suicides among youths took place within four months following another suicide in the same district. During a twelve-month period, a cluster of eight male suicides in the Sami core area alone accounted for about 27 per cent of all male suicides in the Sami core area during the study period 1970–98. It is important to take clustering of suicides into consideration when interpreting time trends using aggregated statistics.[12]

The Sami core area has generally had a high rate of suicide, especially towards the end of the 1980s. During the summer of 1987, five young males committed suicide in a small village of less than 3,000 inhabitants. They all lived in the same village and some of them were even close friends. These suicides were a great trauma and loss for the families and the whole community. The local health services responded to the tragedy by establishing prevention strategies. Unfortunately, the suicide cluster received extensive exposure in the local and national media. As a result, the village became well-known all over Norway and was labelled a 'suicide-village,' reinforcing the stereotype of the 'suicidal Sami.'

The outbreak of suicides was probably triggered by mechanisms other than ethnicity per se; for example, by imitation and contagion. Due to the small population size of Sami communities and the interconnectedness of the inhabitants, any suicide might serve as a role model for others and influence those who are already vulnerable. After the suicide cluster this village continued to experience relatively high suicide rates, averaging about two suicides annually. As a result, there are many bereaved families in this community.

Firearms and hanging tend to be the method of choice for suicide among indigenous people in the Arctic. In Greenland, firearms and hanging accounted for 91 per cent of cases among males and 70 per

Figure 19.2   Trend in suicide mortality among Alaska Natives, Greenlanders, and Canadian Inuit

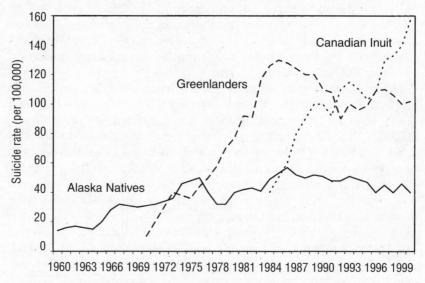

Note: Canadian Inuit refer to Inuit in Baffin Island and Nunavik.
Source: Unpublished data by J. Hicks and P. Bjerregaard.

cent among females. Among Sami males, firearms accounted for 41 per cent and hanging for 37 per cent of suicides. In northern Norway, and Norway in general, there is widespread ownership of firearms for hunting, both as a traditional pursuit and as a form of modern recreation. In northern Canada, despite the widespread ownership of firearms, firearms are used much less frequently in suicides than is hanging. About half of the suicides among Sami females were by hanging, a higher proportion than observed nationally. From a prevention perspective, unlike the use of firearms, little can be done to reduce the frequency of hanging by limiting access to the implements used.[13]

Suicidal Attempts and Thoughts

Suicide mortality represents only the tip of the iceberg. For every successful suicide, there are many more suicide attempts, and for every suicide attempt there are numerous people harbouring suicidal thoughts. Suicide attempts may or may not result in any contact with the health and social service systems, making their true magnitude difficult to estimate. Suicidal thoughts are probably seldom presented to the health care practitioners. Furthermore, there appears in many instances not to be a sharp distinction between overt suicidal behaviour and other self-destructive behaviour like excessive risk-taking or abuse of alcohol and drugs in which the likelihood of dying is high. Many accidental deaths might be the result of a concealed wish to die.

In the Greenland Health Interview Survey, 13 per cent of Greenlandic men and 19 per cent of the women reported having seriously considered committing suicide. The percentage decreased with age from 27 per cent in the eighteen to twenty-four year range to 3 per cent in those 60 and above, but the preponderance of women is found in all age groups. There is a close association between suicidal thoughts and the reporting of mental problems and symptoms. Of those who reported ever having been treated for mental health problems, 39 per cent reported suicidal thoughts compared with only 13 per cent in the rest of the population. However, the majority of those who have had suicidal thoughts have never been treated for mental health problems and do not report current problems. There is an association between relf-reported alcohol misuse and suicidal thoughts but not as pronounced as between mental health problems and suicidal thoughts.

In the Kivalliq region in northern Canada, 20 per cent of adult Inuit answered 'yes' to ever having planned or attempted to commit suicide, with a considerably higher percentage of women among those below the age of forty-five. In Nunavik, 12 per cent of Inuit reported having had serious suicidal thoughts and 14 per cent reported suicide attempts. In Kivalliq the percentage of persons with suicidal behaviour ranged from 13 per cent to 23 per cent in individual communities, but it was not possible to characterize the communities according to acculturation or traditionality.[14]

In northern Norway, there were no ethnic differences in the prevalence of self-reported suicide attempts between Sami adolescents and their majority peers.

Age and Gender Perspectives

Gender and age are two of the most important demographic markers of those at risk of suicide. Worldwide, suicide is more prevalent among males, while suicide attempts in general are more prevalent among females than males, a phenomenon sometimes described as the 'gender paradox' by suicidologists. Among Sami during the period 1970–98 the male/female ratio of completed suicides was 3.7:1. However, Sami adolescent girls (14 per cent) were twice as likely to report a suicide attempt as boys (7 per cent). In a study among adolescents in Greenland, the male/female patterns were similar but the percentages were much higher: 20 per cent of boys and 52 per cent of girls had suicidal ideations, 11 per cent of boys and 33 per cent of girls had attempted suicide. The male/female ratio for completed suicide was 2.2 to 1. However, there are exceptions, for example, among the Inuit in Nunavik, where young males were not only much more likely to complete suicide but also attempted it more frequently. The high rates of suicidal behaviour found among young indigenous males fit with the perception that there has been greater disruption of traditional roles for men, resulting in profound problems of identity and self-esteem. Another hypothesis is that males more often than females are brought up first with too few, but later with too many, demands. Such an upbringing may contribute to an individual having difficulties handling competition on equal terms, conflict, and rejection. Considering the fact that intrapersonal conflicts and the break-up of romantic relationships are two of the primary precipitating events in adolescence, young males can become even more vulnerable to suicidal behaviour.[15]

Suicidal behaviour among indigenous people is primarily a problem among young people. In Greenland the suicide rates in general are high (100 per 100,000), however, the rates among young males aged fifteen to twenty-four years are even higher (450–500 per 100,000). A similar pattern was found among the Sami, with the highest suicide rates among the fifteen to twenty-four years olds, 53 per 100,000 person years for males and 16 for females, respectively. Although the suicide rates are especially high among young indigenous males, the rates found among young indigenous females are also high compared with their majority counterparts. Also the prevalence of suicide attempts among indigenous females have been reported to be high, for example, 33 per cent among Inuit females in Greenland. Consistent with these findings is the fact that Sami females aged fifteen to twenty-four years also had a significant increase in suicide mortality and a higher prevalence of suicide attempts than their majority counterparts (14 per cent versus 10 per cent, respectively). In contrast to the national Norwegian population's suicide rates, which indicate minor differ-

Figure 19.3   Age-sex specific suicide rates among Norwegian Sami

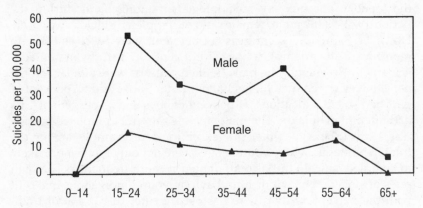

Source: Silviken, Haldorsen, and Kvernmo (2006).

ences between age groups among adults, the age specific rates among
Sami indicate a more variable pattern, especially among males. This
pattern is more consistent with findings among other indigenous populations where suicide rates peak at age fifteen to twenty-four and
then decrease with age.[16] (See fig. 19.3.)

Risk Factors for Suicidal Behaviour

Suicide is a complex phenomenon described as a 'multidimensional
malaise' that is influenced by biological, psychological, and sociocultural factors. Risk of suicidal behaviour depends on a variety of
factors: (1) social and family factors; (2) individual and personality
factors; (3) mental health factors; (4) precipitating circumstances and
stressful life event factors; and (5) environmental and contextual
factors. Affective disorders, disruptive disorders, previous suicide
attempts, and substance abuse are well established suicide risk predictors in adolescence. Similar risk factors also operate among indigenous
peoples. Among Canadian Inuit, risk factors include poverty, childhood separation and loss, accessibility to firearms, alcohol abuse and
dependence, a history of personal or familial health problems, and
past sexual or physical abuse. The increased risk of suicidal behaviour
among indigenous peoples can to some extent be explained by the

high prevalence of risk factors, such as substance use, mental health problems, sexual abuse and family violence. It appears that the high rates of suicidal behaviour among indigenous peoples may be an expression of the accumulation of risk factors across a variety of domains, rather than a single all-important determining factor.[17]

A number of factors have been shown to be associated with suicidal behaviour among adolescents in Greenland. The presence of depressive symptoms were significant for both boys and girls and can probably be viewed as a mediator between social risk factors and suicidal behaviour. In a multivariate analysis, loneliness, termination of a relationship, and suicide of a close friend were independent risk factors for suicidal behaviour among boys, while having experienced a sexual assault, loneliness, problems with parents, and suicide of a close fried were independent risk factors for girls.

Among Sami adolescents in Norway, alcohol intoxication, single-parent homes, and paternal overprotection are associated with suicidal attempts. These risk factors can be considered as diverging from traditional Sami cultural norms. Since the mid-nineteenth century, the strongly anti-alcohol Laestadian movement (discussed in chapters 9 and 12) has had a strong influence in the Sami areas of northern Scandinavia. Alcohol intoxication is a culturally more divergent behaviour among Sami adolescents than among their majority peers. Furthermore, traditional Sami families consist of an extended family that often includes parents, children, and other close relatives like grandparents. In a Sami cultural context, single parent homes are culturally divergent. As a result, single-parent homes may represent a stronger risk factor among Sami adolescents than they do in the Norwegian culture. Sami childrearing practices place strong emphasis on individual autonomy and a parenting style characterized by high permissiveness, low control, and personal warmth. Paternal overprotection thus contrasts with the common childrearing norms in Sami culture, and may therefore increase the risk for conflicts, especially during adolescence. However, it is important to emphasize that individual risk factors do not exert their effect in isolation. The risk of developing suicidal behaviour depends on accumulative exposure to a series of social, family, personality, and mental health factors.[18]

Within a few decades, the suicide rates among several indigenous peoples have increased rapidly (fig. 19.2). Few indigenous communities have been unaffected by the process of rapid social changes brought about by colonization and modernization. In this process of change, many indigenous peoples lost their roots, their beliefs, and their value systems very quickly, and this led to a loss of self-worth, diseases of self-neglect, and suicide. At the level of the community and family life, the rapid social changes led to instability that had severe consequences such as dysfunctional homes (e.g. due to increased alcohol consumption and domestic violence), high rates of crime, delinquency, and imprisonment. The most vulnerable within the changing social and family structures were the children, who belonged to the first generation that had been raised in communities and families affected by normative instability.[19]

The socio-economic status and living conditions among the Sami in Norway are quite different from the situation found in other indigenous populations, while the gap in living conditions between the Sami and their majority population in northern Norway has narrowed considerably. The process of cultural revitalization has resulted in the Sami enjoying a much greater extent of cultural equality and less socio-economic disadvantage compared with other indigenous peoples, which is also reflected in their health status. This explains the large difference in suicide rates between Sami and other circumpolar indigenous communities.

Impact of Acculturation

As described in chapter 9, since the 1970s, a process of integration and increased ethnic revival has gradually replaced a history of forced assimilation and colonization among Norwegian Sami. However, the outcome of the acculturation and the ethnic revitalization processes has varied in the different regions they inhabit. The assimilation process has had the greatest impact on the coastal communities where the Sami became a minority and many lost their Sami identity and their language. In this area, prejudice and ethnic conflicts about land rights and teaching in the Sami language are still present, and there is little structural and practical support for the Sami culture. In the highland communities, however, where the majority of the population is Sami and Sami-speaking, there are several established Sami institutions like the Sami parliament, research and broadcasting centres, and education in the indigenous language is possible up to college level. There is also a well-organized, highly professional indigenous-oriented health and social service network run by Sami medical doctors, social workers, nurses, and so on.[20]

The increased risk of suicide found among Sami males in the Sami core area is thus unexpected. According to the North Norwegian Youth Study from the mid-1990s, Sami adolescents in the Sami core area had the strongest ethnic identity and separation attitudes, but at the same time they also favoured integration more than peers in the other areas. The study also revealed that ethnocultural factors did not have an impact on the mental health of young Sami males in this context at this time. A cluster of suicides in young males in this area had taken place a decade before the study and at the beginning of a strong cultural revival period among an older cohort who possibly did not benefit from the positive sociocultural development in their area. Crossing and mismatching expectations from both the indigenous Sami and the dominant Norwegian societies may possibly have created stress and psychological maladjustment for vulnerable young indigenous males without the necessary bicultural competence and coping strategies. These cultural factors can accumulate other risk factors that are well-known for suicidal behaviour, such as alcohol misuse, depression, and loss of significant others.[21]

Protective Factors against Suicide

Even though suicidal behaviour is a serious problem among many indigenous peoples, the majority of them are not suicidal. Among the Sami in Norway, reindeer-herding households had almost no increased suicide mortality among males and there was a lower risk among Sami females (see table 19.1). In the core region of Sami communities, semi-nomadic reindeer herding is one of the traditional occupations. Although reindeer herding has undergone radical changes during the last decades due, in part, to increased motorization and socio-economic pressures, it is still an important way of living and a significant symbol of Sami culture. This finding is consistent with a study from Sweden, which showed no significant increased risk of suicide among reindeer-herding Sami males. Sami in Norway who are involved in reindeer herding have high status within their culture and have a strong ethnic identity. However, this pattern may change with future pressures and changes in the reindeer-herding occupation and culture.[22]

Suicide Intervention Programs

Suicidal behaviour is a multidimensional phenomenon which can make it both complicated and challenging in creating effective interventions to reduce its occurrence. Different prevention strategies have been implemented, such as appropriate help for suicide attempters, treatment of depression, reduction of substance use, increased problem-solving strategies, and legislation controlling firearms availability. Unfortunately, it is difficult to demonstrate if these strategies have had a significant effect in reducing suicidal behaviours or achieving long-term sustainable results. A past history of suicide attempts represents the strongest known risk factor for future suicide attempts and completions. Hence, an important suicide-prevention strategy is to give appropriate help to individuals who are suicidal, especially after an attempt, and to identify those experiencing suicidal ideation. Only a minority of those attempting suicide go to health facilities for medical attention. Unfortunately, the majority of suicide attempts remain unnoticed and those who come into contact with public health services represent only the tip of the iceberg. There are many plausible factors affecting help-seeking behaviour, such as age, method of attempted suicide, seriousness of an attempt, culture, and accessibility to health care. For some indigenous peoples, access to health care is probably an important factor in this respect, due to long distances and lack of appropriate health services. There is a general tendency for indigenous peoples to refuse to seek help from official mental health services. Adolescents in general prefer to seek help from informal sources, such as friends and parents, rather than from formal agencies. Official mental health services thus have a special responsibility to make their services more accessible and attractive to indigenous youth.[23] After the suicide cluster in the Sami core area in the mid-1980s, the Sami Psychiatric Youth Team was initiated by the local health services to prevent suicidal behaviour and substance use/abuse among adolescents and young adults (see box 19.2).

Focusing on resilience and protective factors may prove to be more effective than individually oriented prevention in the health care system. In a Sami context, good school performance and regular attendance at church, integration of traditional culture, and degree of self-government have been mentioned as examples. Greenland adolescents have advocated better social conditions during childhood and adolescence, more attentive parents, and less alcohol abuse.

Box 19.2 The Sami Psychiatric Youth Team

The Sami Psychiatric Youth Team was started in 1990 with its main office in Karasjok, in northern Norway. The team's catchment's area includes the five largest Sami municipalities located in the inland area of Finnmark county. These municipalities are all within the jurisdiction of the *Sami Language Act of Norway*. The team serves adolescents and young adults aged fifteen to thirty years, and its main tasks are the prevention and treatment of suicidal behaviour problems and substance abuse. The team emphasizes a cultural sensitivity approach and its multidisciplinary staff includes psychologists, social workers, and a medical doctor, who have either indigenous ancestry or Sami-language competency, or who have acquired a formal education in the Sami culture. The adolescent clients have easy access to the treatment facilities and can admit themselves for treatment, so that it is not the sole responsibility of school nurses and social workers. The adolescents are able to receive treatment in their local communities, and there is an extensive use of short message services (SMS), both for arranging appointments and as part of clinical intervention. One-fifth of the clients have admitted themselves for treatment. Extensive use of SMS has increased the team's ability to communicate with Sami adolescents. SMS has been especially useful in cases of intervention with adolescents who report self-harm, suicidal thoughts, and suicide attempts. There has also been a decline in the dropout rates because of SMS.

Two other important aspects in suicide prevention are to increase the awareness of warning signs of suicidality and to develop appropriate ways of responding to people in distress. Unfortunately, an important barrier in reaching adolescents may be the failure of parents and teachers – the traditional gatekeepers to child and adolescent mental health care – to recognize adolescent suicidality. Increased competence among gatekeepers to recognize suicidality is required to overcome this barrier. Since 1998, the Sami Psychiatric Youth Team has been offering the Applied Suicide Intervention Skills Training course (ASIST), developed by LivingWorks Education (www.livingworks.net). The aim of ASIST workshops is to help gatekeepers become more comfortable, confident, and competent in their contact with suicidal youth in order to prevent the immediate risk of suicide.

In designing programs to prevent youth suicide, it is important to recognize the different perspectives on the causes of suicide and to understand that the potential solutions offered by adults may differ to those offered by youths. In a survey of adult and youths in twelve villages in north-west Alaska, for example, adults identified boredom as the main reason for suicide and solutions as programs that offer young people activities, education, and a sense of culture. In contrast, youths attributed suicide to stress and emphasized the need for meaningful everyday communication and interaction.[24]

The Sami Psychiatric Youth Team presents a model of a suicide prevention strategy among adolescents and young adults in the Sami core area. However, it is important that the focus on the prevention of suicidal behaviour includes the entire community and not only those individuals who are at risk. Furthermore, suicide prevention among the Sami in general requires data derived from specific target communities, so that local trends and population characteristics can be identified and appropriate strategies devised from both the Norwegian and Sami society. Although Norway was among the first nations in the world to propose a national suicide prevention plan in 1994, there exists no specific plan for prevention of suicidal behaviour for the Sami people. An important next step appears to be a specific suicide prevention plan in the Sami areas that would implement effective interventions.

NOTES

1   The General Health Questionnaire (GHQ) was originally developed by Goldberg as a screening tool for psychiatric illness and used in many countries. It focuses on changes in normal function during the past two weeks rather than lifelong traits. An abbreviated twelve-question version was developed in Greenland and translated into Greenlandic.

2   Data from the 1993–4 Greenland survey were originally reported in Bjerregaard and Young (1998:163–4). A similar survey was conducted among Greenlandic migrants in Denmark in 1997–8 (Bjerregaard, Curtis, and the Greenland Population Study 2002). Details on the adolescents survey in Greenland are available in Danish in Curtis, Larsen, et al. (2006).

3 The North Norwegian Youth Study was analysed in more detail in Kvernmo (2004).

4 Utilization of psychiatric services by Canadian Inuit was reported by L.T. Young et al. (1991), and Abbey et al. (1991).

5 For a full discussion of mental illness in Greenland, see the comprehensive monograph by Lynge (1997).

6 See for example Leineweber et al. (2001), Borowsky et al. (1999), Thorslund (1991), and Bjerregaard and Lynge (2006) for information about suicide rates among indigenous peoples residing in the Arctic.

7 For definitions of the term suicide attempt see Wagner, Wong, and Jobes (2002).

8 For information about suicide in a historical perspective see T.K. Young (1994), Lester (2006), and Bogoras (1975).

9 Descriptions of traditional Inuit suicide can be found in Leighton and Hughes (1955), Boas (1964:207), and Balikci (1970:163).

10 For data on suicide rates in Norway see Retterstøl, Ekeberg, and Mehlum (2002), Mehlum, Hytten, and Gjertsen (1999), Gjertsen (1995), and the website of the National Register on Causes of Death, Statistics Norway at www.ssb.no.

11 Details of this study are reported by Silviken, Haldorsen, and Kvernmo (2006).

12 For information about suicide cluster see, for example, Kirmayer (1994); Bechtold (1988), Hunter and Harvey (2002); Gould et al. (1990); Stevenson et al. (1998); Thorslund (1991); Wissow et al. (2001); and Silviken, Haldorsen, and Kvernmo (2006).

13 For information about suicide methods among indigenous people see, for example, Hunter and Harvey (2002), Bjerregaard and Lynge (2006), and Boothroyd et al. (2001). Information on suicide methods in Norway are available from the website of the National Register on Causes of Death, Statistics Norway, www.ssb.no, and from Mehlum, Hytten, and Gjertsen (1999).

14 Suicidal behaviour in Kivalliq was reported by O'Neil et al. (1994) and in Nunavik by Boyer et al. (1994).

15 For information and discussion about gender differences among Inuit see Curtis, Larsen, et al. (2006); Kirmayer, Boothroyd, and Hodgins (1998); Kirmayer, Malus, and Boothroyd (1996); Grove and Lynge (1979); Kirmayer, Brass, and Tait (2000); Bjerregaard and Lynge (2006); Lynge (1994); and Javo, Rønning, and Heyerdahl (2004) for data on Sami.

16 Age distribution and age-specific rates of suicidal behaviour are available

in Bjerregaard and Lynge (2006); Blum et al. (1992); Curtis et al. (2006); Silviken and Kvernmo (2007); Gjertsen (2002); and Diekstra (1993).

17 For general information and discussion about risk factors associated with suicidal behaviour, see Brent (1995); Lewinsohn, Rohde, and Seeley (1996); Fergusson, Woodward, and Horwood (2000); Grøholt et al. (2000), Wichstrøm (2000); Marttunen, Aro, and Lönnqvist (1992); and Grøholt et al. (1997). For studies on risk factors for suicidal behaviour among indigenous peoples, see Kirmayer, Brass, and Tait (2000).

18 A recent study by Silviken and Kvernmo (2007) reported on suicide attempts among adolescents from the North Norwegian Youth Study. Javo, Rønning, and Heyerdahl (2004) compared childrearing practices.

19 For more information about the consequence of colonization and modernization among indigenous peoples, see Hunter and Harvey (2002), Bjerregaard and Lynge (2006), and Ferry (2000).

20 Hovland (1996) conducted an anthropological field research on the diverse premises and development of ethnic identity among Sami youth residing in two different Sami societies in northern Norway.

21 See Berry (1985), and Kvernmo and Heyerdahl (2003, 2004) for discussion on the impact of sociocultural conditions and acculturation.

22 For studies reporting protective factors against suicidal behaviour among indigenous peoples, see Kirmayer, Brass, and Tait (2000), Lester (1999), and Chandler and Lalonde (1998). See chapter 9 in this volume for more information about the study by Hassler, Sjölander, et al. (2004).

23 For information about suicide prevention and help-seeking behaviour and suicide prevention, see Krug et al. (2002), Grøholt et al. (1997), and Thompson et al. (2006).

24 Wexler and Goodwin (2006) conducted a five-item, open-ended survey of 382 participants.

20 Maternal and Child Health

JON ØYVIND ODLAND AND LAURA ARBOUR

Circumpolar maternal and child health is a very complex issue. Life conditions and socio-economic status vary considerably between countries, regions, and population groups. A good example is the area along the Norwegian-Russian border, where socio-economic differences have been among the highest in the world between neighbouring nations. Two important international programs have discussed life conditions for pregnant women and children in detail since the 1990s: the Arctic Monitoring and Assessment Programme (AMAP) under the Arctic Council, and the Analysis of Arctic Children and Youth Health Indicators project (AACYHI), an initiative of the Arctic Council's Sustainable Development Working Group. In this chapter, issues important for the health of mothers and children of the Arctic will be reviewed, complementing and updating data available from these two programs.[1]

Health determinants and health outcomes among mothers and children are discussed according to the different stages of the life course: pregnancy, infancy, childhood, and adolescence. While data are not uniformly available in a consistent manner across all regions, much can still be used in formulating guidelines for improving this group's health.

The Child and Childbearing Population

Relatively large numbers of children and youth in a society increase the need for services, including housing, education, health care, and employment. As table 1.2 shows, the youthfulness of the population varies across the circumpolar region. The highest proportion of the

Table 20.1   Distribution of children and youth, and women of childbearing age among circumpolar populations

Country/ Northern regions	Children and youth (% of total pop.)				Women (% of total pop.)
	0–4	5–9	10–14	15–19	15–44
United States[a]	7.0	6.8	7.2	6.8	21.0
State of Alaska	7.7	8.0	8.4	8.4	21.1
Canada[b]	5.7	6.6	6.8	6.8	22.0
Yukon	5.9	7.0	8.1	8.0	24.2
Northwest Territories	8.0	9.6	9.4	7.9	24.5
Nunavut	12.5	12.5	12.1	9.4	23.1
Denmark[c]	6.0	6.3	6.5	5.8	19.4
Greenland[d]	7.7	8.1	9.0	8.0	22.1
Faroe Islands[e]	7.3	7.5	7.9	8.0	18.4
Iceland[c]	7.0	7.2	7.6	7.4	21.2
Norway[c]	6.2	6.6	6.8	6.4	20.0
Finnmark	6.1	7.0	7.3	6.6	19.8
Troms	6.0	6.7	7.1	6.6	19.9
Nordland	5.6	6.6	7.1	6.8	18.7
Sweden[c]	5.5	5.2	6.6	6.6	19.2
Norrbotten	4.8	4.9	6.5	6.9	17.2
Västerbotten	5.1	4.9	6.7	6.9	19.3
Finland[c]	5.4	5.6	6.3	6.1	18.8
Lappi	4.8	5.3	6.5	6.8	17.2
Russian Federation[f]	4.4	4.8	7.2	8.8	23.3
Murmansk Oblast	4.5	4.6	7.1	9.5	24.1
Kareliya Republic	4.4	4.5	7.3	8.9	23.7
Arkhangelsk Oblast	4.6	4.7	7.5	9.1	23.1
[Nenets AO]	6.6	6.8	9.7	8.9	23.4
Komi Republic	4.9	5.1	7.7	9.4	24.9
Yamal-Nenets AO	6.3	6.9	9.5	8.2	27.1
Khanty-Mansi AO	5.8	6.0	8.8	8.9	27.3
Taymyr AO	6.5	6.9	9.9	8.8	25.7
Evenky AO	6.9	7.3	10.1	8.5	23.5
Sakha Republic	6.9	7.6	9.8	9.8	24.9
Magadan Oblast	4.9	4.8	7.4	8.4	24.2
Koryak AO	6.2	6.7	9.4	7.9	22.5
Chukchi AO	6.0	6.3	8.8	9.0	23.3

[a]U.S. age distribution data are from the 2005 *American Community Survey* (U.S. Census Bureau http://factfinder.census.gov).
[b]Canadian age distribution data are from the 2001 Census (Statistics Canada www12.statcan.ca/English/census01/home/index.cfm).
[c]Age distribution data for the Nordic countries are derived from national population registries as of 1 January 2006 for Norway (http://statbank.ssb.no) and Denmark

Table 20.1   (*continued*)

(www.statbank.dk) and 31 December 2005 for Sweden (www.ssd.scb.se), Finland (www.stat.fi), and Iceland (www.statice.is) obtained from the interactive websites of the respective national statistical agencies.

dGreenland data are from Statistics Greenland (www.statgreen.gl); age distribution as of 1 January 2006.

eFaroe Islands data are obtained from Hagstova Føroya, the statistical agency of the territory (www.hagstova.fo); age distribution as of 1 January 2006.

fRussia: age distribution for the country and regions are based on the 2002 Census from the Federal State Statistics Service (www.gks.ru).

under-fifteen population are found in Nunavut and the Northwest Territories in Canada, Greenland, and Alaska, all regions with a high proportion of indigenous peoples in the population. In contrast, the percentages of population under fifteen among the northern regions of Norway, Sweden, and Finland are very similar to their national populations.

The youthfulness of a population depends mainly on the number of women in the age range of fifteen to forty-four years (the most common ages at which women bear children) and their fertility rate. Infant mortality rates have declined greatly during the twentieth century and now have little impact on the population age structure. Population pyramids for various regions have been presented in chapters 2 to 6. Table 20.1 compares the relative sizes of various child and adolescent age groups and women in their childbearing years.

Pregnancy

In some traditional cultures (such as the Inuit), early marriage and childbearing have been the norm. In modern Westernized societies, a lower average maternal age is generally linked to higher rates of teen pregnancies and may indicate high juvenile sexual activity and a lack of understanding about or availability of contraception. Pregnant teens have a higher prevalence of tobacco, alcohol, and other substance use and often delay prenatal care. Teen mothers have increased risks of pre-eclampsia, anemia, urinary tract infection, and postpartum hemorrhage, and their infants have higher risks of low birth weight, preterm birth, certain birth defects, and infant mortality. Despite the fact that indigenous populations generally provide extended family support for teen mothers, early pregnancy places the mothers at risk of

Figure 20.1   Age-specific fertility rates of selected circumpolar populations

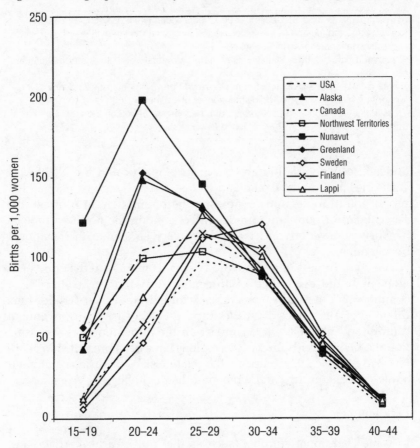

Note: Figures refer to number of live births per 1,000 women in the age group, mean of 2000–4.

Sources: Canadian data are from Statistics Canada (CANSIM Table 102-4503); U.S. data are from the National Center for Health Statistics' VitalStats interactive website (www.cdc.gov/nchs/datawh/vitalstats.htm); Swedish data are from Statistics Sweden (www.ssd.scb.se); Finnish data are from Statistics Finland (www.stat.fi).

not completing secondary or post-secondary education. Male partners of teen mothers tend to be unsuccessful in school and have limited earnings and high rates of substance use. Infants of teen mothers are at risk of physical abuse and neglect; as children they are more likely to drop out of school and become teen mothers or fathers themselves.[2] This indicator is essential for assessing the needs for contraception education and social support for young mothers, and for evaluating the impact of existing programs.

The predominantly Inuit region of Nunavut has the lowest mean maternal age of 25 compared with 29–30 years for the rest of Canada and in Scandinavian countries, yet has the highest proportion of teenage mothers (table 20.2). The age-specific fertility rate of selected circumpolar regions is shown in figure 20.1. It can be seen that Nunavut has the highest birth rate in the 15–19 and 20–24 age groups, about five times that of the Scandinavian countries. However, the situation is reversed at age 30–34, with Denmark and Sweden having the highest rate. Greenland and Alaska also have high fertility in the younger age groups.

Prenatal care is a major predictor of adverse pregnancy outcomes, including low birth weight, stillbirth, and infant mortality. Prenatal care comprises three main activities: screening for health and psychosocial factors likely to increase the possibility of specific adverse outcomes; providing therapeutic interventions known to be beneficial; and educating pregnant women on how to plan for a safe birth and how to deal with emergencies during pregnancy. A study of ten European countries concluded that access to prenatal care was associated with lower perinatal mortality rates. The effectiveness of prenatal care in reducing low birth weight, pre-eclampsia/eclampsia, severe postpartum anemia, and urinary tract infection depends on the efficacy and uptake of interventions and not simply the number of prenatal visits. By enrolling in prenatal care, pregnant women increase their access to preventive programs aimed at improving maternal diets (including the intake of iron, folate, and calcium supplements) and reducing maternal exposure to alcohol, tobacco, and other substances that harm the fetus. Also, participants in prenatal care are more likely to access postnatal preventive health services for themselves and their family. The proportion of women failing to receive adequate prenatal care is an important indicator of society's commitment to providing the most basic preventive services aimed at improving pregnancy outcomes and a healthy start in life for newborn infants. Prenatal care per se is unlikely to account entirely for improved pregnancy outcomes as women in higher educational and socio-economic categories tend to access such care earlier and more frequently.[3]

At least 90 per cent of mothers in Greenland and northern Scandinavia received complete prenatal care. In Alaska, 80 per cent of pregnant women began their prenatal care in the first trimester, whereas only 70 per cent of Alaska Native women did. The prenatal care received was rated inadequate in 29 per cent of Native women's pregnancies, compared with a state average of 17 per cent.[4]

Maternal prenatal smoking causes fetal death, intrauterine growth restriction, preterm birth, and cardiac and possibly other birth defects. Prenatal maternal smoking and postnatal infant exposure to environmental tobacco smoke is a major cause of sudden infant death syndrome and an important cause of asthma. Data from the U.S. Pregnancy Risk Assessment Monitoring System (PRAMS) showed that the prevalence of prenatal smoking tended to be high among young women and those in low socio-economic status.[5]

For alcohol, PRAMS data indicated that it was older women and those with higher income and education who had the highest use rates. Prenatal alcohol use is toxic to the developing fetus and infant and is a major cause of birth defects and developmental disabilities. No safe level of prenatal alcohol consumption has been identified. Severe outcomes include early fetal death (spontaneous abortion) and structural, growth, and functional abnormalities variably categorized as fetal alcohol syndrome (FAS), fetal alcohol effects (FAE), and alcohol-related neurodevelopmental disorder (ARND). Given the difficulty of obtaining accurate data on the incidence of FAS/FAE/ARND, there is an urgent need to monitor prenatal maternal alcohol consumption. This, too, will involve challenges, especially the need to measure alcohol use accurately during early pregnancy when a woman may not be aware of her condition or if she under-reports her consumption.

The prevalence of smoking and alcohol use during pregnancy and their differential impact on infant mortality among Alaska Native and non-Native women is shown in table 20.3. About 40 per cent of Alaska Native women smoke during pregnancy, compared with 16 per cent of non-Native women in the state. In Scandinavia, Sweden reported the lowest rate of 10 per cent, while Norway's was twice that. The smoking prevalence tends to decline towards the end of the pregnancy (to 7 per cent in Sweden and 15 per cent in Norway). Within Norway, rates for the northern counties is generally some 4 per cent higher than the national rate.[6]

In addition to tobacco and alcohol, prenatal maternal volatile substance abuse has been linked to prenatal growth restriction, cognitive, speech and motor deficits, and craniofacial abnormalities similar to those of fetal alcohol syndrome.[7]

Preterm births are an important cause of neonatal deaths. Because preterm infants have immature body systems, they face increased risks of respiratory complications, infections, cerebral palsy and other neurodevelopmental deficits, and visual and other problems that can cause long-term disability. The risk of serious neurobehavioural effects is inversely related to gestational age and is particularly high for very preterm/very low birth weight infants. Risk factors for preterm birth include maternal factors (smoking, alcohol, other substance abuse, medical illness, age thirty-five or older), infant characteristics (multiple birth pregnancy, birth defects, stillbirth, female gender), obstetric history (inadequate prenatal care, no previous pregnancy, previous preterm birth, cervical surgery, therapeutic abortion, short interpregnancy interval), environmental factors (environmental tobacco smoke) and socio-demographic variables (race, socio-economic status, marital status).[8]

The preterm birth rate varied considerably among the circumpolar nations (table 20.2) with Iceland and the Faroe Island having the lowest rate (4–5 per cent) and Alaska Natives and Nunavut (12 per cent) having the highest rates. Women in Greenland, northern Scandinavia, Russia, and the Yukon and Northwest Territories in Canada had intermediate preterm birth rates (6–8 per cent). Within Russia, the rates varied among the various northern regions, ranging from a low of 3 per cent in the Taymyr autonomous *okrug* to 9 per cent in Chukotka.

Many Arctic indigenous populations lack access to early ultrasound examinations. In the absence of uniform estimations of gestational age, preterm birth rates may not be strictly comparable among circumpolar countries. In addition, accurate gestational age data are essential for differentiating preterm births from intrauterine growth retardation. Given that preterm birth is the major cause of perinatal and infant mortality, circumpolar nations should continue to monitor and improve gestational age data. As a first step, it would be useful to estimate the current prevalence of access to prenatal ultrasound in circumpolar countries and their Arctic subpopulations. Such data would facilitate sound interpretation of preterm birth rate data.

Low birthweight (LBW), defined as birthweight lower than 2,500 grams, comprises two distinct subgroups: preterm infants with normal birth weight for their gestational age and infants with intrauterine

Table 20.2   Selected maternal and child health indicators among circumpolar populations

Country/ Northern regions	Mean maternal age (yrs)	% mothers aged 15–19	% pre-term delivery[a]	% LBW births[b]	Perinatal mortality rate[c]
United States[d]	*27.3*	*10.7*	*12.1*	*7.8*	*6.9*
State of Alaska	–	10.8	10.3	5.8	4.9
Alaska Natives	–	17.7	11.0	6.0	5.5
Canada[e]	*29.0*	*4.7*	*7.6*	*5.7*	*6.3*
Yukon	28.3	8.0	7.2	4.7	8.5
Northwest Territories	27.4	11.4	8.3	5.0	8.7
Nunavut	24.7	22.2	11.6	7.5	9.5
Denmark[f]	*29.9*	*1.4*	*6.9*	*5.7*	*6.9*
Greenland[g]	27.0	12.6	8.3	6.0	15.5
Faroe Islands[h]	28.8	3.7	3.5	–	3.6
Iceland[i]	*29.2*	*4.5*	*4.7*	*3.9*	*4.0*
Norway[j]	*29.4*	*2.4*	*7.1*	*5.0*	*5.3*
Finnmark	29.1	4.1	6.7	4.6	4.1
Troms	29.2	3.4	6.9	4.5	4.4
Nordland	28.8	4.3	7.1	5.0	6.2
Sweden[k]	*29.9*	*1.2*	*6.3*	*4.3*	*5.2*
Norrbotten	29.5	1.5	–	–	5.6
Västerbotten	29.6	1.0	–	–	6.3
Finland[l]	*29.9*	*3.0*	*5.3*	*4.4*	*5.4*
Lappi	29.4	4.4	4.8	4.5	5.9
Russian Federation[m]	*26.3*	*12.2*	*5.6*	*6.4*	*11.9*

[a]Pre-term delivery refers to births under 37 weeks of gestation.
[b]Low birthweight (LBW) is defined as birthweight under 2,500 grams.
[c]Perinatal mortality rates refer to the sum of stillbirths and infant deaths under 7 days per 1,000 total births.
[d]United States perinatal mortality data are from National Center for Health Statistics (NCHS) *National Vital Statistics Reports* for relevant years (U.S. 2000–3); LBW, pre-term, and maternal age data are mean of 2000–4 from NCHS's VitalStats website (www.cdc.gov/nchs/datawh/vitalstats.htm). Perinatal mortality data for Alaska and Alaska Natives (2000–3) are by special request from NCHS.
[e]Canadian data are mean of 2000–4, from Statistics Canada: perinatal mortality data from CANSIM Table 102-0508; maternal age data from CANSIM Table 102-4503; pre-term data from CANSIM Table 102-4512; and LBW data from CANSIM Table 102-4509.
[f]Denmark perinatal mortality data are mean of 2002–3, from NOMESCO (2006); LBW and maternal age data (mean of 2000–4) are from Statistics Denmark's StatBank website (www.statbank.dk); pre-term delivery data (mean of 2000–4) are from the Medical Birth Registry of the National Board of Health (Sundhedsstyrelsen [various years]).
[g]Greenland perinatal mortality and pre-term delivery data (mean of 2000–4) are from the annual reports of the Chief Medical Officer (Embedslægeinstitutionen i Grønland

Table 20.2   (*continued*)

[various years]); maternal age and birthweight data are from Statistics Greenland's annual reports.

[h]Faroe Islands data (mean of 2000–4) are from the annual reports of the Chief Medical Officer (Landslaegan på Færøerne [various years]).

[i]Iceland data (mean of 2000–4) on perinatal mortality, maternal age, and birthweight are from Statistics Iceland's interactive website; prematurity data are from Gissler and Vuori (2005).

[j]Norway data (mean of 2000–4) are from the Medical Births Registry of the National Institute of Public Health (www.mfr.no).

[k]Sweden data (mean of 2000–4) are from the Medical Births Registry, National Board of Health and Welfare (Socialstyrelsen [various years]).

[l]Finland data (mean of 2000–4) are from the annual reports of the Medical Births Registry maintained by STAKES, the National Research and Development Centre for Welfare and Health (STAKES [various years]), and special requests from STAKES.

[m]Russian maternal age and perinatal mortality data are from *Demographic Yearbook* (Federal State Statistics Service, 2006a), pre-term delivery data from *Main Indices of Mother and Child Health ...* (2004), and LBW data from *Public Health in Russia 2005* (Federal State Statistics Service 2006c).

growth retardation. Many of the health risks associated with preterm births also apply to LBW. Higher LBW rates among subpopulations reflect disparities in socio-economic status, access to prenatal care, and the prevalence of risk factors that include maternal smoking, inadequate diet, and alcohol consumption.

As table 20.2 shows, the lowest proportion of LBW births was reported in Iceland (<4 per cent), while Nunavut (8 per cent) had the highest. Note that the national all-race LBW rate in the United States was also quite high – however, there was a substantial difference between LBW for blacks and whites, with the former having almost twice the rate of the latter. A study from the province of Quebec in Canada showed that Inuit women had higher risks of preterm birth but their risks of LBW were comparable to women from French or English background. The First Nations or North American Indian population, in contrast, have a problem with high birthweights, possibly attributable to a higher prevalence of maternal gestational glucose intolerance.[9] It is important to differentiate intrauterine growth restriction from preterm births since these outcomes require different preventive health strategies. Because health risks are increased for infants with a low or high birthweight for gestational age, circumpolar nations should monitor birthweight distributions in addition to low birthweight rates.

Figure 20.2   Infant mortality rates in selected circumpolar populations

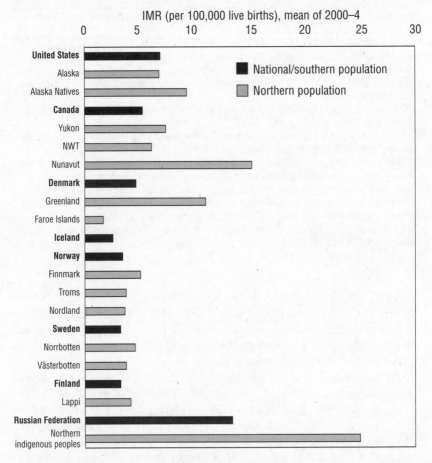

Sources: U.S. data are from National Center for Health Statistics *National Vital Statistics Reports* (various years) and Alaska Bureau of Vital Statistics *Annual Reports* (various years); Canadian data are from Statistics Canada (CANSIM Table 102-0507); Nordic countries (national) data are from EUROSTAT; regional data are from Statistics Sweden, Statistics Norway and Statistics Finland; Faroe Islands data are from Hagstova Føroya; Greenland data are from Statistics Greenland; Russian data are from Federal State Statistics Service; rates for northern indigenous people are calculated from *Economic and Social Indicators* (Federal State Statistics Service 2005).

Another overall measure of pregnancy outcomes is the perinatal mortality rate, which combines stillbirths and early neonatal deaths (under seven days of life). Such a measure is sensitive to the care of the mother during pregnancy and delivery and also to the mother's care of the newborn. As shown in table 20.2, Greenland and northern Canada have the highest rates.

Infancy

Mortality during the first year of life is a sensitive indicator not only of child health but also of the overall health status of a population. It can be divided into two periods: neonatal (first twenty-eight days of life) and post-neonatal (from the twenty-ninth day up to the completion of the first year of life). High infant mortality rates reflect disparities in access to adequate food, shelter, education, sanitation, and preventive and therapeutic health care services. The two leading causes of neonatal deaths are preterm births and birth defects. Leading causes of post-neonatal mortality in economically advantaged countries include sudden infant death syndrome (SIDS), birth defects, infections (especially respiratory, central nervous system, and gastrointestinal infections), and injuries.[10]

Infant mortality rates have varied from less than five in the Nordic countries to over ten in Nunavut and Greenland, and as high as twenty-five among indigenous peoples of Arctic Russia. There is little difference between the northern regions of the Nordic countries and the rest of the country (fig. 20.2).

Box 20.1 Birth Defects among Inuit in northern Canada

Birth defects are an important cause of perinatal and infant mortality. Their impact is particularly significant in communities far from tertiary care centres, such as the Canadian Arctic. In the Nunavik region of northern Quebec in the 1990s, with an infant mortality rates five times that of the rest of the province, about two-thirds of the neonatal deaths were due to birth defects. In Nunavik and Nunavut, a chart review of more than 2,500 Inuit births during 1989–94 was carried out and compared with the Canadian province of Alberta, where a well-established surveillance system exists. This baseline study confirms that the birth prevalence of defects of all types was two times higher among Inuit. For specific defects, the prevalence was 4.2 times higher for congenital heart defects, 4.5 times higher for central nervous system malformations, and 5.5 times for malformations of the gastrointestinal tract.[11]

The causes for excess risk among the Inuit are unclear, but likely involve both nutritional and genetic factors. Since the 1990s, studies have shown that many congenital malformations – such as spina bifida and certain defects of the heart, limbs, and urinary tract – can be prevented by taking supplemental vitamins containing folic acid. Studies have also investigated the role of genetic variants in folate metabolism and the occurrence of spina bifida. Public health efforts are now in place in many jurisdictions to encourage women in the childbearing years to take multivitamins containing 400 µg of folic acid. Since 1998, all enriched flour, rice, pasta, cornmeal, and other grain products have been fortified with folic acid. For low-intake populations such as northern Aboriginal peoples, such measures may still not be sufficient. Folate-rich foods include vegetables and fruits such as broccoli, spinach, and oranges that are sold at exorbitant prices, when they are available, in the North. Even with fortification, Inuit women of childbearing years in Baffin Island were found to consume only 209–263 µg of folic acid per day, well below the recommended intake.[12]

Vitamin A is a nutrient that is important in embryonic development, including the heart septum, and its chronic excess or deficiency has been shown to be associated with congenital heart defects. Low intake of this vitamin has also been demonstrated in the Canadian Inuit.[13]

Research is underway in the Canadian North to assess the impact of folate fortification on dietary intake of folate and folate levels in red blood cells among women of childbearing age and the rates of birth defects in the population. What are also needed are the development of a sustainable and efficient surveillance system and heightened public health efforts directed at dietary interventions.

The control of infectious diseases through the provision of safe drinking water and immunization has contributed much to the dramatic decrease in post-neonatal mortality rates (PNMR). In the Nordic countries, Canada, and the United States, PNMR comprised about 30 per cent of infant deaths in the first half of the year 2000. The proportion was much higher for Alaska Natives and the northern territories

Table 20.3   Comparison of Alaska Natives and non-Native: Proportion of all births and infant mortality rate by selected maternal characteristics, 1992–2001

Characteristics	% of all births		Infant mortality rate (per 1,000 live births)		
	Native	non-Native	Native	non-Native	Ratio
Mother's education					
< grade 12	26.5	10.4	14.3	9.2	1.6
grade 12	55.8	38.2	10.2	6.4	1.6
> grade 12	17.7	51.4	7.4	4.6	1.6
Mother's age					
<20	17.2	9.3	12.2	9.8	1.2
20–24	30.2	26.2	10.8	6.8	1.6
25–34	42.6	50.6	11.3	4.7	2.4
>34	10.0	13.8	12.3	6.8	1.8
Prenatal alcohol/tobacco use					
Yes	40.1	16.3	15.9	10.2	1.6
No	59.9	83.7	8.4	5.2	1.6

Source: Alaska Department of Health and Social Services (2006d).

of Canada, about 50–60 per cent. In northern Quebec, Inuit and First Nations infants had higher rates of SIDS, infectious disease, and post-neonatal mortality than non-Aboriginal infants. Since the implementation of intensive public education programs aimed at young parents instructing them on the safest sleeping positions for their infants, the previously high incidence of SIDS among Alaska Native infants appears to have begun to decrease. Further data gathering will be required to confirm this, but the trend has been observed in many countries in response to this simple intervention.[14]

In Alaska, the disparities between Native and non-Native exist in almost all health indicators. According to the Alaska Maternal-Infant Mortality Review (table 20.3), Native births had poorer outcomes in terms of infant mortality rates. They were also associated with a higher prevalence of risk factors such as low maternal education, young maternal age, and prenatal use of alcohol and tobacco.

Breastfeeding protects the infant from gastrointestinal, respiratory, and middle-ear infections; it appears to enhance cognitive development and to reduce the risk of postpartum bleeding. In addition, prolonged breastfeeding may reduce the risk of pre-menopausal breast

Figure 20.3   Prevalence of breastfeeding in selected northern populations

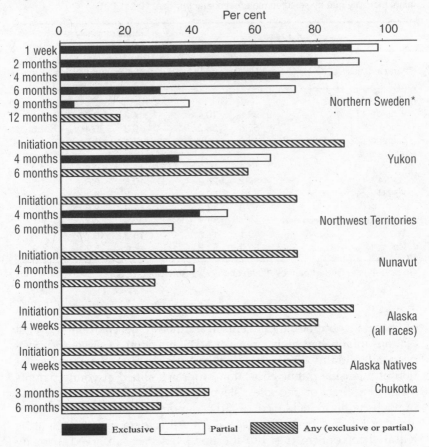

*Northern Sweden: combined data for Västerbotten and Norrbotten
Sources: Canadian data from the 2003 Canadian Community Health Survey
(Statistics Canada CANSIM Table 105-0244); Alaskan data from PRAMS
(Perham-Hester et al. 2005); Swedish data from *Amning av barn fodda 2004*
(Socialstyrelsen 2006); Chukotka data from *Public Health in Russia 2005*
(Federal State Statistics Service 2006c).

cancer. The World Health Organization (WHO) stated that exclusive
breastfeeding should, ideally, be continued until the age of six months.
Breastfeeding rates tend to be higher among women who are older

and have higher socio-economic status. Breastfeeding rates in Scandinavia are very high, and there are little differences between the northern regions and the national average. The example of northern Sweden is shown in figure 20.3. In Canada, the proportion of women who did not breastfeed at all was 15 per cent nationally and 27 per cent in the Northwest Territories and Nunavut. The proportion of northern women who initiated and continued breastfeeding for six months was lower than nationally, although they are comparable in terms of the duration of exclusive breastfeeding.[15]

The immunization status of a population reflects a community's commitment to preventive public health efforts. Low or declining immunization rates increase the risk of infectious disease outbreaks and may reflect changes in policies and program priorities or capacities. This is an essential indicator for assessing the availability and use of an extremely important preventive health service.

Most countries had over 90 per cent coverage for diphtheria, pertussis, tetanus, polio, measles, mumps, rubella, polio, and *Haemophilus influenzae* type B. Immunization rates for children in Arctic Canada were 10–15 per cent lower than national rates. In the United States, 90 per cent of all children and 85 per cent of Alaskan Native children were vaccinated against hepatitis B. Note that immunization schedules varied by country with regard to the type of vaccines included and the target age groups.

Vaccines contributed substantially to reduced infant and childhood infectious disease incidence and death rates during the last century and new vaccines continue this trend. Chapter 15 reviews the tremendous progress that has been undertaken in reducing (and, in some cases, almost eliminating) several serious infectious diseases affecting infants and very young children in the Arctic.

Childhood

With the control of many infectious diseases, chronic diseases are becoming increasingly important health problems for children as they are among adults. Age-standardized cancer incidence rates for children, youth, and young adults show that Greenland had the highest cancer incidence rate whereas northern Canada and Finland had the lowest rates.

Cancer mortality rates for persons age from birth to twenty-four years were obtained from the World Health Organization Cancer Mortality Database. Cancer mortality rates for males and females in this category were relatively high in the Russian Federation (7.9 and 6.3 deaths per 100,000 population per year, respectively) and substantially lower in other populations examined (about two to five deaths per 100,000 population per year). In all countries and regions, cancer mortality rates were higher in males than females (this is true for most populations globally). It should be noted that cancer mortality rates reflect both the risk of developing cancer and survival rates among affected persons. Cancer survival rates in this age range have improved dramatically in countries with high access to modern cancer therapies. Thus, high cancer mortality rates may reflect high incidence rates and/or poor survival rates because of inadequate treatment.

The two types of diabetes, type-1 and type-2, affect Arctic populations differently. Nordic countries are at high risk and Finland has the world's highest incidence of childhood type-1 diabetes. The rate continues to increase. However, within Finland, the highest risk areas are located in central Finland, while Lapland is at relatively low risk. As for type-2 diabetes, it is an increasingly serious problem among the indigenous peoples of North America (see chapter 16). Among the First Nations population in southern Canada, an increasingly lower age of onset in childhood and adolescence has been observed. However, this trend has not been observed in the Arctic.[16]

Childhood is also a vulnerable period for emotional, physical or sexual abuse, and emotional or physical neglect, resulting in immediate or delayed biophysical and psychosocial adverse effects. Child physical abuse is a significant cause of hospitalization, disability, and death. The battered child is a rejected child likely to experience long-term difficulty in mental and emotional development. Children exposed to family and domestic violence also experience problems in emotional development and are at risk of becoming abusers as adults. Child abuse is associated with parental youth/immaturity, poor marital adjustment, mental illness, cultural losses, sexual aberrations, and close birth intervals. There is a strong public health case for monitoring and tracking these relatively common and preventable early life hazards.

The World Health Organization defined child abuse and neglect as all forms of physical or emotional ill-treatment, sexual abuse, neglect or negligent treatment or commercial or other exploitation resulting in actual or potential harm to the child's health, survival, development or dignity in the context of a relationship of responsibility, trust, or power. Greenland reported the highest prevalence of child abuse, but

Table 20.4 Selected health risk behaviours among Alaskan high school students

	Alaska 2003	United States 2001
Safety		
Rarely/never used bicycle helmet	73.9	84.7
Rarely/never used seat belts	19.1	14.1
Drove while drunk	11.3	13.3
Carried weapons		
M	29.8	29.3
F	6.3	6.2
Smoking		
Ever smoker	56.1	63.9
Current (once or more past month)	19.2	28.5
Frequent (20+ past month)	8.0	13.8
Alcohol use		
Ever (at least 1 drink)	75.1	78.2
Current (once or more past month)	38.7	47.1
Binge (5+ drinks within 2 hrs, past month)	26.5	29.9
Other drugs (ever used)		
Marijuana	47.5	42.4
Cocaine	6.6	9.4
Inhalants	10.2	14.7
Steroids	3.5	5.0
Injection drugs	1.7	2.3
Crystal meth	5.9	9.8
Heroin	1.8	3.1
Ecstasy	6.2	–

Source: Alaska Youth Risk Behavior Survey 2003 (Green et al. 2004). Comparative national data are from the CDC, as provided in the Alaska report.

given that the definition of child abuse varies between jurisdictions, meaningful comparisons between countries are not possible. Infant abuse in Alaska, severe enough to result in hospitalization or death, was associated with either parent having less than twelve years of education, the mother being unmarried and maternal prenatal substance abuse.[17]

Adolescence and Youth

Many health risk behaviours – smoking, alcohol and drug use – that have a long-lasting impact on adult health are initiated during adolescence. Comprehensive and comparable data for the circumpolar regions are lacking. Table 20.4 presents some key findings from the 2003 Alaska Youth Risk Behaviour Survey, a school-based survey of Alaskan children in Grades 9 to 12 that shows how they compare with Americans nationally.

Overall, most smokers become addicted as teenagers. Although most countries have conducted surveys of tobacco use, knowledge about smoking behaviour in youth is limited and tobacco use remains the most significant preventable health problem of youth and adults. Modern manufactured tobacco products are strongly addictive and promoted by commercial interests. In Canada in 2005, 12 per cent of teens aged 12–19 were current smokers (either daily or occasional smokers). The prevalence was higher in the North – 15 per cent in the Yukon (13 per cent male, 18 per cent female), 18 per cent in Northwest Territories (20 per cent male, 15 per cent female), and 43 per cent in Nunavut (35 per cent male, 51 per cent female). The Nunavut prevalence is higher than anywhere else in the circumpolar North.[18]

Alcohol consumption, solvent abuse, and illicit drug use have direct adverse effects on the developing nervous system of young children, and they can cause accidental death and markedly lower levels of academic performance and behavioural problems. Affected children and youth may be unable to reach their full potential. Illicit drug use can lead to addiction and to crime to support the drug habit. Given the preventability of these serious health consequences of substance abuse, there is a strong public health case for monitoring this indicator to assess the need for and effectiveness of intervention programs. Alcohol abuse is one component of a cluster of youth risk behaviours that also includes other substance abuse and risky sexual behaviours.[19]

Among males fifteen years of age, the prevalence of consuming alcohol at least weekly was about 50 per cent in Denmark, 25–35 per cent in Canada, Greenland and the Russian Federation, and 18–24 per cent in the U.S.A., Alaska, Norway, Sweden, and Finland. The prevalence among females followed a similar pattern by country/region but was substantially lower than males, except in Alaska, Denmark, Norway, and Finland. No distinction was made as to the type of alcohol used.

Solvent use includes sniffing of gasoline, glue, and aerosol propellants. The prevalence of solvent use was about 20 per cent in Alaska and among Alaska Natives; 10–15 per cent in Arctic Canada, Greenland, and Finland; and 6–8 per cent in Iceland and Norway. Prenatal maternal or childhood solvent abuse can disrupt normal childhood nervous system development, and acute high-dose exposures can cause death.

A review of data from the U.S. Toxic Exposure Surveillance System of the American Association of Poison Control Systems found that volatile substance abuse declined by 37 per cent during the period 1996–2001. Among children six to nineteen years of age, 20 per cent of cases had moderate to serious effects including death. Solvent abuse may be associated with anti-social behaviour, including minor criminal activity. Among Alaska Native children in isolated villages, the prevalence of lifetime inhalant use was 48 per cent; heavy use was associated with the male gender and onset at an early age.[20]

The prevalence of reported illicit drug use was 25–35 per cent among youth in the U.S. (national, Alaska, and Alaska Natives), Arctic Canada and Greenland; 15–24 per cent in Canada (national), Norway, and Arctic Finland; and 10–12 per cent in Iceland and Finland (national). Illicit drug use can lead to addiction and criminal behaviour to support the drug habit.

In terms of causes of mortality, adolescents and youths are particularly vulnerable to injuries, both intentional (suicide and assaults) and unintentional (accidents). Suicide has been described as the ultimate expression of alienation. For those who attempt suicide and fail, the result can be permanent mental or physical disability as well as continuing emotional stress. All methods of suicide carry grave dangers for survivors, including brain damage, spinal cord injury, nerve damage, and major organ failure. Childhood and youth suicides are unnecessary deaths and reflect cultural dislocation and inadequacies in socio-economic conditions, social support systems, and preventive and therapeutic health services. High rates imply a need for intervention programs that include education, improved recognition and treatment of depression, and counselling and support services. The tragic personal, family, and social consequences of suicide and its preventability speak to the importance of monitoring this indicator for targeting and evaluating intervention programs.

Suicide rates were much higher among Alaskan and Canadian Arctic indigenous people and in Greenland compared with their national populations. In contrast, suicide rates in northern Sweden were much lower, although rates among men were higher than their national counterparts. Suicide rates were consistently higher for males compared with females. (See chapter 19 for further discussion on suicide.)

Unintentional injuries are a leading cause of child and adolescent hospitalization, deaths, and disability. Those surviving potentially fatal unintentional injuries may suffer permanent physical and mental disability. Injury death rates reflect the net impact of preventive (e.g., regulatory, educational, and other measures aimed at improving consumer product and environmental safety) and intervention programs (e.g., timely access to emergency and medical care services). High unintentional injury rates among some subpopulations may indicate disparities in income, housing, and education. The tragic personal, family, and social consequences of unintentional injuries and their preventability speak to the importance of monitoring this indicator.

Total unintentional injury death rates were much higher among Alaskan and Canadian Arctic indigenous persons from birth to twenty-four years compared with their national counterparts. Similarly, unintentional injury death rates in Greenland were higher than those in Denmark but appeared to fluctuate, probably because of the small numbers. In the three populations for which unintentional injury death rates were available for infants less than one year old (Canada, Greenland, and Sweden), the rates were higher in Arctic regions and in indigenous subpopulations compared with their national populations.

Within the age range studied, most unintentional injury deaths occurred among those fifteen to twenty-four years of age. Risk-taking behaviours tend to be more prevalent among persons in this age range, and among males in particular. In Arctic regions, other contributory factors likely include extreme climate, type of vehicular transportation (e.g., snowmobiles and all-terrain vehicles), reduced access to health care (for timely treatment of life-threatening injuries), and risk-taking behaviours such as substance abuse. Unintentional injury death rates were consistently higher among males compared with females. (See chapter 18 for further discussion of injuries.)

As chapter 15 has discussed, sexually transmitted diseases are particularly rampant in Greenland, Alaska, and northern Canada. The Alaska Youth Risk Behaviour Survey showed that by the time they reached their final year of high school, 65 per cent of boys and 55 per cent of girls had already experienced sexual intercourse, a minority of whom were engaged in sexual activity with multiple partners (see fig. 20.4). Only 66 per cent of boys and 58 per cent of girls used condoms the last time they had intercourse. In northern Canada, among the

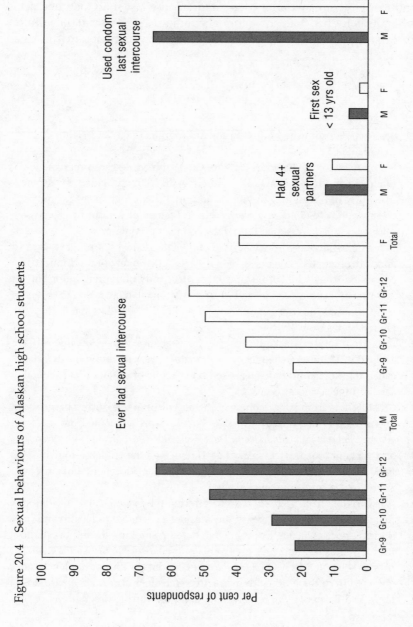

Figure 20.4 Sexual behaviours of Alaskan high school students

Source: Alaska Youth Risk Behaviors Survey 2003 (Green et al. 2004).

fifteen to twenty-four year olds, 60 per cent of men and 73 per cent of women had sexual intercourse at least once, and 72 per cent of men and 69 per cent of women used condoms the last time they had sex, which was higher than the national average. Clearly, sexual health is an important component of health promotion activities in this age group.[21]

NOTES

1 See Arctic Monitoring and Assessment Program (2003) and Health Canada (2005).

2 For a review of the health risks associated with adolescent pregnancy, see Elfenbein and Felice (2003). Westenberg et al. (2002) provided a comparative study of Aboriginal and non-Aboriginal teen pregnancies in Australia. Archibald (2004) interviewed Inuit women of various ages across northern Canada to solicit their views on teen pregnancy.

3 Banta (2003) reviewed the evidence of the effectiveness of prenatal care and Carroli et al. (2001) performed a systematic review of randomized controlled trials. The ten-European country study of perinatal mortality and prenatal care was reported by Richardus et al. (2003). Kogan et al. (1998) tracked the changing pattern of prenatal care utilization in the United States from 1981–95.

4 Data are from the Alaska Bureau of Vital Statistics, *2004 Annual Report*. The APNCU Index (Adequancy of Prenatal Care Utilization Index), also called the Kotelchuk Index, is based on the time of initiation of prenatal care and the services received.

5 PRAMS data from Alaska on smoking and alcohol use during pregnancy, and also other protective and risk behaviours, are available from the *Alaska Maternal and Child Health Data Book 2004* (Perham-Hester, Wiens, and Schoellhorn 2005). O'Leary (2004) reviewed the epidemiology of FAS. Alcohol-induced teratogenesis and neurodevelopmental disorders are reviewed by Sampson et al. (1997, 2000).

6 Alaskan data from 1992–2001 are cited from the *Epidemiology Bulletin: Recommendations and Reports* of the Alaska Department of Health and Social Services (2006d). Scandinavian data on smoking during pregnancy for the years 2000 and 2003 are from *Health Statistics in the Nordic Countries 2004* by NOMESCO (2006). Norwegian data at the county level are obtained from the Norhealth interactive website, http://norgehelsa.no.

7 Jones and Balster (1998) reviewed inhalant use during pregnancy.

8   For reviews of the health consequences of preterm births and/or low birthweights, see Health Canada (2000), Knoches and Doyle (1993), and Robinson, Regan, and Norwitz (2001); and Anderson and Doyle (2003) specifically for neurobehavioural outcomes. Tough et al. (2001) surveyed the characteristics of preterm deliveries and low birthweights in one Canadian province.

9   The study by Luo et al. (2004) covered the whole of Quebec province, with separate data available for the Inuit living in the northern Nunavik region as well as for the more southerly located First Nations living in the subarctic and the St Lawrence valley.

10 The risk factors for post-neonatal mortality are reviewed in Scott et al. (1998).

11 See Hodgins (1997) on neonatal mortality in Nunavik. Arbour, Gilpin, et al. (2004) reported on the baseline chart reviews on birth defects. Description of the Alberta Congenital Anomalies Surveillance System (ACASS) can be found on its website, www.health.gov.ab.ca/resources/publica tions/ACASS_report5.pdf.

12 For a review of folate supplementation and prevention of birth defects, see Botto, Olney, and Erickson (2004). The Canadian experience with folate fortification was evaluated by Ray et al. (2002) and Kapur and Koren (2001). Folate intake data are available from Arbour, Christensen, et al. (2002) on the James Bay Cree; Receveur, Boulay, and Kuhnlein (1997) on Dene and Métis of the Northwest Territories; and Kuhnlein, Receveur, et al. (2004) on Inuit. B. Christensen et al. (1999) investigated genetic polymorphisms of the enzymes MTHFR and methionine synthase involved in folate metabolism.

13 For a review of the association between vitamin A and congenital cardiac defects, see Botto, Loffredo, et al. (2001). Egeland et al. (2004) assessed vitamin A intake among the Inuit.

14 Native-non-Native differences in infant mortality in the United States are discussed in Van Landingham and Hogue (1995) and Baldwin et al. (2002). See Luo et al. (2004) for data from the Quebec study. Sources of data on PNMR and NMR are as listed in the notes to figure 20.2.

15 For a general review of the health benefits of breastfeeding, see World Health Organization (2003b). Lipworth, Bailey, and Trichopoulous (2000) reviewed the evidence for the association with a reduced breast cancer risk.

16 See Green and Patterson (2001) for incidence data for type-1 diabetes in Europe, and Rytkönen et al. (2001) for geographic variation in Finland. The situation of type-2 diabetes among Canadian indigenous peoples has been reviewed by Young, Reading, et al. (2000).

17 The World Health Organization and the International Society for the Prevention of Childhood Abuse and Neglect (2006) has produced a guide to action and data collection. Gessner, Moore, et al. (2004) reviewed data for Alaska.
18 Canadian data are from Statistics Canada, based on the 2005 Canadian Community Health Survey (CANSIM Table 105-0427).
19 High-risk health behaviours among adolescents are reviewed in Melzer-Lange (1998).
20 Spiller (2004) reviewed data from U.S. poison control centres. Mackesy-Amiti and Fendrich (1999) contrasted the profiles of inhalant users and other drug users. Zebrowski and Gregory (1996) provided data on Eskimo school children in western Alaska.
21 Alaska data are from the *Alaska Youth Risk Behaviors Survey 2003* (T. Green et al. 2004). Canadian data were reported by Rotermann (2005).

PART FIVE

Strategies

21 Improving the Health of Arctic Populations

PETER BJERREGAARD, KUE YOUNG, AND JAMES BERNER

The previous chapters of the book have given an overview of the disease patterns of circumpolar peoples with an emphasis on the Inuit, Dene, and Sami and have outlined the main genetic, environmental, and behavioural causes of disease in these populations. Basically, three distinct patterns emerge: that of the Sami, who, in regard to health, are more or less indistinguishable from their non-Sami neighbours; that of the Inuit in North America and Greenland as well as the Dene in Canada and Alaska, who differ from the non-indigenous majority populations; and that of the ethnic minorities in Arctic Russia, who carry a severe disease burden due to poverty and serious economic dislocation. Among the non-indigenous populations of the circumpolar countries, being 'northern' does not appear to be a significant cause of health and socio-economic disparities; rather, these populations tend to fare better than the national averages due to selective migration.

An example of the disparities among the different 'Norths' is evident in figure 21.1, which displays the infant mortality rates of the circumpolar countries and their northern regions/populations when compared with all the countries in the world. The Nordic countries and Canada are among those countries with the lowest infant mortality rates (see also fig. 20.2). Note that the difference among the countries at the low end is extremely small, with many countries sharing the same rank.

Social Change and Health Transition

The indigenous peoples of the circumpolar north have, since the 1950s, undergone profound social changes that have been accompanied by

Figure 21.1 Global ranking of infant mortality rates

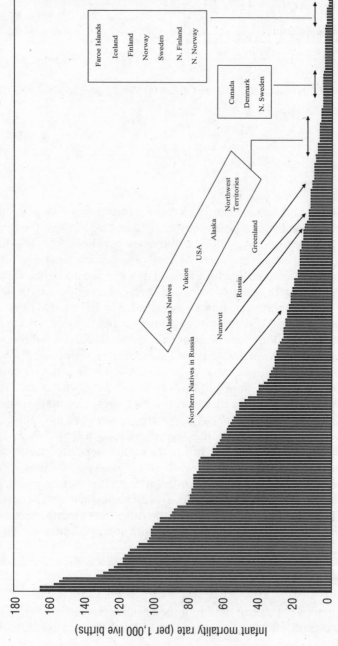

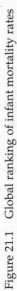

Note: See note to fig. 20.2 for sources of data for circumpolar countries and their northern regions.

Source: World Health Organization online database: Estimates of child and adult mortality and life expectancy at birth by country (www.who.int/healthinfo/statistics/mortlifeexpectancy/en/index.html).

an unprecedented health transition. The health transition has been more or less pronounced among the different populations. In 1950, the health and disease pattern of the circumpolar indigenous peoples, with the Scandinavian Sami as a possible exception, was characterized by very high morbidity and mortality rates from acute and chronic infectious diseases such as tuberculosis and acute respiratory infections, as well as from accidents. This disease pattern has changed for the better regarding infectious diseases, but the post–Second World War period witnessed an increase in suicides, alcohol-related conditions, and tobacco-induced diseases and the new millennium saw an increase in chronic diseases such as diabetes and heart disease, which threaten to place a substantially increased demand on the health care sector. This latter development is partly due to an aging population and partly due to an increased reliance on imported junk food, a decreased level of physical activity, and an increased prevalence of obesity.

The impacts of social changes on health have mostly been positive, if we focus only on physical health. The life expectancy has increased substantially in all regions and modern health care has been made accessible to the greater part of the population, but at a tremendous cost. Regarding mental health, the situation is not as positive. The rapid social change from a society made up of small, self-reliant hunting communities to modern towns with several thousand inhabitants and the relegation of hunting to a leisurely pastime has been accompanied by rates of youth suicides and suicidal behaviour that are among the highest of any population in the world. Misuse of alcohol and illegal drugs is also recognized as a major problem along with dropping out of school and a lack of education. It is obvious that while some circumpolar residents are able to face the challenges and grasp the opportunities of a changing society, a disquietingly large minority is not.

In our previous book, *The Circumpolar Inuit*, we identified eight main causes of changing health among the Inuit. Ten years later, the list still stands with a few modifications and an addition, and is broadly applicable to the other populations:

1 *Change from an economy based on hunting to modern wage earning.*
   This change has had a major impact on the importance of education and on the appropriateness of the traditional upbringing of children. The change has also resulted in a decreased mortality

from accidents. The traditional life in the North was extremely per-
ilous and many hunters died at an early age. Although mortality
from accidents is still high, it has decreased considerably. Alcohol
now plays a major role in accident causation.

2 *Improved housing conditions, sanitation, and food security.* Household
sizes are smaller and houses are bigger, with more rooms, thus
decreasing the transmission of infectious diseases, in particular
tuberculosis and other respiratory infections. Sanitation has
improved in towns and most villages, decreasing the exposure to
several microorganisms. Nutrition has generally improved, if not
qualitatively then at least with respect to reliability – seasonal starvation has disappeared from all communities thus increasing
general resistance to infections.

3 *Increased contact with the rest of the world.* Increased contact through
travel and migration has brought a number of infectious diseases
to the circumpolar communities – measles, gonorrhea, syphilis,
AIDS – but has also brought new ideas to the previously isolated
communities.

4 *Demographic change.* The influx of non-indigenous peoples, rapid
growth of the population, and increasing concentration in larger
communities of up to several thousand inhabitants have pro-
foundly altered the social structure of the northern communities.

5 *Political culture.* The power balance between indigenous and non-
indigenous peoples has changed. Before 1950, the indigenous
people were the absolute majority and, although subject to colonial
rule, were able to manage their day-to-day life on their own. From
the 1950s onward, an overwhelming arrival of non-indigenous
skilled labour who often gave indigenous peoples little respect
eventually led to strong feelings of ethnic identity and a wish for
self-determination on the part of the indigenous peoples. A new
ruling class has emerged, that is, those who can speak and navi-
gate equally well in indigenous and non-indigenous circles.

6 *Dietary changes and reduced physical activity.* The change to an
increased reliance on store-bought food and an increasingly sedentary lifestyle have played a major role in the emergence of chronic
diseases well-known in Western societies: obesity, diabetes, atherosclerotic heart disease, and dental caries.

7 *Increased access to alcohol and tobacco.* The use of these drugs has
become excessive in many circumpolar communities. The still very
high prevalence of smoking has resulted in record-high mortality

from lung cancer in women. Tobacco use is a causative factor in many other cancers as well as in chronic heart and lung disease.

8 *Improved health care*. Along with infrastructural and sociocultural changes, the circumpolar peoples have achieved general access to a modern health care system. Although there is less accessibility for indigenous peoples living in villages than for predominantly urban populations in southern countries, and although tertiary level care usually involves travel to hospitals in the south, the health care services have been an important factor in the reduction of morbidity and mortality from tuberculosis and several other infectious diseases, in the reduction of perinatal mortality, and in the improvement of dental health. The health care services have furthermore played a substantial role in improving the quality of life of many people due to early treatment of disabling diseases.

On the political front, substantial and largely positive changes have occurred in the Arctic, with the indigenous peoples achieving considerable though variable degrees of political autonomy and cultural revival. Notable changes include the establishment of Alaska Native regional corporations; successful land claims negotiations in northern Canada and the creation of Nunavut; the achievement of Home Rule in Greenland; Sami cultural revival and the strengthening of Sami institutions in Scandinavia; and the loosening of central totalitarian control and the emergence of indigenous peoples' rights organizations in Russia. Outright assimilationist policies and colonial practices that were once prevalent, although sometimes with benevolent intent if not outcomes, have largely been reversed or halted. We do not subscribe to the simplistic view that colonialism or post-colonialism is the root of all ill health (if not evils) and that political self-determination will automatically bring about health for all. We do, however, see political freedom and cultural integrity as preconditions for bringing about much needed changes in health policies, programs, and practices.

Disease Prevention and Health Promotion

Improvement of the health of all subgroups of the population is the general goal of all health policies in the circumpolar countries. This goal can be furthered by placing emphasis on the indigenous population and focusing on reducing social inequalities. While Greenland has developed a national health policy, there are no comparable health plans in the other regions, which is not to say they lack effective and successful interventions. We highlight here the Greenland policy as a model of how a coherent strategy that is unique to the Arctic can be developed.

The Greenland national health policy targets the whole population, including the majority Inuit population and the minority (10 per cent) European population. During the early 2000s, the total budget for health care was approximately 870 million Danish kroner (U.S.$145 million) of which an estimated 98.5 per cent was spent on curative services and the rest on prevention and research. After three years of preparation, a new public health program was approved by the parliament in 2006.

The Greenland public health program was named *Inuuneritta*, which means 'Let us have a good life.' It is the first comprehensive health program since the tuberculosis campaigns of the 1950s, but it builds on a number of existing preventive initiatives such as a national strategy for suicide prevention, preventive care for pregnant women and young children, and preventive dental care. The following themes were included in the program:

- alcohol and drug abuse
- violence and sexual violence
- diet and physical activity
- smoking
- reproductive health
- suicides
- dental health
- children and youth
- the elderly

It is obvious that the themes cover a wide span of health problems and target a large proportion of the population. The recommendations for action are still not explicitly described and the coming years will show how the allotted budget will be spent. The additional budget of 8 million Danish kroner (U.S.$1.35 million) is evidently not enough to cover a comprehensive set of initiatives in all areas. A systematic evaluation of the program and its impact on health will be given high priority.

It was originally the aim to develop a public health program with participation from all sectors of society, including schools, municipalities, physical planning, and social security, but the final program is led by the health sector alone. It is hoped that cross-sectoral activities will emanate once the actual work begins.

At the same time, there are plans to revise the structure of the health care services in Greenland. Presently, each of sixteen small municipalities has a hospital/health centre staffed with at least one physician. Because of the increasing difficulties of recruiting physicians with sufficient skills into general surgery, internal medicine, psychiatry, pediatrics, and obstetrics, the need for larger units staffed with several physicians is becoming increasingly acute. It is furthermore believed that larger units will make it easier to attract skilled staff.

The increased weight on primary prevention is in line with the research results that we have presented in this book. Individual behaviours such as smoking, alcohol abuse, eating too much, and lack of physical activity are responsible for a large disease burden and a heavy drain on the health care system. Successful prevention will eventually reduce this burden and make it possible to reduce the health care expenditure or at least maintain it at its present level. Unfortunately, the reduction in health care expenditure will take place sometime in the future while the investment in prevention is needed now. It is important to make this clear to the politicians and health administrators and not to market prevention as a cost-reducing initiative.

Furthermore, it is important to create a dynamic health care sector based on the needs of today and of the future, and not those of forty years ago. The community has changed and so has its disease pattern. Given its inborn torpidity, a large health care system will lag behind if appropriate action is not taken. The need for changes to the infrastructure, staff, and education must be continuously appraised and reappraised in order to meet the requirements of an ever-changing community. Given the huge investments in buildings and education, and the importance of a hospital/health centre as a major place of work in any given community, this is no minor task and has great political significance.

Health Care Delivery in Remote Areas

Sustainable circumpolar communities, no matter how small, require access to some level of health care. In general, the smaller and more isolated the community, the greater the difficulty in providing on-site health care. The challenge for national and regional jurisdictions has

Figure 21.2   Total health expenditures in the circumpolar countries
(amount per capita, per cent of GDP, and share of private and public sectors)

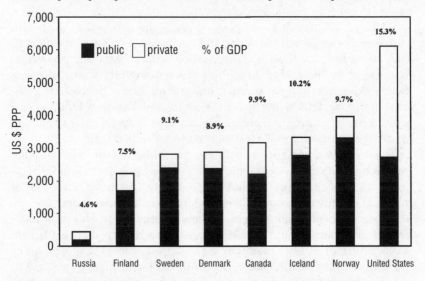

Note: Expenditures refer to the year 2004, converted from national currencies
to US$ PPP (purchasing power parities); PPPs are computed by OECD to allow
for more meaningful comparison across different economies by equalising the
purchasing power of different currencies by eliminating the differences in price
levels between countries. Total health expenditures are defined by OECD's
System of Health Accounts, and include curative, rehabilitative, long-term
nursing, and ancillary services, medical goods and drugs, prevention and
public health, health administration and insurance, and capital investments;
but excludes health research, education and training, food hygiene, environmental health and sanitation, public safety and social services.
Source: Data except Russia from Organization of Economic Cooperation and
Development (OECD) *Health Data 2006*. Russian data from OECD *Economic
Surveys: Russian Federation* (2006/17, ch. 5).

been the provision of basic services in the smallest, most isolated
communities.

Northern health care must be discussed in the context of the
respective national health systems of which it is a part. Across the circumpolar world, there is substantial variation in how health care is

organized, financed, and delivered. A detailed comparison of national health systems is beyond the scope of this book. Key differences, and similarities, exist in terms of the per capita national health expenditures, the per cent of gross domestic product (GDP) consumed by health care, and the share of health care financing between the public and private sectors. As figure 21.2 shows, the United States and Russia are at the two extremes in terms of per cent of GDP and per capita expenditures. Canada and the Nordic countries, all characterized by a predominantly publicly financed health care system, have largely similar per capita expenditures and share of GDP, with the exception of Finland, which spends less than the others on health care. The private sector is proportionately more important in both the United States and Russia.

On a per capita basis, more health care resources are devoted to some, but not all, northern regions relative to the rest of the country. Total health expenditures in the Yukon, Northwest Territories, and Nunavut were 1.3, 1.7, and 2.5 times that of Canada nationally, whereas Greenland's was only 0.65 times that of Denmark's. In Alaska, per capita expenditures on personal health services were on par with the United States as a whole. The importance of health care in the economy is particularly evident in Nunavut, where as much as 29 per cent of GDP was consumed by health care alone.[1]

Over much of the most remote regions of the Arctic, systems of care have slowly evolved. The steady advances in medical care, transportation, and communication technology have greatly improved health services in regional hub communities. A competent remote primary health care system is critical for sustainability, and it is also needed to facilitate economic opportunities such as eco-tourism, university science installations, fishing lodges, and air-charter services.

The desired level of services must be balanced against available resources and population characteristics. At the most basic level, comprehensive health care includes preventive, curative, and rehabilitative services. It requires a communication and transportation infrastructure to link the regional hubs with the peripheral service centres in terms of logistical support, technical advice, and the movement of patients and health personnel.

Two basic constraints tend to shape regional solutions to providing basic care. The first constraint is the limitation of financial resources to build, equip, and maintain the health care, communication, and transportation infrastructure. The second constraint is the limitation of human resources to carry out the scope of health care that can be supported by the financial resources available. The development of the rural health care system for Alaska Natives, which is characterized by several important innovations, is discussed here in some detail.

With over 140 small isolated Alaska Native villages, ranging in population from 25 to 1,500, a primary care system that is based on non-traditional provider clinics has developed. The provider in these clinics, the Community Health Aide (CHA), is unique in the United States. The typical CHA is an Alaska Native village resident, a high school graduate, appointed by the village tribal council, and employed and supported by the regional tribal health corporation providing care in a small village-built clinic. Training is provided in a twenty-week course conducted in one of four tribal training centres, in four-week blocks separated by months of supervised practice. The CHA uses the regional tribal health organization's physicians and dentists for consultation and referral and receives on-site training and quality assurance oversight from the regional tribal health organization.

U.S. congressional legislation created the legal authority for the expanded scope of CHA practice, with oversight authority of all activities invested in the federal CHA Certification Board, based in Anchorage. CHA training covers all three components of medical care and is based on a comprehensive CHA manual (CHAM), which has been in use for over forty years. It is a step-by-step protocol for the evaluation of all common symptoms and conditions, so that the CHA can gather all needed information to transmit to the referral physician or dentist. Simple complaints, such as a middle-ear infection or an upper-respiratory infection, can be evaluated and treated according to a protocol, with medications pre-packaged in the clinic, and without consultation. A unified, simple medical record system has been developed and is essential for quality assurance and continuity of care.

The village-based provider concept has been extended to include a Dental Health Aide (DHA) and a Behavioral Health Aide (BHA). These two new categories of provider were established to address primary prevention in oral health and behavioural health, areas of disparity in Alaska Native health status. In addition, villages have also trained emergency response workers to assist in initial treatment, stabilization, and transport of injured patients.

Since the majority of the Alaska Native population (approximately 60 per cent) live in villages served by CHA clinics, the remote care system in Alaska has been a major contribution to the improvement in the health of the populations, which is evident from several indicators (see chapter 4). There has been positive economic outcomes as well. Employment as a village-based provider is often a significant economic asset in a very small community. Associated services, such as village residents being trained as home-based care attendants and specially modified homes for three to four disabled elders, can further contribute to the village economy. This reduces relocating elders to regional nursing care facilities, lowers the cost of care, and strengthens the community's cultural connections and knowledge.

The Alaska Native experience amply demonstrates that it is possible to deliver a reasonably high standard of medical care even in very small, remote communities. The critical component of such a system is a well-trained, village-based provider, preferably a resident who speaks the language and is selected by, and accountable to, the village. He/she must be supported by a regional infrastructure and protected by authorizing legislation that allows for an expanded scope of practice outside of standard professional practice regulations.

Health care services in remote areas is an important component of any comprehensive stategy to improve health status, address health disparities, and contribute to community sustainability.

The Role of Health Research

In the long term, beyond public health and health care delivery, health research will play an important role in improving the health of Arctic populations. Research is the cornerstone of evidence-based prevention and treatment. While some research can be better – and more cheaply – conducted outside the Arctic itself and subsequently applied to circumpolar peoples' health, other research can only be carried out in the circumpolar communities.

Research to identify the causes of and risk factors for prevalent diseases is important in order to establish locally tailored prevention. One example is the ongoing Inuit Health in Transition project, in which researchers in Greenland, Canada, and Alaska are cooperating to identify risk factors for diabetes and cardiovascular disease among the Inuit. In this book we have raised numerous relevant and scientifically interesting research questions that could contribute to future projects. For instance:

- What are the modifiable causes of suicidal behaviour?
- How can alcohol and smoking behaviour be influenced?
- What factors contribute towards good health?
- What are the risk factors for diabetes and cardiovascular disease in the circumpolar populations?
- What are the benefits and risks associated with traditional foods and environmental contaminants and how do we balance them?
- How do we further reduce the lingering 'old' infectious diseases such as tuberculosis, pneumonia, meningitis, and sexually transmitted diseases, while instituting early warning systems for new emerging infections?
- How do we apply cancer prevention programs that have been shown to be effective to the realities and constraints of health care delivery systems in the Arctic?
- What are emerging health issues related to climate change?

Research on how to implement the preventive initiatives in the local communities is also important. In order to succeed, prevention must take into consideration the social conditions, education, and culture of the target group. It is highly improbable that an intervention developed, for example, in Copenhagen will work in the villages in northern Greenland. It should, however, be kept in mind that distinct differences also exist within the circumpolar regions. An intervention that works well in one of the towns in the North is not guaranteed to work at all at the village level.

Research with circumpolar peoples is made difficult by two factors. In the first place, the populations are so small that for statistical reasons it is difficult to discover risk factors and establish causal associations beyond what is immediately obvious. Second, the small, scattered communities and the high cost of transportion contribute towards making research in the circumpolar region much more expensive than research anywhere else. The first obstacle can be overcome by international cooperation; the second obstacle by focusing on research that can best or only be conducted in the circumpolar north and by convincing funding agencies that this is the case.

The greatest challenges for health care in the circumpolar north are to provide health care to small, scattered populations, to maintain uninterrupted care despite frequent shortages of staff, and to do this within a given budget. The solution to these challenges is political. Research faces other challenges. One is to develop viable partnerships with a sound balance between, on the one hand, local knowledge and influence and, on the other, scientific expertise, which is most often provided by non-local non-indigenous university-affiliated researchers. Each side must acknowledge that the other can make valuable contributions to the research process. A final challenge is to increase research cooperation among indigenous peoples globally through the exchange of ideas and expertise.

NOTE

1 Canadian data are for 2004 from Canadian Institute for Health Information (2006); U.S. data are for 1998 from Centers for Medicare and Medicaid Services, Office of the Actuary, 'National Health Expenditures Data,' available online from www.cms.hhs.gov/NationalHealthExpendData; Greenland data are for 2004 from NOMESCO (2006).

References

Note: The titles of Russian language publications were translated into English by the authors; the transliteration of the original titles from Cyrillic script was not provided. Such references are indicated by (in Russian). Titles of publications in other languages were not translated unless an English version was provided in the original or in the bibliographic database (such as PubMed). In such cases, only the English translation of the title is provided, enclosed in parentheses, and the citations are indicated by, for example (in Danish).

Abbey, S.E., E. Hood, L.T. Young, and S. Malcolmson. 1991. 'New perspectives on mental health problems in Inuit women.' In B.D. Postl, P. Gilbert, J. Goodwill, M.E.K. Moffatt, J.D. O'Neil, P.A. Sarsfield, and T.K. Young, eds., *Circumpolar Health 90*, 285–7. Winnipeg: University of Manitoba Press.
Abildsnes, A.K., A.J. Søgaard, and A. Hafstad. 1998. 'Hvem stumper røyken?' *Tidsskrift for den Norske Lægeforeningen* 14:2170–5.
Adamson, J.D., J.P. Moody, A.F. Peart, R.A. Smillie, J.C. Wilt, and W.J. Wood. 1949. 'Poliomyelitis in the Arctic.' *Canadian Medical Association Journal* 61:339–48.
Alaska Area Native Health Service. 2001a. *2000 Census Counts for Alaska Natives*. Anchorage: AANHS.
– 2001b. *Alaska Native Births and Infant Deaths, 1980–1997*. Anchorage: AANHS.
Alaska Bureau of Vital Statistics. (various years). *Annual Report*. Anchorage: Department of Health and Social Services.
Alaska Department of Health and Social Services. (various years). *Health Risks in Alaska Among Adults: Annual Report of the Behavioral Risk Factor Surveillance System*. Anchorage: DHSS.
– 2006a. 'HIV infection in Alaska, 2005.' *Epidemiology Bulletin*, no. 9: n.p.

– 2006b. 'Chlamydia trachomatis – Alaska, 2005.' *Epidemiology Bulletin*, no. 10: n.p.

– 2006c. 'Gonorrhea – Alaska, 2005.' *Epidemiology Bulletin*, no. 11: n.p.

– 2006d. 'Findings of the Alaska Maternal-Infant Mortality Review, 1992–2001.' *Epidemiology Bulletin: Recommendations and Reports* 10, no. 3:1–17.

Alaska Native Health Board. 2004. *Selected Results from the Behavioral Risk Factor Surveillance System for Alaska Natives, 2001–2003*. Anchorage: ANHB.

Albeck, H., J. Bentzen, H.H. Ockelmann, N.H. Nielsen, P. Bretlau, and H.S. Hansen. 1993. 'Familial clusters of nasopharyngeal carcinoma and salivary gland carcinomas in Greenland natives.' *Cancer* 72:196–200.

Alberg, A.J., M.V. Brock, and J.M. Samet. 2005. 'Epidemiology of lung cancer: Looking to the future.' *Journal of Clinical Oncology* 23:3175–85.

Allen, J.A. 1877. 'The influence of physical conditions in the genesis of species.' *Radical Review* 1:108–40.

American Psychiatric Association. 2000. *Diagnostic and Statistical Manual of Mental Disorders. DSM-IV-Text Revision*. Washington, DC: APA.

Amft, A. 2000. *Sápmi in a Time of Change: A Study of Swedish Sami Living Conditions during the Twentieth Century from a Gender and Ethnic Perspective*. Umeå, Sweden: Department of Archaeology and Sami Studies, Umeå University.

Andersen, K.L., Y. Loyning, J.D. Nelms, O. Wilson, R.H. Fox, and A. Bolstad. 1960. 'Metabolic and thermal responses to a moderate cold exposure in nomadic Lapps.' *Journal of Applied Physiology* 15:649–53.

Anderson, P., and L.W. Doyle. 2003. 'Neurobehavioral outcomes of school-age children born extremely low birth weight or very preterm in the 1990s.' *Journal of the American Medical Association* 289:3264–72.

Anttonen, H., H. Virokannas, and M. Sorri. 1994. 'Noise and hearing loss in reindeer herders.' *Arctic Medical Research* 53 (Suppl. 3):35–40.

Arbour, L., B. Christensen, T. Delormier, R. Platt, B. Gilfix, P. Forbes, I. Kovitch, J. Morel, and R. Rozen. 2002. 'Spina bifida, folate metabolism, and dietary folate intake in a northern Canadian aboriginal population.' *International Journal of Circumpolar Health* 61:341–51.

Arbour, L., C. Gilpin, V. Millor-Roy, G. Pekeles, G.M. Egeland, S. Hodgins, and P. Eydoux. 2004. 'Increased incidence of heart defects and other malformations in the Inuit of Baffin Island and Arctic Quebec: A baseline study.' *International Journal of Circumpolar Health* 63:251–66.

Archibald, L. 2004. *Teen Pregnancy in Inuit Communities: Issues and Perspectives*. Ottawa: Pauktuutit – Inuit Women's Association.

Arctic Climate Impact Assessment (ACIA). 2005. Cambridge: Cambridge University Press.

Arctic Human Development Report (AHDR). 2004. Akureyri, Iceland: Stefans-son Arctic Institute.

Arctic Monitoring and Assessment Program (AMAP). 1997. *Arctic Pollution Issues: A State of the Arctic Environment Report*. Oslo: AMAP.

– 1998. *AMAP Assessment Report: Arctic Pollution Issues*. Oslo: AMAP.

– 2003. *AMAP Assessment 2002: Human Health in the Arctic*. Oslo: AMAP.

– 2004. *Persistent Toxic Substances, Food Security and Indigenous Peoples of the Russian North: Final Report*. Oslo: AMAP.

Auvinen, A., T. Haldorsen, P. Hall, S. Hassler, E. Pukkala, P. Sjölander, and T. Tynes. 2002. 'Cancer incidence among reindeer-herding Saami in the Nordic countries.' Paper presented at Nordisk konferens om Samisk hälsa och livskvalitet, Vilhelmina, Sweden.

Baggett, H.C., T.W. Hennessy, K. Rudolph, D. Bruden, A. Reasonover, A. Parkinson, R. Sparks, R.M. Donlan, P. Martinez, K. Mongkolrattanothai, and J.C. Butler. 2004. 'Community-onset methicillin-resistant Staphylococcus aureus associated with antibiotic use and the cytotoxin Panton-Valentine leukocidin during a furunculosis outbreak in rural Alaska.' *Journal of Infectious Diseases* 189:1565–73.

Baggett, H.C., A.J. Parkinson, P.T. Muth, B.D. Gold, and B.D. Gessner. 2006. 'Endemic iron deficiency associated with *Helicobacter pylori* infection among school-aged children in Alaska.' *Pediatrics* 117:e396–404.

Balikci, A. 1970. *The Netsilik Eskimo*. Garden City, NY: Natural History Press.

Baldwin, L.M., D.C. Grossman, S. Casey, W. Hollow, J.R. Sugarman, W.L. Freeman, and L.G. Hart. 2002. 'Perinatal and infant health among rural and urban American Indians/Alaska Natives.' *American Journal of Public Health* 92:1491–7.

Banerji, A., A. Bell, E.L. Mills, J. McDonald, K. Subbarao, G. Stark, N. Eynon, and V.G. Loo. 2001. 'Lower respiratory tract infections in Inuit infants on Baffin Island.' *Canadian Medical Association Journal* 164:1847–50.

Banta, D. 2003. *What Is the Efficacy/Effectiveness of Antenatal Care and Its Financial and Organizational Implications?* Copenhagen: World Health Organization Regional Office for Europe (Health Evidence Network Report E82996).

Barker, D.J.P., J.G. Eriksson, T. Forsén, and C. Osmond. 2002. 'Fetal origins of adult disease: Strength of effects and biological basis.' *International Journal of Epidemiology* 31:1235–9.

Barrett, D.H., J.M. Burks, B. McMahon, S. Elliott, K.R. Berquist, T.R. Bender, and J.E. Maynard. 1977. 'Epidemiology of hepatitis B in two Alaska communities.' *American Journal of Epidemiology* 105:118–22.

Barss, P., G.S. Smith, S.P. Baker, and D. Mohan. 1998. *Injury Prevention: An International Perspective. Epidemiology, Surveillance, and Policy*. New York: Oxford University Press.

Batal M., K. Gray-Donald, H.V. Kuhnlein, and O. Receveur. 2005. 'Estimation of traditional food intake in indigenous communities in Denendeh and the Yukon.' *International Journal of Circumpolar Health* 64:46–54.

Baxter, J.D. 1999. 'Otitis media in Inuit children in the Eastern Canadian Arctic: An overview, 1968 to date.' *International Journal of Pediatric Otorhinolaryngology* 49 (Suppl. 1):S165–8.

Bechtold, D.W. 1988. 'Cluster suicide in American Indian adolescents.' *American Indian and Alaska Native Mental Health Research* 1:26–35.

Benedetti, J.L., E. Dewailly, F. Turcotte, and M. Lefebvre. 1994. 'Unusually high blood cadmium associated with cigarette smoking among three subgroups of the general population, Quebec, Canada.' *Science of the Total Environment* 152:161–7.

Berger, T.R. 1985. *Village Journey: The Report of the Alaska Native Review Commission.* New York: Hill and Wang.

Bergmann, C. 1847. 'Über die Verhältnisse der wärmeökonomie der Thiere zu ihrer Grösse.' *Göttinger Studien* 3(1):595–708.

Berkman, L.F., and I. Kawachi, eds. 2000. *Social Epidemiology.* New York: Oxford University Press.

Berry, J.W. 1985. 'Acculturation among circumpolar people: Implications for health status.' *Arctic Medical Research* 40:21–7.

– 1990. 'Acculturation and adaptation: Health consequences of culture contact among circumpolar people.' *Arctic Medical Research* 49:142–50.

Bertelsen, A. 1904. 'Om forekomsten af Cancer i Grønland.' *Hospitalstidende* 4(12):209–14.

– 1937. 'Grønlandsk medicinsk statistik og nosografi.' *Meddelelser om Grønland* 117(2):1–248.

Berthelsen, A. 1943. 'Grønlandsk medicinsk statistik og nosografi: Undersøgelser og erfaringer fra 30 aars grønlandsk lægevirksomhed.' *Meddelelser om Grønland* 117(4):1–244.

Biery, A.J., S.O. Ebbesson, A.R. Shuldiner, and B.B. Boyer. 1997. 'The beta(3)-adrenergic receptor TRP64ARG polymorphism and obesity in Alaskan Eskimos.' *International Journal of Obesity and Related Metabolic Disorders* 21:1176–9.

Bittel, J. 1992. 'The different types of general cold adaptation in man.' *International Journal of Sports Medicine* 13 (Suppl. 1):S172–6.

Bjerregaard, P. 1990. 'Geographic variation of mortality in Greenland: Economic and demographic correlations.' *Arctic Medical Research* 49:16–24.

– 2004. *Folkesundhed i Grønland.* Nuuk: Grønlands Hjemmestyre.

Bjerregaard, P., and B. Bjerregaard. 1985. 'Disease patterns in Upernavik in relation to housing conditions and social group.' *Meddelelser om Grønland: Man and Society* 8:1–18.

Bjerregaard, P., T. Curtis, K. Borch-Johnsen, G. Mulvad, U. Becker, S. Andersen, and V. Backer. 2003. 'Inuit health in Greenland: A population survey of life style and disease in Greenland and among Inuit living in Denmark.' *International Journal of Circumpolar Health* 62 (Suppl. 1):3–79.

Bjerregaard, P., T. Curtis, and the Greenland Population Study. 2002. 'Cultural change and mental health in Greenland: The association of childhood conditions, language, and urbanization with mental health and suicidal thoughts among the Inuit of Greenland.' *Social Science and Medicine* 54:33–48.

Bjerregaard, P., E. Dewailly, T.K. Young, C. Blanchet, R.A. Hegele, S.E. Ebbesson, P.M. Risica, and G. Mulvad. 2003. 'Blood pressure among the Inuit (Eskimo) populations in the Arctic.' *Scandinavian Journal of Public Health* 31:92–9.

Bjerregaard, P., and J. Dyerberg. 1988. 'Mortality from ischemic heart disease and cerebrovascular disease in Greenland.' *International Journal of Epidemiology* 17:514–9.

Bjerregaard, P., M.E. Jørgensen, S. Andersen, G. Mulvad, K. Borch-Johnsen, and the Greenland Population Study. 2002. 'Decreasing overweight and central fat patterning with Westernization among the Inuit in Greenland and Inuit migrants.' *International Journal of Obesity and Related Metabolic Disorders* 26:1503–10.

Bjerregaard, P., M.E. Jørgensen, and K. Borch-Johnsen. 2004. 'Serum lipids of Greenland Inuit in relation to Inuit genetic heritage, westernisation and migration.' *Atherosclerosis* 174:391–8.

Bjerregaard, P., and I. Lynge. 2006. 'Suicide: A challenge in modern Greenland.' *Archives of Suicide Research* 10:209–20.

Bjerregaard, P., and J. Misfeldt. 1992. 'Infant mortality in Greenland: Secular trend and regional variation.' *Arctic Medical Research* 51:126–35.

Bjerregaard, P., G. Mulvad, and H.S. Pedersen. 1997. 'Cardiovascular risk factors in Inuit of Greenland.' *International Journal of Epidemiology* 26:1182–90.

Bjerregaard, P., H.S. Pedersen, and G. Mulvad. 2000. 'The associations of a marine diet with plasma lipids, blood glucose, blood pressure and obesity among the Inuit in Greenland.' *European Journal of Clinical Nutrition* 54:732–7.

Bjerregaard, P., and T.K. Young. 1998. *The Circumpolar Inuit: Health of a Population in Transition.* Copenhagen: Munksgaard.

Bjerregaard, P., T.K. Young, and R.A. Hegele. 2003. 'Low incidence of cardiovascular disease among the Inuit. What is the evidence?' *Atherosclerosis* 166:351–7.

Blot, W.J., A. Lanier, J.F. Fraumeni, Jr., and T.R. Bender. 1975. 'Cancer mortality among Alaskan natives, 1960–69.' *Journal of the National Cancer Institute* 55:547–54.

Blum, R.W., B. Harmon, L. Harris, L. Bergeisen, and M.D. Resnick. 1992. 'American Indian–Alaska Native youth health.' *Journal of the American Medical Association* 267:1637–44.

Boas F. 1964. *The Central Eskimo*. Lincoln: University of Nebraska Press. Reprinted from the 6th Annual Report of the Bureau of Ethnology, Smithsonian Institution, 1888.

Boffetta, P., and M. Hashibe. 2006. 'Alcohol and cancer.' *Lancet Oncology* 7:149–56.

Bogoras, W. 1975. *The Chukchee*. New York: AMS.

Bogoyavlensky, D. 2004. 'Les peuples du Nord disparaissent-ils?' *Population and Society: Informational Bulletin of Human Demography and Ecology Center of the Institute of National Economy Forecasting* (Russian Academy of Sciences) 83:1–4.

Bogoyavlensky, D., and A. Siggner. 2004. 'Arctic demography.' In: *Arctic Human Development Report*, 27–41. Akureyi, Iceland: Stefansson Arctic Institute.

Bone, R.M. 1992. *The Geography of the Canadian North: Issues and Challenges.* Toronto: Oxford University Press.

– 2002. *The Regional Geography of Canada*. 2nd ed. Toronto: Oxford University Press.

Boothroyd, L.J., L.J. Kirmayer, S. Spreng, M. Malus, and S. Hodgins. 2001. 'Completed suicides among the Inuit of northern Quebec, 1982–1996: A case-control study.' *Canadian Medical Association Journal* 165:749–55.

Boreman, P. 1953. *Læstadianismen Fennoskandiens märkligste väckelse och dess förhållande till kyrkan*. Stockholm: Svenska Kyrkans Daikonistyrelses Bokförlag.

Borneman, W.R. 2003. *Alaska: Saga of a Bold Land*. New York: HarperCollins.

Borowsky, I.W., M.D. Resnick, M. Ireland, and R.W. Blum. 1999. 'Suicide attempts among American Indian and Alaska Native youth: Risk and protective factors.' *Archives of Pediatrics and Adolescent Medicine* 153:573–80.

Bosch, E., F. Calafell, Z.H. Rosser, S. Nørby, N. Lynnerup, M.E. Hurles, and M.A. Jobling. 2003. 'High level of male-biased Scandinavian admixture in Greenlandic Inuit shown by Y chromosomal analysis.' *Human Genetics* 112:353–63.

Botto, L.D., C. Loffredo, K.S. Scanlon, C. Ferencz, M.J. Khoury, D. Wilson, and A. Correra. 2001. 'Vitamin A and cardiac outflow tract defects.' *Epidemiology* 12:491–6.

Botto, L.D., R.S. Olney, and J.D. Erickson. 2004. 'Vitamin supplements and the risk for congenital anomalies other than neural tube defects.' *American Journal of Medical Genetics. Part C, Seminars in Medical Genetics* 125C:12–21.

Boudreau, D.A., W.D. Scheer, G.T. Malcom, G. Mulvad, H.S. Pedersen, and E. Jul. 1999. 'Apolipoprotein E and atherosclerosis in Greenland Inuit.' *Atherosclerosis* 145:207–19.

Bowen, H.M. 1968. 'Diver performance and the effects of cold.' *Human Factors* 10(5):445–64.

Boyer, R., R. Dufour, M. Préville, and L. Bujold-Brown. 1994. 'State of mental health.' In M. Jetté, ed., *Santé Québec: A Health Profile of the Inuit*. Vol. 2, 117–50. Montreal: Ministère de la Santé et des Services sociaux.

Brems, C. 1996. 'Substance use, mental health, and health in Alaska: Emphasis on Alaska Native peoples.' *Arctic Medical Research* 55:135–47.

Brenna, W. 1997. 'The Sami of Norway.' Available online at Norwegian Ministry of Foreign Affairs, http://odin.dp.no/odin/english/p30008168/history.

Brent, D.A. 1995. 'Risk factors for adolescent suicide and suicidal behavior: Mental and substance abuse disorders, family environmental factors, and life stress.' *Suicide and Life-Threatening Behavior* 25 (Suppl.):52–63.

Brown, M.O., A.P. Lanier, and T.M. Becker. 1998. 'Colorectal cancer incidence and survival among Alaska Natives, 1969–1993.' *International Journal of Epidemiology* 27:388–96.

Brox, J., E. Bjornstad, and K. Olaussen. 2003. 'Hemoglobin, iron, nutrition and life-style among adolescents in a coastal and an inland community in northern Norway.' *International Journal of Circumpolar Health* 62:130–41.

Bruce, M.G., D.L. Bruden, B.J. McMahon, T.W. Hennessy, A. Reasonover, J. Morris, D.A. Hurlburt, H. Peters, F. Sacco, P. Martinez, M. Swenson, D.E. Berg, D. Parks, and A.J. Parkinson. 2006. 'Alaska sentinel surveillance for antimicrobial resistance in *Helicobacter pylori* isolates from Alaska Native persons, 1999–2003.' *Helicobacter* 11:581–8.

Bruce, M.G., T. Cottle, S. Deeks, M. Lovgreen, L. Jette, and T. Hennessy. 2006. 'The International Circumpolar Surveillance System for population-based surveillance of invasive pneumococcal disease 1999–2004.' *Clinical Microbiology and Infection* 12 (S4):O220.

Bulkow, L.R., R.J. Singleton, R.A. Karron, and L.H. Harrison. 2002. 'Risk factors for severe respiratory syncytial virus infection among Alaska native children.' *Pediatrics* 109:210–6.

Bulterys M, H. Morgenstern, T.K. Welty, and J.F. Kraus. 1990. 'The expected impact of a smoking cessation program for pregnant women on infant mortality among Native Americans.' *American Journal of Preventive Medicine* 6:267–73.

Bunker, J.P., H.S. Frazier, and F. Mosteller. 1994. 'Improving health: Measuring effects of medical care.' *Milbank Quarterly* 72:225–58.

Butler, J.C., A.J. Parkinson, E. Funk, M. Beller, G. Hayes, and J.M. Hughes. 1999. 'Emerging infectious diseases in Alaska and the Arctic: A review and a strategy for the 21st century.' *Alaska Medicine* 41:35–43.

Bye, E.K., ed. 2003. *Rusmidler i Norge.* Oslo: Statens Institutt for Alkohol- og Narkotika Forskning.

Campbell, L. 1997. *American Indian Languages: The Historical Linguistics of Native America.* New York: Oxford University Press.

Canadian Institute for Health Information. 2006. *National Health Expenditure Trends, 1975–2006.* Ottawa: CIHI.

Carroli, G., J. Villar, G. Piaggio, D. Khan-Neelofur, M. Gulmezoglu, M. Mugford, P. Lumbiganon, U. Farnot, P. Bersgjo, and the WHO Antenatal Care Trial Research Group. 2001. 'WHO systematic review of randomised controlled trials of routine antenatal care.' *Lancet* 357:1565–70.

Carter, E.A., J.W. MacCluer, B. Dyke, B.V. Howard, R.B. Devereux, E.O. Ebbesson, and H.E. Resnick. 2006. 'Diabetes mellitus and impaired fasting glucose in Alaska Eskimos: The Genetics of Coronary Artery Disease in Alaska Natives (GOCADAN) study.' *Diabetologia* 49:29–35.

Castellani, J.W., and C. O'Brien. 2005. 'Peripheral vasodilation responses to prevent local cold injuries.' In *Prevention of Cold Injuries,* KN2:1-KN2:14. Proceedings of a NATO Meeting RTO-MP-HFM-126.

Castrodale, L., B. Gessner, L. Hammitt, M. Chimonas, and T. Hennessy. 2007. 'Invasive early-onset neonatal Group B streptococcal cases – Alaska 2000–2004.' *Maternal and Child Health Journal* 11:91–5.

Caulfield, R.A. 1997. *Greenlanders, Whalers and Whaling: Sustainability and Self-Determination in the Arctic.* Hanover: University Press of New England.

Cavalli-Sforza, L.L., P. Menozzi, and A. Piazza. 1994. *The History and Geography of Human Genes.* Princeton, NJ: Princeton University Press.

Centers for Disease Control and Prevention. 1997. 'Recommended framework for presenting injury mortality data.' *Morbidity and Mortality Weekly Report* 46 (RR-14):1–30.

Chan, H.M., K. Fediuk, S. Hamilton, L. Rostas, A. Caughey, H. Kuhnlein, G. Egeland, and E. Loring. 2006. 'Food security in Nunavut, Canada: Barriers and recommendations.' *International Journal of Circumpolar Health* 65:416–31.

Chan, K.C., and Y.M. Lo. 2002. 'Circulating EBV DNA as a tumor marker for nasopharyngeal carcinoma.' *Seminars in Cancer Biology* 12:489–96.

Chandler, M.J., and C. Lalonde. 1998. 'Cultural continuity as a hedge against suicide in Canada's First Nations.' *Transcultural Psychiatry* 35:191–219.

Chang, C.K., and C.M. Ulrich. 2003. 'Hyperinsulinaemia and hyperglycaemia: Possible risk factors of colorectal cancer among diabetic patients.' *Diabetologia* 46:595–607.

Chaussonnet, V. 1995. *Crossroads Alaska: Native Cultures of Alaska and Siberia.* Washington, DC: Arctic Studies Center, National Museum of Natural History, Smithsonian Institution.

Check, E. 2006. 'Bird flu: On border patrol.' *Nature* 442:348–50.

Cheshko, S. 2000. *Disintegration of the USSR: Ethnopolitical Analysis* (in Russian). Moscow: Institute of Ethnology and Anthropology, Russian Academy of Sciences.

Chesnais, J.C. 1992. *The Demographic Transition: Stages, Patterns, and Economic Implications. A Longitudinal Study of Sixty-Seven Countries Covering the Period 1720–1984.* Translated by E. Kreager and P. Kreager. Oxford: Clarendon Press.

Chiou, L.A., T.W. Hennessy, A. Horn, G. Carter, J.C. Butler. 2002. 'Botulism among Alaska natives in the Bristol Bay area of southwest Alaska: A survey of knowledge, attitudes, and practices related to fermented foods known to cause botulism.' *International Journal of Circumpolar Health* 61:50–60.

Christensen, B., L. Arbour, P. Tran, D. Leclerc, N. Sabbaghian, R. Platt, B.M. Gilfix, D.S. Rosenblatt, R.A. Gravel, P. Forbes, and R. Rozen. 1999. 'Genetic polymorphisms in methylenetetrahydrofolate reductase and methionine synthase, folate levels in red cells and risk of neural tube defects.' *American Journal of Medical Genetics* 84:151–7.

Christensen, H.P., H. Schmidt, and H.O. Bang. 1954. 'Measles in virgin soil: Greenland 1951.' *Danish Medical Bulletin* 1:2–6.

Christiansen, J., P. Poulsen, and K. Ladefoged. 2004. 'Invasive pneumococcal disease in Greenland.' *Scandinavian Journal of Infectious Diseases* 36:325–9.

Clark, A.M. 1974. 'The Athapaskans: Strangers of the North.' In *The Athapaskans: Strangers of the North*, 17–42. Ottawa: National Museum of Man.

Clark, G.A., M.A. Kelly, J.M. Grange, and M.C. Hill. 1987. 'The evolution of mycobacterial disease in human populations.' *Current Anthropology* 28:45–62.

Coates, K.S. 2004. *A Global History of Indigenous Peoples: Struggle and Survival.* New York: Palgrave Macmillan.

Coble, J.D., and R.E. Rhodes. 2006. 'Physical Activity and Native Americans.' *American Journal of Preventive Medicine* 31:36–46.

Coleshaw, S.R.K., R.N.M. Van Someren, A.H. Wolff, H.M. Davis, and W.R.

Keatinge. 1983. 'Impaired memory registration and speed of reasoning caused by low body temperature.' *Journal of Applied Physiology* 55:27–31.

Colgrove, J. 2002. 'The McKeown thesis: A historical controversy and its enduring influence.' *American Journal of Public Health* 92:725–9.

Comstock, G.W., C. Baum, and D.E. Snider. 1979. 'Isoniazid prophylaxis among Alaskan Eskimos: A final report of the Bethel isoniazid studies.' *American Review of Respiratory Diseases* 119:827–30.

Cottle, T., M. Bruce, and S. Deeks. 2006. 'International circumpolar surveillance of invasive bacterial diseases.' Paper presented at the 13th International Congress on Circumpolar Health, June 2006, Novosibirsk, Russia.

Curriero, F.C., K.S. Heiner, J.M. Samet, S.L. Zeger, L. Strug, and J.A. Patz. 2002. 'Temperature and mortality in 11 cities of the eastern United States.' *American Journal of Epidemiology* 155:80–7.

Curtis, T., S. Kvernmo, and P. Bjerregaard. 2005. 'Changing living conditions, life style and health.' *International Journal of Circumpolar Health* 64:442–50.

Curtis, T., H.B. Larsen, K. Helweg-Larsen, C.P. Pedersen, I. Olesen, K. Sørensen, M. Jørgensen, and P. Bjerregaard. 2006. *Unges trivsel i Grønland 2004.* Nuuk: Grønlands Hjemmestyre.

Daerga, L., A. Edin-Liljegren, and P. Sjölander. 2004. 'Work-related musculoskeletal pain among reindeer herding Sami in Sweden – a pilot study on causes and prevention.' *International Journal of Circumpolar Health* 63 (Suppl. 2):343–8.

Damas, D., ed. 1984. *Handbook of North American Indians.* Vol. 5. *Arctic.* Washington, DC: Smithsonian Institution.

– 1996. 'The Arctic from Norse contact to modern times.' In B.G. Trigger and W.E. Washburn, eds., *The Cambridge History of the Native Peoples of the Americas.* Vol. 1, 329–99. Cambridge: Cambridge University Press.

Danet, S., F. Richard, M. Montaye, S. Beauchant, B. Lemaire, C. Graux, D. Cottel, N. Marecaux, and P. Amouyel. 1999. 'Unhealthy effects of atmospheric temperature and pressure on the occurrence of myocardial infarction and coronary deaths: A 10–year survey.' *Circulation* 100(1):E1–7.

Davidson, M., A.J. Parkinson, L.R. Bulkow, M.A. Fitzgerald, H.V. Peters, and D.J. Parks. 1994. 'The epidemiology of invasive pneumococcal disease in Alaska, 1986–1990: Ethnic differences and opportunities for prevention.' *Journal of Infectious Diseases* 170:368–76.

Davis, F.M., A.D. Baddeley, and T.R. Hancock. 1975. 'Diver performance: The effect of cold.' *Undersea Biomedical Research* 2:195–213.

Davydova, G.M. 1989. *Anthropology of Mansi.* Moscow: Institute of Ethnography, USSR Academy of Sciences.

Day, G.E., and A.P. Lanier. 2003. 'Alaska Native mortality, 1979–1998.' *Public Health Reports* 118:518–30.

de Knijff, P., L.G. Johansen, M. Rosseneu, R.R. Frants, J. Jespersen, and L.M. Havekes. 1992. 'Lipoprotein profile of a Greenland Inuit population.' *Arteriosclerosis and Thrombosis* 12:1371–9.

de Maat, M.P., E.M. Bladbjerg, L.G. Johansen, J. Bentzen, and J. Jespersen. 1997. 'PlA1/A2 polymorphism of platelet glycoprotein IIIa and risk of cardiovascular disease.' *Lancet* 349:1099–100.

de Maat, M.P., E.M. Bladbjerg, L.G. Johansen, P. de Knijff, J. Gram, C. Kluft, and J. Jespersen. 1999. 'DNA-polymorphisms and plasma levels of vascular disease risk factors in Greenland Inuit – is there a relation with the low risk of cardiovascular disease in the Inuit?' *Thrombosis and Haemostasis* 81:547–52.

de Maat, M.P., P. de Knijff, F.R. Green, A.E. Thomas, J. Jespersen, and C. Kluft. 1995. 'Gender-related association between beta-fibrinogen genotype and plasma fibrinogen levels and linkage disequilibrium at the fibrinogen locus in Greenland Inuit.' *Arteriosclerosis, Thrombosis and Vascular Biology* 15:856–60.

de Maat, M.P., F. Green, P. de Knijff, J. Jespersen, and C. Kluft. 1997. 'Factor VII polymorphisms in populations with different risks of cardiovascular disease.' *Arteriosclerosis, Thrombosis and Vascular Biology* 17:1918–23.

Demina, M.N., E.L. Lensky, E.P. Petrenko, and O.E. Sokolenko. 1998. 'The analysis of the death rate connected to alcoholic abuse, in the Chukotka Autonomous Area (1980–1994).' In: *Chukotka: Nature and Man* (in Russian), 118–23. Magadan: Scientific Information Center 'Chukotka,' North-Eastern Scientific Centre, Far Eastern Department of the Russian Academy of Sciences.

Demura, S., T. Kitabayashi, A. Kimura, and J. Matsuzawa. 2005. 'Body sway characteristics during static upright posture in health and disordered elderly.' *Journal of Physiology, Anthropology, and Applied Human Sciences* 24:551–5.

Desrochers, F., and M.A. Curtis. 1987. 'The occurrence of gastrointestinal helminths in dogs from Kuujjuaq (Fort Chimo, Quebec, Canada).' *Canadian Journal of Public Health* 78:403–6.

Dewailly, E., C. Blanchet, S. Lemieux, L. Sauvé, S. Gingras, P. Ayotte, and B.J. Holub. 2001. 'N-3 fatty acids and cardiovascular disease risk factors among the Inuit of Nunavik.' *American Journal of Clinical Nutrition* 74:464–73.

Dewailly, E., G. Mulvad, H. Sloth Pedersen, J.C. Hansen, N. Behrendt, and J.P. Hart Hansen. 2003. 'Inuit are protected against prostate cancer.' *Cancer Epidemiology, Biomarkers and Prevention* 12:926–7.

Dewhurst, S., P.E. Riches, M.A. Nimmo, and G. De Vito. 2005. 'Temperature dependence of soleus h-reflex and M wave in young and older women.' *European Journal of Applied Physiology* 94:491–9.

Diamond, J. 2004. *Collapse: How Societies Choose to Fail or Succeed.* New York: Viking.

Diekstra, R.F. 1993. 'The epidemiology of suicide and parasuicide.' *Acta Psychiatrica Scandinavica* 371 (Suppl.):9–20.

Dippe, S.E., M. Miller, P.H. Bennett, J.E. Maynard, and K.R. Berquist. 1975. 'Lack of causal association between Coxsackie B4 virus infection and diabetes.' *Lancet* 1:1314–7.

Dixon, E.J. 2006. 'Paleo-Indian: Far Northwest.' In D.H. Ubelaker, ed., *Handbook of North American Indians.* Vol. 3, *Environment, Origins, and Population,* 129–47. Washington, DC: Smithsonian Institution.

Donaldson, G.C., S.P. Ermakov, Y.M. Komarov, C.P. McDonald, and W.R. Keatinge. 1998. 'Cold related mortalities and protection against cold in Yakutsk, eastern Siberia: Observation and interview study.' *British Medical Journal* 317:978–82.

Donaldson, G.C., H. Rintamäki, and S. Näyhä. 2001. 'Outdoor clothing: Its relationship to geography, climate, behaviour and cold-related mortality in Europe.' *International Journal of Biometeorology* 45:45–51.

Donaldson, G.C., V.E. Tchernjavskii, S.P. Ermakov, K. Bucher, and W.R. Keatinge. 1998. 'Winter mortality and cold stress in Yekaterinburg, Russia: Interview survey.' *British Medical Journal* 316:514–8.

Dupouy-Camet, J. 2000. 'Trichinellosis: A worldwide zoonosis.' *Veterinary Parasitology* 93:191–200.

Duval, L., L. MacDonald, L. Lugtig, J. Mollins, and R. Tate. 1994. 'Otitis media in the Keewatin: 20 years of experience 1970–1991.' *Arctic Medical Research* 53 (Suppl. 2):676–9.

Dyerberg, J. 1989. 'Coronary heart disease in Greenland Inuit: A paradox. Implications for western diet patterns.' *Arctic Medical Research* 48:47–54.

Ebbesson, S.O., C.D. Schraer, P.M. Risica, A.I. Adler, L. Ebbesson, A.M. Mayer, E.V. Shubnikof, J. Yeh, O.T. Go, and D.C. Robbins. 1998. 'Diabetes and impaired glucose tolerance in three Alaskan Eskimo populations: The Alaska-Siberia Project.' *Diabetes Care* 21:563–9.

Ebbesson, S.O.E., P.M. Risica, L.O. Ebbesson, and J. Kennish. 2005. 'Eskimos have CHD despite high consumption of omega-3 fatty acids: The Alaska Siberia Project.' *International Journal of Circumpolar Health* 64:387–95.

Edin-Liljegren, A., S. Hassler, P. Sjölander, and L. Daerga. 2004. 'Risk factors for cardiovascular diseases among Swedish Sami: A controlled cohort study.' *International Journal of Circumpolar Health* 63 (Suppl. 2):292–7.

Egeland, G.M., P. Berti, R. Soueida, L. Arbour, O. Receveur, and H. Kuhnlein. 2004. 'Age differences in vitamin A intake among Canadian Inuit.' *Canadian Journal of Public Health* 95:465–9.

Elfenbein, D.S., and M.E. Felice. 2003. 'Adolescent pregnancy.' *Pediatric Clinics of North America* 50:781–800.

Ellis, H.D. 1982. 'The effects of cold on the performance of serial choice reaction time and various discrete tasks.' *Human Factors* 24:589–98.

Ellis, H.D., S.E. Wilcock, and S.A. Zaman. 1985. 'Cold and performance: The effects of information load, analgesics, and the rate of cooling.' *Aviation, Space and Environmental Medicine* 56:233–7.

Elsner, R.W., K.L. Andersen, and L. Hermansen. 1960. 'Thermal and metabolic responses of Arctic Indians to moderate cold exposure at the end of winter.' *Journal of Applied Physiology* 15:659–61.

Elsner, R.W., J.D. Nelms, and L. Irving. 1960. 'Circulation of heat to the hands of Arctic Indians.' *Journal of Applied Physiology* 15:662–6.

Embedslægeinstitutionen i Grønland. (various years). *Årsberetning.* Nuuk: Directoratet for Sundhed.

– 2004. 'HIV/AIDS 2003.' *Embedslægeinstitutionens Nyhedsbrev*, no. 1.

Enander, A. 1984. 'Performance and sensory aspects of work in cold environments: A review.' *Ergonomics* 27:365–78.

– 1987. 'Effects of moderate cold on performance of psychomotor and cognitive tasks.' *Ergonomics* 30:1431–45.

Eng, H., and J.B. Mercer. 1998. 'Seasonal variations in mortality caused by cardiovascular diseases in Norway and Ireland.' *Journal of Cardiovascular Risk* 5:89–95.

Eriks-Brophy, A., and H. Ayukawa. 2000. 'The benefits of Sound Field Amplification in classrooms of Inuit students of Nunavik: A pilot project.' *Language, Speech and Hearing Services in Schools* 31:324–35.

Eriksson, A.W., W. Lehman, and N.E. Simpson. 1980. 'Genetic studies on circumpolar populations.' In F.A. Milan, ed., *The Human Biology of Circumpolar Populations*, 81–168. Cambridge: Cambridge University Press.

Ervasti, O., K. Juopperi, P. Kettunen, J. Remes, H. Rintamaki, J. Latvala, R. Pihlajaniemi, T. Linna, and J. Hassi. 2004. 'The occurrence of frostbite and its risk factors in young men.' *International Journal of Circumpolar Health* 63:71–80.

Eshleman, J.A., R.S. Malhi, and D.G. Smith. 2003. 'Mitochondrial DNA studies of Native Americans: Conceptions and misconceptions of the population prehistory of the Americas.' *Evolutionary Anthropology* 12:7–18.

Eskesen, B., and B. Glahn. 1955. 'The epidemic of poliomyelitis in Greenland, 1953.' *Danish Medical Bulletin* 2:46–51.

Eurowinter Group. 1997. 'Cold exposure and winter mortality from ischaemic heart disease, cerebrovascular disease, respiratory disease, and all causes in warm and cold regions of Europe.' *Lancet* 349:1341–6.

Expert Committee on the Diagnosis and Classification of Diabetes Mellitus. 2003. 'Follow-up report on the diagnosis of diabetes mellitus.' *Diabetes Care* 26:3160–7.

Ezzati, M., A.D. Lopez, A. Rodgers, and C.J.L. Murray, eds. 2004. *Comparative Quantification of Health Risks: Global and Regional Burden of Diseases Attributable to Selected Major Risk Factors.* Geneva: World Health Organization.

Fandrick, B. 2005. 'Water management issues in Inuit communities.' *Inuit Tapiriit Kanatami Environment Bulletin* 3:9–11.

Fanella, S., S.B. Harris, T.K. Young, A.J. Hanley, B. Zinman, P.W. Connelly, and R.A. Hegele. 2000. 'Association between PON1 L/M55 polymorphism and plasma lipoproteins in two Canadian aboriginal populations.' *Clinical Chemistry and Laboratory Medicine* 38:413–20.

Faulkner, J.A., E. Zerba, and S.V. Brooks. 1990. 'Muscle temperature of mammals: cooling impairs most functional properties.' *American Journal of Physiology* 28:259–65.

Federal State Statistics Service. 2003. *Russian Statistics Yearbook 2000* (in Russian). Moscow: Novosti Press.

– 2005. *Economic and Social Indicators for the Districts of Residence of Indigenous Numerically Small Peoples of the North 2004* (in Russian). Moscow: Rosstat.

– 2006a. *The Demographic Yearbook of Russia 2006* (in Russian and English). Moscow: Rosstat.

– 2006b. *Regions of Russia: Main Characteristics of Subjects of the Russian Federation* (in Russian). Moscow: Rosstat.

– 2006c. *Public Health in Russia* (in Russian). Moscow: Rosstat.

Fergusson, D.M., L.J. Woodward, and L.J. Horwood. 2000. 'Risk factors and life processes associated with the onset of suicidal behaviour during adolescence and early adulthood.' *Psychological Medicine* 30:23–39.

Ferry, J. 2000. 'No easy answer to high native suicide rates.' *Lancet* 355:906.

Feschbach, M., ed. 1995. *Environmental and Health Atlas of Russia* (in Russian). Moscow: PAIMS Press.

Fibiger, J. 1923. 'Über das Vorkommen von Krebs und Geswülsten in Grönland.' *Zeitschrift für Krebsforschung* 20:148–87.

Fisher, E.B., D. Haire-Joshu, G.D. Morgan, H. Rehberg, and K. Rost. 1990. 'Smoking and smoking cessation.' *American Review of Respiratory Diseases* 142:702–20.

Fitzhugh, W.W., and A. Crowell, eds. 1988. *Crossroads of Continents: Cultures of Siberia and Alaska*. Washington, DC: Smithsonian Institution.

Fog-Poulsen, M. 1955. 'Poliomyelitis in Greenland.' *Danish Medical Bulletin* 2:241–6.

– 1957. 'Mæslingeepidemier i Grønland.' *Ugeskrift for Læger* 119:509–20.

Forsyth, J. 1992. *A History of the Peoples of Siberia: Russia's North Asian Colony, 1581–1990*. Cambridge: Cambridge University Press.

Fortuine, R. 1989. *Chills and Fever: Health and Disease in the Early History of Alaska*. Fairbanks: University of Alaska Press.

– 2005. *'Must We All Die?' Alaska's Enduring Struggle with Tuberculosis*. Fairbanks: University of Alaska Press.

– 2006. *A Century of Adventure in Northern Health: The Public Health Service Commissioned Corps in Alaska, 1879–1978*. Andover, MD: PHS Commissioned Officers Foundation for the Advancement of Public Health.

Friborg, J., A. Koch, J. Wohlfarht, H.H. Storm, and M. Melbye. 2003. 'Cancer in Greenlandic Inuit 1973–1997: A cohort study.' *International Journal of Cancer* 107:1017–22.

Friborg, J., J. Wohlfahrt, A. Koch, H. Storm, O.R. Olsen, and M. Melbye. 2005. 'Cancer susceptibility in nasopharyngeal carcinoma families: A population-based cohort study.' *Cancer Research* 65:8567–72.

Friesen, T.M. 2004. 'Contemporaneity of Dorset and Thule cultures in the North American Arctic: New radiocarbon dates from Victoria Island, Nunavut.' *Current Anthropology* 45:685–91.

Fumoleau, R. 1975. *As Long as This Land Shall Last: A History of Treaty 8 and Treaty 11, 1870–1939*. Toronto: McClelland and Stewart.

Furnham, A., and P. Baguma. 1994. 'Cross-cultural differences in the evaluation of male and female body shapes.' *International Journal of Eating Disorders* 15:81–9.

Gad, F. 1971–82. *The History of Greenland*. 3 vols. Montreal: McGill-Queen's University Press.

Gadjiev, Y., and V.I. Akopov. 2005. 'Evaluation of economic development levels of the Russian North regions.' In V.N. Lazhencev, ed., *The North as an Object for Complex Regional Research* (in Russian), 197–225. Syktyvkar: Komi Scientific Centre.

Galloway, V.A., W.R. Leonard, and E. Ivakine. 2000. 'Basal metabolic adaptation of the Evenki reindeer herders of Central Siberia.' *American Journal of Human Biology* 12:75–87.

Gao, C., and J. Abeysekera. 2004. 'A systems perspective of slip and fall accidents on icy and snowy surfaces.' *Ergonomics* 47:573–98.

Gerasimova, E., N. Perova, I. Ozerova, V. Polessky, V. Metelskaya, I.

Sherbakova, M. Levachev, S. Kulakova, Y. Nikitin, and A. Astakhova A. 1991. 'The effect of dietary n-3 polyunsaturated fatty acids on HDL cholesterol in Chukot residents vs Muscovites.' *Lipids* 26:261–5.

Gessner, B.D., H.C. Baggett, P.T. Muth, E. Dunaway, B.D. Gold, Z. Feng, and A.J. Parkinson. 2006. 'A controlled, household-randomized, open-label trial of the effect that treatment of *Helicobacter pylori* infection has on iron deficiency in children in rural Alaska.' *Journal of Infectious Diseases* 193:537–46.

Gessner, B.D., M. Moore, B. Hamilton, and P.T. Muth. 2004. 'The incidence of infant physical abuse in Alaska.' *Child Abuse and Neglect* 28:9–23.

Gessner, B.D., and T.M. Wickizer. 1997. 'The contribution of infectious diseases to infant mortality in Alaska.' *Pediatric Infectious Disease Journal* 16:773–9.

Geurts, C.L., G.G. Sleivert, and S.S. Cheung. 2005. 'Local cold acclimation of the hand impairs thermal responses of the finger without improving hand neuromuscular function.' *Acta Physiologica Scandinavica* 183:117–24.

Gielen, A.C., and D. Sleet. 2003. 'Application of behaviour-change theories and methods to injury prevention.' *Epidemiologic Reviews* 25:65–76.

Giesbrecht, G.G., J.L. Arnett, E. Vela, and G.K. Bristow. 1993. 'Effect of task complexity on mental performance during immersion hypothermia.' *Aviation, Space and Environmental Medicine* 64:206–11.

Gilberg, R. 1984. 'Polar Eskimo.' In D. Damas, ed., *Handbook of North American Indians*. Vol. 5., *Arctic*, 577–94. Washington, DC: Smithsonian Institution.

Gissler, M., and E. Vuori. 2005. *Perinatal Statistics in the Nordic Countries*. Helsinki: STAKES.

Gjertsen, F. 1995. 'Variations of suicide rate in the population: Historical perspectives with special reference to the 1970s and 1980s' (in Norwegian). *Tidsskrift for den Norske Laegeforening* 115:18–22.

– 2002. 'Cause of death registry: An important data source for medical research' [in Norwegian]. *Tidsskrift for den Norske Laegeforening* 122: 2551–4.

Godel, J.C., T.K. Basu, H.F. Pabst, R.S. Hodges, P.E. Hodges, and M.L. Ng. 1996. 'Perinatal vitamin A (retinol) status of northern Canadian mothers and their infants.' *Biology of the Neonate* 69:133–9.

Goldsmith, S., J. Angvik, L. Howe, A. Hill, and L. Leask. 2004. *The Status of Alaska Natives Report 2004*. Anchorage: University of Alaska Anchorage Institute of Social and Economic Research.

Gordon, R.G., Jr., ed. 2005. *Ethnologue: Languages of the World*. 15th ed. Dallas: SIL International.

Gould, M.S., S. Wallenstein, M.H. Kleinman, P. O'Caroll, and J. Mercy. 1990. 'Suicide clusters: An examination of age-specific effects.' *American Journal of Public Health* 80:211–2.

Green, A., and C.C. Patterson on behalf of the EURODIAB TIGER Study Group. 2001. 'Trends in the incidence of childhood-onset diabetes in Europe 1989–1998.' *Diabetologia* 44 (Suppl. 3):B3–8.

Green, T., J. Middaugh, S. Saxon, and C.J. Utermohle. 2004. *Alaska Youth Risk Behavior Survey 2003.* Anchorage: Department of Health and Social Services.

Greenberg, J.H., C.G. Turner, and S.L. Zegura. 1986. 'The settlement of the Americas: A comparison of the linguistic, dental, and genetic evidence.' *Current Anthropology* 27:477–97.

Gribble, J.N., and S. Preston, eds. 1993. *The Epidemiological Transition: Policy and Planning Implications for Developing Countries.* Washington, DC: National Academy Press.

Grøholt, B., O. Ekeberg, L. Wichstrom, and T. Haldorsen. 1997. 'Youth suicide in Norway, 1990–1992: A comparison between children and adolescents completing suicide and age- and gender-matched controls.' *Suicide and Life-Threatening Behavior* 27:250–63.

– 2000. 'Young suicide attempters: A comparison between a clinical and an epidemiological sample.' *Journal of the American Academy of Child and Adolescent Psychiatry* 39:868–75.

Grønlands Statistik. 2006. *Tilgangen af boliger og bolighestand 2005.* Nuuk: Grønlands Statistik.

Grønlands Statistik. (various years). *Befolkningens bevægelser.* Nuuk: Grønlands Statistik.

Grønnow, B., and I. Pind, eds. 1996. *The Paleo-Eskimo Cultures of Greenland: New Perspectives on Greenlandic Archaeology.* Copenhagen: Danish Polar Centre.

Grove, O., and I. Lynge. 1979. 'Suicide and attempted suicide in Greenland: A controlled study in Nuuk (Godthaab).' *Acta Psychiatrica Scandinavica* 60:375–91.

Grzybowski, S., K. Styblo, and E. Dorken. 1976. 'Tuberculosis in Eskimos.' *Tubercle* 57 (Suppl. 4):S1–58.

Guettier, J.M., A. Georgopoulos, M.Y. Tsai, V. Radha, S. Shanthirani, R. Deepa, M. Gross, G. Rao, and V. Mohan. 2005. 'Polymorphisms in the fatty acid-binding protein 2 and apolipoprotein C-III genes are associated with the metabolic syndrome and dyslipidemia in a South Indian population.' *Journal of Clinical Endocrinology and Metabolism* 90:1705–11.

Guyot, M., C. Dickson, C. Paci, C. Furgal, and H.M. Chan. 2006. 'Local observations of climate change and impacts on traditional food security in two northern Aboriginal communities.' *International Journal of Circumpolar Health* 65:403–15.

Gyllerup, S., J. Lanke, L.H. Lindholm, and B. Schersten. 1992. 'Socioeconomic factors in the community fail to explain the high coronary mortality in cold parts of Sweden.' *European Heart Journal* 13:878–81.

Haddon, W. 1980. 'Advances in the epidemiology of injuries as a basis for public policy.' *Public Health Rep.* 95:411–21.

Håglin, L. 1991. 'Nutrient intake among Saami people today compared with an old, traditional Saami diet.' *Arctic Medical Research* Suppl.1:741–6.

– 1999. 'The nutrient density of present-day and traditional diets and their health aspects: The Sami and lumberjack families living in rural areas of Northern Sweden.' *International Journal of Circumpolar Health* 58:30–43.

Hahn, G.H., A. Koch, M. Melbye, and K. Molbak. 2005. 'Pattern of drug prescription for children under the age of four years in a population in Greenland.' *Acta Paediatrica* 94:99–106.

Haines, A., and J.A. Patz. 2004. 'Health effects of climate change.' *Journal of the American Medical Association* 291:99–103.

Hajat, S., W. Bird, and A. Haines. 2004. 'Cold weather and GP consultations for respiratory conditions of elderly people in 16 locations in the UK.' *European Journal of Epidemiology* 19:959–68.

Haldorsen, T., and T. Tynes. 2005. 'Cancer in the Sami population of North Norway, 1970–1997.' *European Journal of Cancer Prevention* 14:63–8.

Hallman, T., G. Burell, S. Setterlind, A. Oden, and J. Lisspers. 2001. 'Psychosocial risk factors for coronary heart disease, their importance compared with other risk factors and gender differences in sensitivity.' *Journal of Cardiovascular Risk* 8:39–49.

Hamilton, S., J. Martin, M. Guyot, M. Trifonopoulos, A. Caughey, and H.M. Chan. 2004. 'Healthy living in Nunavut: an on-line nutrition course for Inuit communities in the Canadian Arctic.' *International Journal of Circumpolar Health* 63:243–50.

Hammel, H.T., K.L. Andersen, P.F. Scholander, C.S. Coon, A. Medina, L. Strozzi, F.A. Milan, and R.J. Hock. 1960. 'Thermal and metabolic responses of the Alacuf Indians to moderate cold exposure.' *WADD Technical Report*, 60–633.

Hankins, G.W. 2000. *'Sunrise over Pangnirtung': The Story of Otto Schaefer, MD.* Calgary: Arctic Institute of North America.

Hansen, J.C., B. Deutch, and H.S. Pedersen. 2004. 'Selenium status in Greenland Inuit.' *Science of the Total Environment* 331:207–14.

Hansen, J.P.H., J. Melgaard, and J. Nordquist. 1985. 'The mummies of Qilakitsoy.' *National Geographic* 167:191–207.

Harpaz, R., B.J. McMahon, H.S. Margolis, C.N. Shapiro, D. Havron, G. Carpenter, L.R. Bulkow, and R.B. Wainwright. 2000. 'Elimination of new chronic hepatitis B virus infections: Results of the Alaska immunization program.' *Journal of Infectious Diseases* 181:413–8.

Hart, J.S., H.B. Sabean, J.A. Hildes, F. Depocas, H.T. Hammel, K.L. Andersen, L. Irving, and G. Foy. 1962. 'Thermal and metabolic responses of coastal Eskimos during a cold night.' *Journal of Applied Physiology* 17:953–60.

Hassi, J. 2005. 'Cold extremes and impact on health.' In W. Kirch, B. Menne, and R. Bertollini, eds., *Extreme Weather Events and Public Health Responses*, 59–67. Berlin: Springer-Verlag, published on behalf of the WHO Regional Office for Europe.

Hassi, J., L. Gardner, S. Hendricks, and J. Bell. 2000. 'Occupational injuries in the mining industry and their association with statewide cold ambient temperatures in the USA.' *American Journal of Industrial Medicine* 38:49–58.

Hassi, J. and T.M. Mäkinen. 2000. 'Frostbites: occurrence, risk factors and consequences.' *International Journal of Circumpolar Health* 59:92–8.

Hassi, J., T.M. Mäkinen, and H. Rintamäki H. 2005. 'Prediction and prevention of frostbite.' In *Prevention of Cold Injuries*, KN1:1–KN1:10. Proceedings of a NATO Meeting RTO-MP-HFM-126.

Hassi, J., J. Remes, J.T. Kotaniemi, P. Kettunen, and S. Näyhä. 2000b. 'Dependence of cold-related coronary and respiratory symptoms on age and exposure to cold.' *International Journal of Circumpolar Health* 59:210–15.

Hassi, J., K. Sikkilä, A. Ruokonen, and J. Leppäluoto. 2001. 'The pituitary-thyroid axis in health men living under subarctic climatological conditions.' *Journal of Endocrinology* 169:195–203.

Hassler, S. 2005. 'The Health Condition in the Sami Population of Sweden, 1961–2002.' PhD diss., Umeå University, Sweden (Umeå University Medical Dissertations, New Series No. 962).

Hassler, S., R. Johansson, P. Sjölander, H. Grönberg, and L. Damber. 2005. 'Causes of death in the Sami population of Sweden, 1961–2000.' *International Journal of Epidemiology* 34:623–9.

Hassler, S., P. Sjölander, M. Barnekow-Bergkvist, and A. Kadesjö. 2001. 'Cancer risk in the reindeer breeding Saami population of Sweden, 1961–1997.' *European Journal of Epidemiology* 17:969–76.

Hassler, S., P. Sjölander, and A.J. Ericsson. 2004. 'Construction of a database on health and living conditions of the Swedish Sami population.' In P. Lantto and P. Skld, eds., *Befolkning och Bosättning I Norr – etnicitet, identitet och gränser I historiens sken*, 107–24. Umeå, Sweden: Centre for Sami Research.

Hassler, S., P. Sjölander, R. Johansson, H. Grönberg, and L. Damber. 2004. 'Fatal accidents and suicide among reindeer herding Sami in Sweden.' *International Journal of Circumpolar Health* 63 (Suppl. 2):384–8.

Havenith, G. 1995. 'The hand in the cold, performance and risk.' *Arctic Medical Research* 54 (Suppl. 2):37–47.

Healey, S., D. Plaza, and G. Osborne. 2003. *A Ten-Year Profile of Cancer in*

Nunavut, 1992–2001. Iqaluit: Nunavut Department of Health and Social Services.

Health Canada. 2000. *Perinatal Health Indicators for Canada: A Resource Manual.* Ottawa: Health Canada (Cat. No. H49-135/2000E).

– 2001. *Unintentional and Intentional Injury Profile for Aboriginal People in Canada, 1990–1999.* Ottawa: Health Canada (Cat. No. H35-4/8-1999).

– 2005. *Analysis of Arctic Children and Youth Health Indicators.* Produced for the Arctic Council Sustainable Development Working Group. Ottawa: Health Canada (Cat. No. H34-129/2005E).

Health and Welfare Canada. (various years). *Report on Health Conditions in the Northwest Territories.* Yellowknife: Medical Services Branch, Northwest Territories Region.

– 1991. *Health Status of Canadian Indians and Inuit, 1990.* Ottawa: Health and Welfare Canada, Medical Services Branch (Cat. No. H34-48/1991E).

Healy, J.D. 2003. 'Excess winter mortality in Europe: A cross country analysis identifying key risk factors.' *Journal of Epidemiology and Community Health.* 57:784–9.

Hegele, R.A. 1999. 'Genetic prediction of atherosclerosis: Lessons from studies in native Canadian populations.' *Clinica Chimica Acta* 286:47–61.

Hegele, R.A., C. Anderson, T.K. Young, and P.W. Connelly. 1999. 'G-protein beta3 subunit gene splice variant and body fat distribution in Nunavut Inuit.' *Genome Research* 9:972–7.

Hegele, R.A., M.R. Ban, and T.K. Young. 2001. 'Serum C-reactive protein in Canadian Inuit and its association with genetic variation on chromosome 1q21.' *Clinical Chemistry* 47:1707–9.

Hegele, R.A., C.P. Busch, T.K. Young, P.W. Connelly, and H. Cao. 1999. 'Mannose-binding lectin gene variation and cardiovascular disease in Canadian Inuit.' *Clinical Chemistry* 45:1283–5.

Hegele, R.A., S.B. Harris, J.H. Brunt, T.K. Young, A.J. Hanley, B. Zinman, and P.W. Connelly. 1999. 'Absence of association between genetic variation in the LIPC gene promoter and plasma lipoproteins in three Canadian populations.' *Atherosclerosis* 146:153–60.

Hegele, R.A., M.W. Huff, and T.K. Young. 2001. 'Common genomic variation in LMNA modulates indexes of obesity in Inuit.' *Journal of Clinical Endocrinology and Metabolism* 86:2747–51.

Hegele, R.A., C. Tully, T.K. Young, and P.W. Connelly. 1997. 'V677 mutation of methylenetetrahydrofolate reductases and cardiovascular disease in Canadian Inuit.' *Lancet* 349:1221–2.

Hegele, R.A., J. Wang, S.B. Harris, J.H. Brunt, T.K. Young, A.J. Hanley, B. Zinman, P.W. Connelly, and C.M. Anderson. 2001. 'Variable association between genetic variation in the CYP7 gene promoter and plasma lipoproteins in three Canadian populations.' *Atherosclerosis* 154:579–87.

Hegele, R.A., Young, T.K., and P.W. Connelly. 1997. 'Are Canadian Inuit at increased genetic risk for coronary heart disease?' *Journal of Molecular Medicine* 75:364–70.

Helander, E. 1992. 'The Sami of Norway.' In *Nytt fra Norge*. Oslo: Ministry of Foreign Affairs.

Helm, J., ed. 1981. *Handbook of North American Indians*, Vol. 16, *Subarctic*. Washington, DC: Smithsonian Institution.

– 2000. *The People of Denendeh: Ethnohistory of the Indians of Canada's Northwest Territories*. Montreal: McGill-Queen's University Press.

Hennessy, T.W., R.J. Singleton, L.R. Bulkow, D.L. Bruden, D.A. Hurlburt, D. Parks, M. Moore, A.J. Parkinson, A. Schuchat, and J.C. Butler. 2005. 'Impact of heptavalent pneumococcal conjugate vaccine on invasive disease, antimicrobial resistance and colonization in Alaska Natives: Progress towards elimination of a health disparity.' *Vaccine* 23:5464–73.

Hensel, M.R., T. Cavanagh, A.P. Lanier, T. Gleason, B. Bouwens, H. Tanttila, A. Reimer, R.L. Dinwiddie, and J.C. Hayes. 1995. 'Quit rates at one year follow-up of Alaska Native Medical Center Tobacco Cessation Program.' *Alaska Medicine* 37:43–7.

Hermansen, R., I. Njølstad, and V. Fonnebo. 2002. 'Physical activity according to ethnic origin in Finnmark County, Norway. The Finnmark Study.' *International Journal of Circumpolar Health* 61:189–200.

Hetta, O.M., P. Somby, Ø. Vandbakk, A. Nordsletta, R. Solbakk, and A.I. Keskitalo. 1978. 'Alcoholism in the Sàmi (Lappis) areas of Indre-Finnmark.' Paper presented at the International Council of Alcohol and Addictions meeting in Fairbanks, Alaska, 15–20 April 1978.

Heus, R., H.A. Daanen, and G. Havenith. 1995. 'Physiological criteria for functioning of hands in the cold: A review.' *Applied Ergonomics* 26:5–13.

Heyerdahl, S., S. Kvernmo, and L. Wichstrøm L. 2004. 'Self-reported behavioural/emotional problems in Norwegian adolescents from multiethnic areas.' *European Child and Adolescent Psychiatry* 13:64–72.

Hildes, J.A., and O. Schaefer. 1984. 'The changing picture of neoplastic disease in the western and central Canadian Arctic (1950–1980).' *Canadian Medical Association Journal* 130:25–32.

Hildesheim, A., L.M. Anderson, C.J. Chen, Y.J. Cheng, L.A. Brinton, A.K. Daly, C.D. Reed, I.H. Chen, N.E. Caporaso, M.M. Hsu, J.Y. Chen, J.R. Idle, R.N. Hoover, C.S. Yang, and S.K. Chhabra. 1997. 'CYP2E1 genetic polymorphisms and risk of nasopharyngeal carcinoma in Taiwan.' *Journal of the National Cancer Institute* 89:1207–12.

Hildesheim, A., R.J. Apple, C.J. Chen, S.S. Wang, Y.J. Cheng, W. Klitz, S.J. Mack, I.H. Chen, M.M. Hsu, C.S. Yang, L.A. Brinton, P.H. Levine, and H.A. Erlich. 2002. 'Association of HLA class I and II alleles and extended haplotypes with nasopharyngeal carcinoma in Taiwan.' *Journal of the National Cancer Institute* 94:1780–9.

Hisdal, J., and R.E. Reinertsen. 1998. 'Seasonal changes in finger blood flow in urban citizens.' In I. Holmér and K. Kuklane, eds., *Problems with Cold Work* (*Arbete och hälsa*) 18:172–4.

Hobart, C.W. 1975. 'Socioeconomic correlates of mortality and morbidity among Inuit infants.' *Arctic Anthropology* 12(1):37–48.

Hodgins, S. 1997. 'Infant and child health' In: *Health and What Affects It in Nunavik: How Is the Situation Changing?* Kuujjuaq, Quebec: Department of Public Health, Nunavik Regional Board of Health and Social Services.

Hodgins, S., R.W. Peeling, S. Dery, F. Bernier, A. LaBrecque, J.F. Proulx, J. Joly, M. Alary, and D. Mabey. 2002. 'The value of mass screening for chlamydia control in high prevalence communities.' *Sexually Transmitted Infections* 78 (Suppl. 1):i64–8.

Hoeppner, V.H., and D.D. Marciniuk. 2000. 'Tuberculosis in aboriginal Canadians.' *Canadian Respiratory Journal* 7(2):141–6.

Hoffecker, J.F. 2005. *A Prehistory of the North: Human Settlement of the Higher Latitudes*. New Brunswick, NJ: Rutgers University Press.

Hoffecker, J.F., and S.A. Elias. 2003. 'Environment and archeology in Beringia.' *Evolutionary Anthropology* 12:34–49.

Hoffman, R.G. 2001. 'Human psychological performance in cold environments.' In K.B. Pandolf and R.E. Burr, eds., *Textbook of Military Medicine: Medical Aspects of Harsh Environments*, 384–410. Washington, DC: Borden Institute of the Walter Reed Army Medical Center.

Holmér, I. 1994. 'Cold stress: Part II. The scientific basis (knowledge base) for the guide.' *International Journal of Industrial Ergonomics* 14:151–9.

Homøe, P. 1997. 'Pneumatization of the temporal bone and otitis media in ancient and modern Greenlanders.' *Meddelelser om Grønland* 22:1–42.

Homøe, P., R.B. Christensen, and P. Bretlau. 1996. 'Prevalence of otitis media in a survey of 591 unselected Greenlandic children.' *International Journal of Pediatric Otorhinolaryngology* 36:215–30.

– 1999a. 'Acute otitis media and age at onset among children in Greenland.' *Acta Otolaryngologica* 119:65–71.

– 1999b. 'Acute otitis media and sociomedical risk factors among unselected children in Greenland.' *International Journal of Pediatric Otorhinolaryngology* 49:37–52.

Homøe P. J. Prag, S. Farholt, J. Henrichsen, A. Hornsleth, M. Kilian, and J.S.

Jensen. 1996. 'High rate of nasopharyngeal carriage of potential pathogens among children in Greenland: Results of a clinical survey of middle-ear disease.' *Clinical Infectious Diseases* 23:1081–90.

Hordvin, O., ed. 2005. *The Drug Situation in Norway 2005: Annual Report to the European Monitoring Centre for Drugs and Drug Addiction.* Oslo: Norwegian Institute for Alcohol and Drug Research.

Hovland, A. 1996. *Moderne urfolk – samisk ungdom i bevegelse.* Oslo: Cappelen akademiske forlag.

Howard, B.V., R.B. Devereux, S.A. Cole, M. Davidson, B. Dyke, S.O. Ebbesson, S.E. Epstein, D.R. Robinson, B. Jarvis, D.J. Kaufman, S. Laston, J.W. MacCluer, P.M. Okin, M.J. Roman, T. Romenesko, G. Ruotolo, M. Swenson, C.R. Wenger, S. Williams-Blangero, J. Zhu, C. Saccheus, R.R. Fabsitz, and D.C. Robbins. 2005. 'A genetic and epidemiologic study of cardiovascular disease in Alaska natives (GOCADAN): Design and methods.' *International Journal of Circumpolar Health* 64:206–21.

Hunter, E., and D. Harvey. 2002. 'Indigenous suicide in Australia, New Zealand, Canada, and the United States.' *Emergency Medicine* (Fremantle, WA) 14:14–23.

Iafrate, A.J., L. Feuk, M.N. Rivera, M.L. Listewnik, P.K. Donahoe, Y. Qi, S.W. Scherer, and C. Lee. 2004. 'Detection of large-scale variation in the human genome.' *Nature Genetics* 36:949–51.

Iburg, K.M., H. Brønnum-Hansen, and P. Bjerregaard. 2001. 'Health expectancy in Greenland.' *Scandinavian Journal of Public Health* 29:5–12.

Intergovernmental Panel on Climate Change. 2001. *Climate Change 2001: The Scientific Basis. Contribution of Working Group I to the Third Assessment Report of the IPCC.* Cambridge: Cambridge University Press.

– *Climate Change 2007: The Physical Science Basis. Contribution of Working Group I to the Fourth Assessment Report of the IPCC.* Cambridge: Cambridge University Press.

International Agency for Research on Cancer. 2003. *World Cancer Report.* Lyon: IARC.

International Diabetes Federation. 2005. *The IDF Consensus Worldwide Definition of the Metabolic Syndrome.* Brussels: IDF.

International Organization of Standardization. 2005. *Ergonomics of the Thermal Environment. Working Practices in Cold: Strategy for Risk Assessment and Management.* (ISO DIS 15743) Geneva: IOS.

International Union of Physiological Sciences. Thermal Commission. 2001. 'Glossary of terms for thermal physiology.' *Japanese Journal of Physiology* 51:245–80.

Ireland, J., V.E. Carlton, M. Falkowski, M. Moorhead, K. Tran, F. Useche, P.

Hardenbol, A. Erbilgin, R. Fitzgerald, T.D. Willis, and M. Faham. 2006. 'Large-scale characterization of public database SNPs causing non-synonymous changes in three ethnic groups.' *Human Genetics* 119:75–83.

Irving, L., K.L. Andersen, A. Bolstand, R.W. Elsner, J.A. Hildes, Y. Loyning, J.D. Nelms, L.J. Peyton, and R.D. Whaley. 1960. 'Metabolism and temperature of Arctic Indian men during a cold night.' *Journal of Applied Physiology* 15:635–44.

Jamison, D.T., W.H. Mosley, A.R. Measham, and J.L. Bobadilla, eds. 1993. *Disease Control Priorities in Developing Countries.* New York: Oxford University Press.

Javo, C., J.A. Rønning, and S. Heyerdahl. 2004. 'Child-rearing an indigenous Sami population in Norway: A cross-cultural comparison of parental attitudes and expectations.' *Scandinavian Journal of Psychology* 45:67–78.

Jenkins, A.L., T.W. Gyorkos, L. Joseph, K.N. Culman, B.J. Ward, G.S. Pekeles, and E.L. Mills. 2004. 'Risk factors for hospitalization and infection in Canadian Inuit infants over the first year of life: A pilot study.' *International Journal of Circumpolar Health* 63:61–70.

Jetté, M. 1994. *Santé Québec: A Health Profile of the Inuit.* Montreal: Ministère de la Santé et des Services sociaux.

Jones, H.E., and R.L.Balster. 1998. 'Inhalant abuse in pregnancy.' *Obstetrics and Gynecology Clinics of North America* 25:153–67.

Jones, V.H., and S.L. Dunavan. 2006. 'Tobacco.' In D.H. Ubelaker, ed., *Handbook of North American Indians*, Vol. 3, *Environment, Origins, and Population*, 447–51. Washington, DC: Smithsonian Institution.

Jørgensen, M.E., P. Bjerregaard, and K. Borch-Johnsen. 2002. 'Diabetes and impaired glucose tolerance among the Inuit population of Greenland.' *Diabetes Care* 25:1766–71.

Jørgensen, M.E., P. Bjerregaard, F. Gyntelberg, K. Borch-Johnsen, and the Greenland Population Study. 2004. 'Prevalence of the metabolic syndrome among the Inuit in Greenland: A comparison between two proposed definitions.' *Diabetic Medicine* 21:1237–42.

Jørgensen, M.E., P. Bjerregaard, J.J. Kjærgaard, and K. Borch-Johnsen. In press. 'High prevalence of markers of coronary heart disease among Greenland Inuit.' *Atherosclerosis.*

Jørgensen, M.E., K. Borch-Johnsen, and P. Bjerregaard. 2006. 'Lifestyle modifies obesity-associated risk of cardiovascular disease in a genetically homogeneous population.' *American Journal of Clinical Nutrition* 84:29–36.

Jørgensen, M.E., Glumer, C., P. Bjerregaard, F. Gyntelberg, T. Jørgensen, and K. Borch-Johnsen. 2003. 'Obesity and central fat pattern among Greenland

Inuit and a general population of Denmark (Inter99): Relationship to metabolic risk factors.' *International Journal of Obesity* 27:1507–15.

Jørgensen, M.E., H. Moustgaard, P. Bjerregaard, and K. Borch-Johnsen. 2006. 'Gender differences in the association between westernization and metabolic risk among Greenland Inuit.' *European Journal of Epidemiology* 21:741–8.

Juopperi, K., J. Hassi, and O. Ervasti. 2002. 'Incidence of frostbite and ambient temperature in Finland, 1986–1995: A national study based on hospital admissions.' *International Journal of Circumpolar Health* 61:352–62.

Kaessmann, H., S. Zollner, A.C. Gustafsson, V. Wiebe, M. Laan, J. Lundeberg, and Pääbo S. 2002. 'Extensive linkage disequilibrium in small human populations in Eurasia.' *American Journal of Human Genetics* 70:673–85.

Kaplan, S.D., A.P. Lanier, R.K. Merritt, and P.Z. Siegel. 1997. 'Prevalence of tobacco use among Alaska Natives : A review.' *Preventive Medicine* 26:460–5.

Kapur, B., and G. Koren. 2001. 'Folic acid fortification of flour three years later.' *Canadian Journal of Clinical Pharmacology* 8:91–2.

Karron, R.A., R.J. Singleton, L. Bulkow, A. Parkinson, D. Kruse, I. DeSmet, C. Indorf, K.M. Petersen, D. Leombruno, D. Hurlburt, M. Santosham, and L.H. Harrison. 1999. 'Severe respiratory syncytial virus disease in Alaska native children: RSV Alaska Study Group.' *Journal of Infectious Diseases* 180:41–9.

Katzmarzyk, P.T., and W.R. Leonard. 1998. 'Climatic influences on human body size and proportions: Ecological adaptations and secular trends.' *American Journal of Physical Anthropology* 106:483–503.

Keatinge, W.R., S.R. Coleshaw, and F. Cotter. 1984. 'Increases in platelet and red cell counts, blood viscosity, and arterial pressure during mild surface cooling: Factors in mortality from coronary and cerebral thrombosis in winter.' *British Medical Journal (Clinical Research)* 289:1405–8.

Keatinge, W.R., G.C. Donaldson, and K. Bucher. 2000. 'Winter mortality in relation to climate.' *International Journal of Circumpolar Health* 59:154–9.

Kelly, J.J., A.P. Lanier, S. Alberts, and C.L. Wiggins. 2006. 'Differences in cancer incidence among Indians in Alaska and New Mexico and U.S. Whites, 1993–2002.' *Cancer Epidemiology, Biomarkers and Prevention* 15:1515–19.

Kharamzin, N.G., and N.G. Khairullina. 2002. *Traditional Social-Economic Structure and Way of Life among the Ob Ugrians (Based on Sociological Research)* (in Russian). Moscow: IKAR.

Kinney, P. 2005. 'Firearm deaths in the NWT.' *EpiNorth* 17(2):1–3.

Kirmayer, L.J. 1994. 'Suicide among Canadian aboriginal peoples.' *Transcultural Psychiatric Research Review* 31:3–58.

Kirmayer, L.J., L.J. Boothroyd, and S. Hodgins. 1998. 'Attempted suicide among Inuit youth: Psychosocial correlates and implications for prevention.' *Canadian Journal of Psychiatry* 43:816–22.

Kirmayer, L.J., G.M. Brass, and C.L. Tait. 2000. 'The mental health of Aboriginal peoples: Transformations of identity and community.' *Canadian Journal of Psychiatry* 45:607–16.

Kirmayer, L.J., M. Malus, and L.J. Boothroyd. 1996. 'Suicide attempts among Inuit youth: A community survey of prevalence and risk factors.' *Acta Psychiatrica Scandinavica* 94:8–17.

Kleivan, I. 1984. 'West Greenland before 1950.' In D. Damas, ed., *Handbook of North American Indians*. Vol. 5, *Arctic*, 595–621. Washington, DC: Smithsonian Institution.

Kloner, R.A. 2006. 'Natural and unnatural triggers of myocardial infarction.' *Progress in Cardiovascular Diseases* 48:285–300.

Kloner, R.A., W.K. Poole, and R.L. Perritt. 1999. 'When throughout the year is coronary death most likely to occur? A 12–year population-based analysis of more than 220,000 cases.' *Circulation* 100:1630–4.

Knoches, A.M., and L.W. Doyle. 1993. 'Long-term outcome of infants born preterm.' *Baillieres Clin Obstet Gynaecol* 7:633–51.

Koch, A., T.G. Krause, K.A. Krogfelt, O.R. Olsen, T.K. Fischer, and M. Melbye. 2005. 'Seroprevalence and risk factors for Helicobacter pylori infection in Greenlanders.' *Helicobacter* 10:433–42.

Koch, A., M. Melbye, P. Sørensen, P. Homøe, H.O. Madsen, K. Mølbak, C.H. Hansen, L.H. Andersen, G.W. Hahn, and P. Garred. 2001. 'Acute respiratory tract infections and mannose-binding lectin insufficiency during early childhood.' *Journal of the American Medical Association* 285:1316–21.

Koch, A., K. Mølbak, P. Homøe, P. Sorensen, T. Hjuler, M.E. Olesen, J. Pejl, F.K. Pedersen, O.R. Olsen, and M. Melbye. 2003. 'Risk factors for acute respiratory tract infections in young Greenlandic children.' *American Journal of Epidemiology* 158:374–84.

Koch, A., P. Sørensen, P. Homøe, K. Molbak, F.K. Pedersen, T. Mortensen, H. Elberling, A.M. Eriksen, O.R. Olsen, and M. Melbye. 2002. 'Population-based study of acute respiratory infections in children, Greenland.' *Emerging Infectious Diseases* 8:586–93.

Kogan, M.D., J.A. Martin, G.R. Alexander, M. Kotelchuck, S.J. Ventura, and F.D. Frigoletto. 1998. 'The changing pattern of prenatal care utilization in the United States, 1981–1995, using different prenatal care indices.' *Journal of the American Medical Association* 279:1623–8.

Kotaniemi, J.T., J. Latvala, B. Lundbäck, A. Sovijärvi, J. Hassi, and K. Larsson. 2003. 'Does living in a cold climate or recreational skiing increase the risk for obstructive respiratory diseases or symptoms?' *International Journal of Circumpolar Health* 62:142–57.

Kotaniemi, J.T., P. Pallasaho, A. Sovijärvi, L. A. Laitinen, and B. Lundbäck. 2002. 'Respiratory symptoms and asthma in relation to cold climate, inhaled allergens and irritants.' *Journal of Asthma* 39:649–58.

Kovesi, T., D. Creery, N.L. Gilbert, R. Dales, D. Fugler, B. Thompson, N. Randhawa, and J.D. Miller. 2006. 'Indoor air quality risk factors for severe lower respiratory tract infections in Inuit infants in Baffin region, Nunavut: A pilot study.' *Indoor Air* 16:266–75.

Kozlov, A. 2004. 'Impact of economic changes on the diet of Chukotka natives.' *International Journal of Circumpolar Health* 63:235–42.

– 2006. 'Alcohol consumption and alcohol-related problems in indigenous populations of northern Russia' (in Russian). *Narcology* 10(58):22–9.

Kozlov, A., and G. Vershubsky. 1999. *Medical Anthropology of the Native Inhabitants of the North of Russia* (in Russian). Moscow: MNEPU.

Kozlov, A., G. Vershubsky, and M. Kozlova. 2003. 'Stress under modernization in indigenous populations of Siberia.' *International Journal of Circumpolar Health* 62:158–66.

Kozlov, A.I., and E.V. Zdor. 2003. 'Whaling products as an element of indigenous diet in Chukotka.' *Anthropology of East Europe Review,* 21:127–37.

Kraemer, L.D., J.E. Berner, and C.M. Furgal. 2005. 'The potential impact of climate on human exposure to contaminants in the Arctic.' *International Journal of Circumpolar Health* 64:498–508.

Krarup, H.B., S. Andersen, P. Madsen, and P. Laurbjerg. 2005. 'Hepatitis B among Inuit in East and West Greenland: A population study.' *Hepatology* 42 (Suppl. 1):726A.

Krauss, M.E. 1997. 'The indigenous languages of the north: A report on their present state.' In H. Shoji and J. Janhunen, eds., *Northern Minority Languages: Problems of Survival,* 1–34. Osaka: National Museum of Ethnology.

Krauss, M.E., and V.K. Golla. 1981. 'Northern Athapaskan languages.' In J. Helm, ed., *Handbook of North American Indians*, Vol. 6, *Subarctic*, 67–85. Washington, DC: Smithsonian Institution.

Kriska, A.M., A.J. Hanley, S.B. Harris, and B. Zinman. 2001. 'Physical activity, physical fitness, and insulin and glucose concentrations in an isolated Native Canadian population experiencing rapid lifestyle change.' *Diabetes Care* 24:1787–92.

Krog, J., B. Folkow, R.H. Fox, and K.L. Andersen. 1960. 'Hand circulation in the cold of Lapps and North Norwegian fishermen.' *Journal of Applied Physiology* 15:654–8.

Krug, E.G., L.C. Dahlberg, J.A. Mercy, A.B. Zwi, and R. Lozano, eds. 2002. *World Report on Violence and Health*. Geneva: World Health Organization.

Kuh, D., and Y. Ben-Shlomo. 2004. *A Life Course Approach to Chronic Disease Epidemiology*. 2nd ed. New York: Oxford University Press.

Kuhnlein, H.V. 1995. 'Benefits and risks of traditional food for indigenous peoples: Focus on dietary intakes of Arctic men.' *Canadian Journal of Physiology and Pharmacology* 73:765–71.

Kuhnlein, H.V., S.A. Kubow, and R. Soueida. 1991. 'Lipid components of traditional Inuit foods and diets of Baffin Island.' *Journal of Food Composition and Analysis* 4:227–36.

Kuhnlein, H.V., O. Receveur, R. Soueida, and G. Egeland. 2004. 'Arctic Indigenous peoples experience the nutrition transition with changing dietary patterns and obesity.' *Journal of Nutrition* 134:1447–53.

Kuhnlein, H.V., R. Soueida, and O. Receveur. 1996. 'Dietary nutrient profiles of Canadian Baffin Island Inuit differ by food source, season, and age.' *Journal of the American Dietetic Association* 96:155–62.

Kunitz, S.J. 1996. 'The history and politics of U.S. health care policy for American Indians and Alaska Natives.' *American Journal of Public Health* 86:1464–73.

Kunst, A.E., C.W. Looman, and J.P. Mackenbach. 1993. 'Outdoor air temperature and mortality in the Netherlands: A time-series analysis.' *American Journal of Epidemiology* 137:331–41.

Kurilovitsch, S.A., A.V. Avksentyuk, I.A. Yakuschenko, and M.I. Voevoda. 1994. 'Alcohol drinking among Chukotka Natives: The myths and reality.' In G. Pétursdottir, G., S.B. Sigurdsson, M.M. Karlsson, and J. Axelsson, eds., *Circumpolar Health 93*. Proceedings of the 9th International Congress on Circumpolar Health. *Arctic Medical Research* 53 (Suppl. 2):545–65.

Kusters, J.G., A.H. van Vliet, and E.J. Kuipers. 2006. 'Pathogenesis of *Helicobacter pylori* infection.' *Clinical Microbiology Reviews* 19:449–90.

Kvernmo, S. 1995. 'Preventive health programs among Sami adolescents in a Sami community.' *Arctic Medical Research* 54 (Suppl. 1):107–12.

– 2000. 'North Norwegian Adolescents in a Multiethnic Context: A Study of Emotional and Behavioural Problems, Ethnic Identity and Acculturation Attitudes in Sami, Kven and Norwegian Adolescents.' PhD diss., University of Tromsø.

– 2004. 'Mental health of Sami youth.' *International Journal of Circumpolar Health* 63:221–34.

Kvernmo, S., and S. Heyerdahl. 1996. 'Ethnic identity in aboriginal Sami adolescents: The impact of the family and the ethnic community context.' *Journal of Adolescence* 19:453–63.

– 1998. 'Influence of ethnic factors on behavior problems in indigenous Sami and majority Norwegian adolescents.' *Journal of the American Academy of Child and Adolescent Psychiatry* 37:743–51.

– 2003. 'Acculturation strategies and ethnic identity as predictors of behavior problems in arctic minority adolescents.' *Journal of the American Academy of Child and Adolescent Psychiatry* 42:57–65.

– 2004. 'Ethnic identity and acculturation attitudes among indigenous Norwegian Sami and ethnocultural Kven adolescents.' *Journal of Adolescent Research* 19:512–32.

Kvernmo, S., Y. Johansen, A.R. Spein, and A.C. Silviken. 2003. 'Ung in Sàpmi: Helse, identitet og levekår blant samisk ungdom.' *Oaidnil: Tidsskriftserie for senter for samisk helseforskning* 1:1–65.

Kvist, R. 1986. 'Samerna och alkoholen – Jokkmokks socken 1760–1860.' *Tidsskrift for Nordisk Alkoholforskning* 3:122–8.

Lambden, J., O. Receveur, J. Marshall, and H.V. Kuhnlein. 2006. 'Traditional and market food access in Arctic Canada is affected by economic factors.' *International Journal of Circumpolar Health* 65:331–40.

Lander, E.S., and N.J. Schork. 1994. 'Genetic dissection of complex traits.' *Science* 265:2037–48.

Landslægeembedet. 1992. *Sundhedstilstanden i Grønland. Årsberetning for 1991.* Nuuk: Landslægeembedet.

Landslaegan på Færøerne. (various years). *Medicinalberetning for Færøerne.* Tórshavn: Landslaegan på Færøerne.

Langdon, S.J. 1987. *The Native People of Alaska.* Anchorage: Greatland Graphics.

Lange, A. 1998. *Samer om diskriminering.* Stockholm: Centrum för invandringsforskning, Stockholm University.

Langer, B.C., G.G. Frosner, and A. von Brunn. 1997. 'Epidemiological study of viral hepatitis types A, B, C, D and E among Inuits in West Greenland.' *Journal of Viral Hepatitis* 4:339–49.

Lanier, A.P., and S.R. Alberts. 1996. 'Cancers of the buccal cavity and pharynx in circumpolar Inuit.' *Acta Oncologica* 35:545–52.

Lanier, A.P., T. Bender, M. Talbot, S. Wilmeth, C. Tschopp, W. Henle, G. Henle, D. Ritter, and P. Terasaki. 1980. 'Nasopharyngeal carcinoma in Alaskan Eskimos Indians, and Aleuts: A review of cases and study of Epstein-Barr virus, HLA, and environmental risk factors.' *Cancer* 46:2100–6.

Lanier, A.P., G.W. Bornkamm, W. Henle, G. Henle, T.R. Bender, M.L. Talbot, and P.H. Dohan. 1981. 'Association of Epstein-Barr virus with nasopharyngeal carcinoma in Alaskan native patients: Serum antibodies and tissue EBNA and DNA.' *International Journal of Cancer* 28:301–5.

Lanier, A.P., L.R. Bulkow, T.E. Novotny, G.A. Giovino, and R.M. Davis. 1990. 'Tobacco use and its consequences in northern population.' *Arctic Medical Research* 49 (Suppl. 2):17–22.

Lanier, A.P., P. Holck, J. Kelly, B. Smith, and T. McEvoy. 2001. 'Alaska Native cancer survival.' *Alaska Medicine* 43:61–9.

Lanier, A.P., J.J. Kelly, P. Holck, B. Smith, T. McEvoy, and J. Sandidge. 2001. 'Cancer incidence in Alaska Natives: Thirty-year report 1969–1998.' *Alaska Medicine* 43:87–115.

Lanier, A.P., J.J. Kelly, J. Maxwell, T. McEvoy, and C. Homan. 2006. *Cancer in Alaska Natives, 1969–2003: 35–Year Report.* Anchorage: Alaska Native Tribal Health Consortium.

Lantto, P. 2000. 'Tiden börjar på nytt: En analys av samernas etnopolitiska mobilisering i Sverige 1900–1950.' *Kulturens Frontlinjer* 32:36–56.

– 2004. 'Nationell symbol, etnisk markör eller utdöende näring? Bilden av renskötseln och dess betydelse inom samerörelsen i Sverige 1900–1960.' In P. Lantto and P. Sköld, eds., *Befolkning och Bosättning i Norr – etnicitet, identitet och gränser i historiens sken,* 279–97. Umeå, Sweden: Centre for Sami Research.

Larke, R.P., G.J. Froese, R.D. Devine, and M.W. Petruk. 1987. 'Extension of the epidemiology of hepatitis B in circumpolar regions through a comprehensive serologic study in the Northwest Territories of Canada.' *Journal of Medical Virology* 22:269–76.

Larsen, S. 1992. 'Saami and Norwegian clients' use of a treatment facility for drug and alcohol problems in northern Norway.' *Arctic Medical Research* 51:81–6.

– 1993. 'The origin of alcohol-related social norms in the Saami minority.' *Addiction* 88:501–8.

Larsen, S., and R. Nergård. 1990. 'Cultural background and drinking patterns in problem drinkers in northern Norway.' *British Journal of Addictions* 85:1469–73.

Larsen, S., and J. Saglie. 1996. 'Alcohol use in Saami and non-Saami areas in northern Norway.' *European Addiction Research* 2:78–82.

Larsson, K., G. Tornling, D. Gavhed, C. Muller-Suur, and L. Palmberg. 1998. 'Inhalation of cold air increases the number of inflammatory cells in the lungs in healthy subjects.' *European Respiratory Journal* 12:825–30.

Leamon, A. 2005. 'A descriptive study of motor vehicle land transportation injuries in the NWT.' *EpiNorth* 17(2):15–18.

LeBlanc, J. 1962. 'Local adaptation to cold of Gaspé fishermen.' *Journal of Applied Physiology* 17:950–2.

Ledrou, I., and J. Gervais. 2005. 'Food insecurity.' *Health Reports* 16:47–51.

Lehtola, V.P. 2004. *The Sámi People: Traditions in Transition.* 2nd rev. ed. Translated by L.W. Müller-Wille. Inari, Finland: Kustannus-Puntsi.

Leighton, A.H., and C.C. Hughes. 1955. 'Notes on Eskimo patterns of suicide.' *Southwestern Journal of Anthropology* 11:327–8.

Leineweber, M., P. Bjerregaard, C. Baerveldt, and P. Voestermans. 2001. 'Suicide in a society in transition.' *International Journal of Circumpolar Health* 60:280–7.

Lensky, E.L., T.V. Chernobrovkina, I.V. Arkavyj, and M.I. Litovka. 1998. 'Prospective analysis of death rate connected with alcoholism in the Chukotka Autonomous Area between 1980 and 1994' (in Russian). *Alcoholism* 10:1–10.

Leonard, W.R., M.V. Sorensen, V.A. Galloway, G.J. Spencer, M.J. Mosher, L. Osipova, and V.A. Spitsyn. 2002. 'Climatic influences on basal metabolic rates among circumpolar populations.' *American Journal of Human Biology* 14:609–20.

Leppäluoto, J., I. Korhonen, and J. Hassi. 2001. 'Habituation of thermal sensations, skin temperatures, and norepinephrine in men exposed to cold air.' *Journal of Applied Physiology* 90:1211–8.

Leppäluoto, J., T. Pääkkönen, I. Korhonen, and J. Hassi. 2005. 'Pituitary and autonomic responses to cold exposures in man.' *Acta Physiologica Scandinavica* 184:255–64.

Leppäluoto, J., K. Sikkilä, and J. Hassi. 1998. 'Seasonal variation of serum TSH and thyroid hormones in males living in subarctic environmental conditions.' *International Journal of Circumpolar Health* 57:383–5.

Lester, D. 1999. 'Native American suicide rates, acculturation stress and traditional integration.' *Psychological Reports* 84:398.

– 2006. 'Suicide in Siberian aboriginal groups.' *Archives of Suicide Research* 10:221–4.

Levin, M.G., and L.P. Potapov. 1964. *The Peoples of Siberia.* Chicago: University of Chicago Press.

Levine, M., L. Duffy, D.C. Moore, and L.A. Matej. 1995. 'Acclimation of a non-indigenous sub-Arctic population: Seasonal variation in thyroid function in interior Alaska.' *Comparative Biochemistry and Physiology Part A* 111:209–14.

Lewinsohn, P.M., P. Rohde, and J.R. Seeley. 1996. 'Adolescent suicidal ideation and attempts: Prevalence, risk factors, and clinical implications.' *Clinical Psychology -Science and Practice* 3:25–46.

Lipworth, L., L.R. Bailey, and D. Trichopoulos. 2000. 'History of breast-feeding in relation to breast cancer risk: A review of the epidemiologic literature.' *Journal of the National Cancer Institute* 92:302–12.

Liu, J., A.J.G. Hanley, T.K. Young, S.B. Harris, and B. Zinman. 2006. 'Characteristics and prevalence of the metabolic syndrome among three ethnic groups in Canada.' *International Journal of Obesity* 30:669–76.

Livingston, S.E., J.P. Simonetti, B.J. McMahon, L.R. Bulkow, K.J. Hurlburt, C.E. Homan, M.M. Snowball, H.H. Cagle, J.L. Williams, and V.P. Chulanov. 2007. 'Hepatitis B virus genotypes in Alaska native people with hepatocellular carcinoma: Preponderance for genotype F.' *Journal of Infectious Diseases* 195:5–11.

Logan, S., and N. Spencer. 1996. 'Smoking and other health related behaviours in the social and environmental context.' *Archives of Disease in Childhood* 74:176–9.

Lohse, N., K. Ladefoged, L. Pedersen, S. Jensen-Fangel, H.T. Sorensen, and N. Obel. 2004. 'Low effectiveness of highly active antiretroviral therapy and high mortality in the Greenland HIV-infected population.' *Scandinavian Journal of Infectious Diseases* 36:738–42.

Long, W.B., III, R.F. Edlich, K.L. Winters, and L.D. Britt. 2005. 'Cold injuries.' *Journal of Long-Term Effects of Medical Implants* 15:67–78.

Lorenz, J.G., and D.G. Smith. 1996. 'Distribution of four founding mtDNA haplogroups among Native North Americans.' *American Journal of Physical Anthropology* 101:307–23.

Lund, M., and R. Lindbak. 2004. *Tall om tobakk 1973–2003*. Oslo: Statens Institutt for Rusmiddelforskning.

Lundmark, L. 2002. *'Lappen är ombytlig, ostadig och obekväm' – Svenska statens samepolitik i rasismens tidevarv*. Umeå, Sweden: Norrlands Universitetsförlag.

Luo, Z.C., R. Wilkins, R.W. Platt, and M.S. Kramer. 2004. 'Risks of adverse pregnancy outcomes among Inuit and North American Indian women in Quebec, 1985–97.' *Paediatric and Perinatal Epidemiology* 18:40–50.

Luoma, P., S. Näyhä, and J. Hassi. 1995. 'High serum concentrations of vitamin E and cholesterol and low mortality from ischaemic heart disease in northern Finland.' *Arctic Medical Research* 54 (Suppl. 2):26–8.

Luoma, P.V., S. Näyhä SL. Pyy, H. Korpela, and J. Hassi. 1992. 'Blood mercury and serum selenium concentrations in reindeer herders in the arctic area of northern Finland.' *Archives of Toxicology* 15:172–5.

Lynge, I. 1994. 'Suicide in Greenland.' In G. Pétursdottir, S.B. Sigurdsson, M.M. Karlsson, and J. Axelsson, eds., *Circumpolar Health 93*. Proceedings of the 9th International Congress on Circumpolar Health. *Arctic Medical Research* 53 (Suppl. 2):551–4.

– 1997. 'Mental disorders in Greenland: Past and present.' *Meddelelser om Grønland. Man and Society* 21:3–73.

Lynnerup, N. and S. Nørby. 2004. 'The Greenland Norse: Bones, graves, computers, and DNA.' *Polar Record* 40:107–11.

Macey, J.F., A. Roberts, L. Lior, T.W. Tam, and P. VanCaeseele. 2002. 'Outbreak of community-acquired pneumonia in Nunavut, October and November, 2000.' *Canada Communicable Diseases Reports* 28:131–8.

Mackenbach, J.P. 1996. 'The contribution of medical care to mortality decline: McKeown revisited.' *Journal of Clinical Epidemiology* 49:1207–13.

Mackesy-Amiti, M.E., and M. Fendrich. 1999. 'Inhalant use and delinquent behavior among adolescents: A comparison of inhalant users and other drug users.' *Addiction* 94:555–64.

Madsen, M.H., M. Grønbaek, P. Bjerregaard, U. Becker, and the Greeland Population Study. 2005. 'Urbanization, migration and alcohol use in a population of Greenland Inuit.' *International Journal of Circumpolar Health* 64:234–45.

Mahley, R.W. 1988. 'Apolipoprotein E: Cholesterol transport protein with expanding role in cell biology.' *Science* 240:622–30.

Maillard, V., P. Bougnoux, P. Ferrari, M.L. Jourdan, M. Pinault, F. Lavillonnière, G. Body, O. Le Floch, and V. Chajès. 2002. 'N-3 and N-6 fatty acids in breast adipose tissue and relative risk of breast cancer in a case-control study in Tours, France.' *International Journal of Cancer* 98:78–83.

Main Indices of Mother and Child Health and Functioning of Birth and Child Care Services in Russian Federation in 2003. 2004. Moscow: GEOTAR-MED.

Mäkinen, T.M. 2007. 'Human cold exposure, adaptation, and performance in high latitude environments.' *American Journal of Human Biology* 19:155–64.

Mäkinen, T.M., L.A. Palinkas, D.L. Reeves, T. Pääkkönen, H. Rintamäki, J. Leppäluoto, and J. Hassi. 2006. 'Effects of repeated exposures to cold on cognitive performance in humans.' *Physiology and Behaviour* 87:166–76.

Mäkinen, T.M., T. Pääkkönen, L.A. Palinkas, H. Rintamäki, J. Leppäluoto, and J. Hassi. 2004. 'Seasonal changes in thermal response of urban residents to cold exposure. *Comparative Biochemistry and Physiology Part A* 139:229–38.

Mäkinen, T.M., V.P. Raatikka, M. Rytkönen, J. Jokelainen, H. Rintamäki, R. Ruuhela, S. Näyhä, and J. Hassi. 2006. 'Factors affecting outdoor exposure in winter: Population-based study. *International Journal of Biometeorology* 51:27–36.

Mäkinen, T.M., H. Rintamäki, J.T. Korpelainen, V. Kampman, T. Pääkkönen, J. Oksa, L.A. Palinkas, J. Leppäluoto, and J. Hassi. 2005. 'Postural sway during single and repeated cold exposures.' *Aviation, Space, and Environmental Medicine* 76:947–53.

Maksimova, T.M. 2005. *Social Gradient in Promoting Health among Populations* (in Russian). Moscow: Per Se Publishers.

Mallet, M.L. 2002. 'Pathophysiology of accidental hypothermia.' *Quarterly Journal of Medicine* 95:775–85.

Mandelcorn, R., P.W. Connelly, A. Boright, T.K. Young, and R.A. Hegele.1998. 'F5 Q506 mutation and the low prevalence of cardiovascular disease in Canadian Inuit.' *Journal of Investigative Medicine* 46:232–5.

Mangerud, J., J.I. Svendsen, and V.I. Astakhov. 1999. 'The age and extent of the Barents and Kara Sea ice sheets in northern Russia.' *BOREAS.* 28:46–80.

Marchand, J.F. 1943. 'Tribal epidemics in the Yukon.' *Journal of the American Medical Association* 123:1019–20.

Martin, B.D., W.L. Smith, P. Orr, and F. Guijon. 1998. 'Follow-up of a decentralized colposcopy program for the investigation and management of cervical intraepithelial neoplasia in the central Canadian Arctic.' *International Journal of Circumpolar Health* 57 (Suppl. 1):406–9.

Martin, D. 2005. 'Quality of drinking water in Nunavik: How a changing climate affects disease.' *Inuit Tapiriit Kanatami Environment Bulletin* 3:13–15.

Martinsen, N., M.E. Jørgensen, P. Bjerregaard, A. Krasnik, B. Carstensen, and K. Borch-Johnsen. 2006. 'Predictions of type 2 diabetes and complications in Greenland in 2014.' *International Journal of Circumpolar Health* 65:243–52.

Marttunen, M.J., H.M. Aro, and J.K. Lönnqvist. 1992. 'Adolescent suicide: Endpoint of long-term difficulties.' *Journal of the American Academy of Child and Adolescent Psychiatry* 31:649–54.

Mason, R. 2004. 'Overview of the Social Transition in the North Project, 1995–1998.' *International Journal of Circumpolar Health* 63 (Suppl. 1):5–12.

McDonald, J.C., T.W. Gyorkos, B. Alberton, J.D. MacLean, G. Richer, and D. Juranek. 1990. 'An outbreak of toxoplasmosis in pregnant women in northern Quebec.' *Journal of Infectious Diseases* 61:769–74.

McGhee, R. 1996. *Ancient People of the Arctic.* Vancouver: UBC Press.

McKeown, I., P. Orr, S. Macdonald, A. Kabani, R. Brown, G. Coghlan, M. Dawood, J. Embil, M. Sargent, G. Smart, and C.N. Bernstein. 1999. '*Helicobacter pylori* in the Canadian arctic: Seroprevalence and detection in community water samples.' *American Journal of Gastroenterology* 94:1823–9.

McKeown, T. 1979. *The Role of Medicine: Dream, Mirage or Nemesis.* 2nd ed. Oxford: Basil Blackwell.

– 1988. *The Origins of Human Disease.* Oxford: Basil Blackwell.

McLaughlin, J.B. 2004. 'Botulism type E outbreak associated with eating a beached whale, Alaska.' *Emerging Infectious Diseases* 10:1685–7.

McLaughlin, J.B., A. DePaola, C.A. Bopp, K.A. Martinek, N.P. Napolilli, C.G. Allison, S.L. Murray, E.C. Thompson, M.M. Bird, and J.P. Middaugh. 2005. 'Outbreak of *Vibrio parahaemolyticus* gastroenteritis associated with Alaskan oysters.' *New England Journal of Medicine* 353:1463–70.

McMahon, B.J. 2004. 'Viral hepatitis in the Arctic.' *International Journal of Circumpolar Health* 63 (Suppl. 2):41–8.

McMahon, B.J., W.L. Alward, D.B. Hall, W.L. Heyward, T.R. Bender, D.P. Francis, and J.E. Maynard. 1985. 'Acute hepatitis B virus infection: relation of age to the clinical expression of disease and subsequent development of the carrier state.' *Journal of Infectious Diseases* 151:599–603.

McMahon, B.J., M. Beller, J. Williams, M. Schloss, H. Tanttila, and L. Bulkow. 1996. 'A program to control an outbreak of hepatitis A in Alaska by using an inactivated hepatitis A vaccine.' *Archives of Pediatrics and Adolescent Medicine* 150:733–9.

McMahon, B.J., M.G. Bruce, T.W. Hennessy, D.L. Bruden, F. Sacco, H. Peters, D.A. Hurlburt, J.M. Morris, A.L. Reasonover, G. Dailide, D.E. Berg, and A.J. Parkinson. 2006. 'Reinfection after successful eradication of *Helicobacter pylori*: A 2–year prospective study in Alaska Natives.' *Alimentary Pharmacology and Therapeutics* 23:1215–23.

McMahon, B.J., L. Bulkow, A. Harpster, M. Snowball, A. Lanier, F. Sacco, E. Dunaway, and J. Williams. 2000. 'Screening for hepatocellular carcinoma in Alaska natives infected with chronic hepatitis B: A 16–year population-based study.' *Hepatology* 32 (4 Pt 1):842–6.

McMahon, B.J., T.W. Hennessy, J.M. Bensler, D.L. Bruden, A.J. Parkinson, J.M. Morris, A.L. Reasonover, D.A. Hurlburt, M.G. Bruce, F. Sacco, and J.C. Butler. 2003. 'The relationship among previous antimicrobial use, antimicrobial resistance, and treatment outcomes for *Helicobacter pylori* infections.' *Annals of Internal Medicine* 139:463–9.

McMahon, B.J., A.P. Lanier, and R.B. Wainwright. 1998. Hepatitis B and hepatocellular carcinoma in Eskimo/Inuit population. *International Journal of Circumpolar Health* 57 (Suppl. 1):414–9.

McMahon, B.J., E.R. Rhoades, W.L. Heyward, E. Tower, D. Ritter, A.P. Lanier, R.B. Wainwright, and C. Helminiak. 1987. 'A comprehensive programme to reduce the incidence of hepatitis B virus infection and its sequelae in Alaskan natives.' *Lancet* 2 (8568):1134–6.

McNabb, S. 1992. 'Native claims in Alaska: A twenty-year review.' *Etudes/Inuit/Studies* 16(1–2):85–95.

Mehli, H., L. Skuterud, A. Mosdol, and A. Tonnessen. 2000. 'The impact of Chernobyl fallout on the Southern Saami reindeer herders of Norway in 1996.' *Health Physics* 79:682–90.

Mehlum, L., K. Hytten, and F. Gjertsen. 1999. 'Epidemiological trends of youth suicide in Norway.' *Archives of Suicide Research* 5:193–205.

Meldorf, G. 1907. 'Epidemiske Sygdomme i Grønland: Influenza og Epidemiske Katarrhalske Affektioner af Luftvejs-Slimhinderne.' *Meddelelser om Grønland* 33:129–305.

Melzer-Lange, M.D. 1998. 'Violence and associated high-risk health behavior in adolescents: Substance abuse, sexually transmitted diseases, and pregnancy of adolescents.' *Pediatric Clinics of North America* 45:307–17.

Menne, B., and L.E. Kristie, eds. 2006. *Climate Change and Adpatation Strategies for Human Health*. Geneva: WHO.

Mercer, J. 2003. 'Cold: An underrated risk factor for health.' *Environmental Research* 92:8–13.

Merriwether, D.A., F. Rothhammer, and R.R. Ferrell. 1995. 'Distribution of the four founding lineage haplotypes in Native Americans suggests a single wave of migration for the New World.' *American Journal of Physical Anthropology* 98:411–30.

Merriwether, D.A. 2006. 'Mitochondrial DNA.' In D.H. Ubelaker, ed., *Handbook of North American Indians*. Vol. 3, *Environment, Origins, and Population*, 817–30. Washington, DC: Smithsonian Institution.

Mersch, P.P.A., H.M. Middendorp, A.L. Bouhuys, D.G.M. Beersma, and R.H. van den Hoofdakker. 1999. 'Seasonal affective disorder and latitude: A review of the literature.' *Journal of Affective Disorders* 53:35–48.

Michael, M.P. 1984. 'Effects of Municipal Services and Housing on Public Health in the Northwest Territories.' PhD diss., University of Toronto.

Michalon, M., G.A. Eskes, and C.C. Mate-Kole. 1997. 'Effects of light therapy on neuropsychological function and mood in seasonal affective disorder.' *Journal of Psychiatry and Neuroscience* 22:19–28.

Middaugh, J.P. 1990. 'Cardiovascular deaths among Alaskan Natives, 1980–86.' *American Journal of Public Health* 80:282–5.

Millar, W.J. 1990a. 'Smoking prevalence in the Canadian Arctic.' *Arctic Medical Research* 49 (Suppl. 2):23–8.

– 1990b. 'Smokeless tobacco use by youths in the Canadian Arctic.' *Arctic Medical Research* 49 (Suppl. 2):39–47.

Miller, B.A., M. Davidson, D. Myerson, J. Icenogle, A.P. Lanier, J. Tan, and A.M. Beckmann AM. 1997. 'Human papillomavirus type 16 DNA in esophageal carcinomas from Alaska Natives.' *International Journal of Cancer* 71:218–22.

Minuk, G.Y., N. Ling, B. Postl, J.G. Waggoner, L.E. Nicolle, and J.H. Hoofnagle. 1985. 'The changing epidemiology of hepatitis B virus infection in the Canadian north.' *American Journal of Epidemiology* 121:598–604.

Minuk, G.Y., and J. Uhanova. 2003. 'Viral hepatitis in the Canadian Inuit and First Nations populations.' *Canadian Journal of Gastroenterology* 17:707–12.

Minuk, G.Y., J.G. Waggoner, R. Jernigan, L.E. Nicolle, B. Postl, and J.H. Hoofnagle. 1982. 'Prevalence of antibody to hepatitis A virus in an isolated Canadian Inuit community.' *Canadian Medical Association Journal* 127:850–2.

Mo, D. 2001. 'Injury mortality risk assessment and targeting the subpopulations for prevention in the Northwest Territories, Canada.' *International Journal of Circumpolar Health* 69:391–9.

Moffatt, M.E.K., J.D. O'Neil, and T.K. Young. 1994. 'Nutritional patterns of Inuit in the Keewatin region of Canada.' In G. Pétursdottir, S.B. Sigurdsson, M.M. Karlsson, and J. Axelsson, eds., Circumpolar Health 93. Proceedings of the 9th International Congress on Circumpolar Health. *Arctic Medical Research* 53 (Suppl. 2):722–5.

Mohatt, G.V, R. Plaetke, J. Klejka, B. Luick, C. Lardon, A. Bersamin, S. Hopkins, M. Dondanville, J. Herron, B. Boyer, and the CANHR Research team. 2007. 'The Center for Alaska Native Health Research Study: A community-based participatory research study of obesity and chronic disease-related protective and risk factors.' *International Journal of Circumpolar Health* 66:8–18.

Molchanov, Y.A. 1977. *The Earliest Stages of the Human Population of the North-Eastern Asia* (in Russian). Novosibirsk, Russia: Nauka.

Moller, L.N. 2006. *Epidemiology of Trichinella in Greenland: Occurrence in Animals and Man and Observations on Anisakidae Infections in Man.* Copenhagen: The Royal Veterinary and Agricultural University and Statens Serum Institut.

Moller, L.N., E. Petersen, C.M. Kapel, M. Melbye, and A. Koch. 2005. 'Outbreak of trichinellosis associated with consumption of game meat in West Greenland.' *Veterinary Parasitology* 132:131–6.

Mollersen, S., H.C. Sexton, and A. Holte. 2005. 'Ethnic variations in the initial phase of mental health treatment: A study of Sami and non-Sami clients and therapists in northern Norway.' *Scandinavian Journal of Psychology* 46:447–57.

Monsalve, M.V., G. Edin, and D.V. Devine. 1998. 'Analysis of HLA class I and class II Na-Dene and Amerindian populations from British Columbia, Canada.' *Human Immunology* 59:48–55.

Monsalve, M.V., A.C. Stone, C.M. Lewis, A. Rempel, M. Richards, D. Straathof, and D.V. Devine. 2002. 'Molecular analysis of the Kwäday Dän Ts'ìnchi ancient remains found in a glacier in Canada.' *American Journal of Physical Anthropology* 119:288–91.

Morrison, W.R. 1998. *True North: The Yukon and Northwest Territories*. Toronto: Oxford University Press.

Mouratoff, G.J., M.D. Berkeley, N.V. Carroll, and E.M. Scott. 1969. 'Diabetes mellitus in Athabascan Indians in Alaska.' *Diabetes* 18:29–32.

Mouratoff, G.J., N.V. Carroll, and E.M. Scott. 1967. 'Diabetes mellitus in Eskimos.' *Journal of the American Medical Association* 199:107–12.

Mouratoff, G.J., and E.M. Scott. 1973. 'Diabetes mellitus in Eskimos after a decade.' *Journal of the American Medical Association* 226:1345–6.

Mulligan, C.J., K. Hunley, S. Cole, and J.C. Long. 2004. 'Population genetics, history and health patterns in Native Americans.' *Annual Review of Genomics and Human Genetics* 5:295–315.

Murphy, N.J., C.D. Schraer, L.R. Bulkow, E.J. Boyko, and A.P. Lanier. 1992. 'Diabetes mellitus in Alaskan Yup'ik Eskimos and Athabascan Indians after 25 years.' *Diabetes Care* 15:1390–2.

Murphy, N.J., C.D. Schraer, M.C. Thiele, E.J. Boyko, L.R. Bulkow, B.J. Doty, and A.P. Lanier. 1995. 'Dietary change and obesity associated with glucose intolerance in Alaska Natives.' *Journal of the American Dietetic Association* 95:676–82.

– 1997. 'Hypertension in Alaska Natives: Association with overweight, glucose intolerance, diet and mechanized activity.' *Ethnicity and Health* 2:267–75.

Must, A., and S.E. Anderson. 2006. 'Body mass index in children and adolescents: Considerations for population-based applications.' *International Journal of Obesity* 30:590–4.

Nakano, T., K. Fediuk, N. Kassi, G.M. Egeland, and H.V. Kuhnlein. 2005. 'Dietary nutrients and anthropometry of Dene/Metis and Yukon children.' *International Journal of Circumpolar Health* 64:147–56.

Nakano, T., K. Fediuk, N. Kassi, and H.V. Kuhnlein. 2005. 'Food use of Dene/Metis and Yukon children.' *International Journal of Circumpolar Health* 64:137–46.

National Center for Health Statistics. (various years). *National Vital Statistics Reports*. Hyattsville, MD: NCHS, Department of Health and Human Services.

National Cholesterol Education Program (NCEP) Expert Panel on Detection, Evaluation, and Treatment of High Blood Cholesterol in Adults (Adult Treatment Panel III). 2001. 'The Third Report: Executive summary.' *Journal of the American Medical Association* 285:2486–97.

Näyhä, S. 1997. 'Low mortality from ischemic heart disease in the Sami district of Finland.' *Social Science and Medicine* 44:123–31.

- 2002. 'Cold and the risk of cardiovascular diseases: A review.' *International Journal of Circumpolar Health* 61:373–80.
- 2005. 'Environmental temperature and mortality.' *International Journal of Circumpolar Health* 64:451–9.

Näyhä, S., and J. Hassi, eds. 1993. *Lifestyle, Work and Health of Finnish Reindeer Herders.* Helsinki: Publications of the Social Insurance Institutions (ML 127).

Näyhä, S., and M.R. Järvelin. 1998. 'Health trends in northern Finland.' *International Journal of Circumpolar Health* 57:94–103.

Näyhä, S., K. Sikkilä, and J. Hassi. 1994. 'Cardiovascular risk factor patterns and their association with diet in Saami and Finnish Reindeer herders.' *Arctic Medical Research* 53 (Suppl. 2):301–4.

Naylor, J.L., C.D. Schraer, A.M. Mayer, A.P. Lanier, C.A. Treat, and N.J. Murphy. 2003. 'Diabetes among Alaska Natives: A review.' *International Journal of Circumpolar Health* 62:363–87.

Neel, J.V., A.B. Weder, and S. Julius. 1998. 'Type II diabetes, essential hypertension, and obesity as a 'syndrome of impaired genetic homeostasis': The 'thrifty genotype' hypothesis enters the twenty-first century.' *Perspectives in Biology and Medicine* 42:44–74.

Newman, M.T. 1960. 'Adaptations in the physique of American aborigines to nutritional factors.' *Human Biology* 32:288–313.

Nguyen, D., J.F. Proulx, J. Westley, L. Thibert, S. Dery, and M.A. Behr. 2003. 'Tuberculosis in the Inuit community of Quebec, Canada.' *American Journal of Respiratory and Critical Care Medicine* 168:1353–7.

Nickels, S., C. Furgal, M. Buell, and H. Moquin. 2005. *Unikkaaqatigiit: Putting the Human Face on Climate Change: Perspectives from Inuit in Canada.* Ottawa: Inuit Tapariit Kanatami.

Nielsen, N.H. 1986. *Cancer Incidence in Greenland.* Oulu: Nordic Council for Arctic Medical Research (Report 43/86).

Nielsen, N.H., H.H. Storm, L.A. Gaudette, and A.P. Lanier. 1996. 'Cancer in Circumpolar Inuit 1969–1988. A summary.' *Acta Oncologica* 35:621–8.

Nilsen, H., E. Utsi, K.H. Bønaa. 1999. 'Dietary and nutrient intake of a Sami population living in traditional Reindeer herding areas in north Norway: Comparisons with a group of Norweigians.' *International Journal of Circumpolar Health* 58:120–33.

Njølstad, I., E. Arnesen, and P.G. Lund-Larsen. 1996. 'Smoking, serum lipids, blood pressure, and sex differences in myocardial infarction: A 12–year follow-up of the Finnmark Study.' *Circulation* 93:450–6.
- 1998. 'Cardiovascular diseases and diabetes mellitus in different ethnic groups: The Finnmark Study.' *Epidemiology* 9:550–6.

NOMESCO. 2006. *Health Statistics in the Nordic Countries 2004*. Copenhagen: Nordic Medico-Statistical Committee.

Northwest Territories Department of Health and Social Services. 2003. *Cancer in the Northwest Territories 1990–2000*. Yellowknife: DHSS.

– 2004a. *NWT School Tobacco Survey 2002*. Yellowknife: DHSS.

– 2004b. *Injury in the Northwest Territories: A Descriptive Report*. Yellowknife: DHSS.

– 2005. *The NWT Health Status Report 2005*. Yellowknife: DHSS.

Nuttall, M. 1992. *Arctic Homeland: Kinship, Community and Development in Northwest Greenland*. Toronto: University of Toronto Press.

– ed. 2005. *Encyclopedia of the Arctic*. New York: Routledge.

Nuttall, M., and T.V. Callaghan, eds. 2000. *The Arctic: Environment, People, Policy*. Amsterdam: Harwood Academic Publishers.

O'Brien, J.T., B.J. Sahakian, and S. Checkley. 1993. 'Cognitive impairments in patients with seasonal affective disorders.' *British Journal of Psychiatry* 163:338–43.

Odland, J.Ø., J.C. Hansen, B. Deutch, and I.C. Burkow. 2003. 'The importance of diet on exposure and effects of persistent organic pollutants on human health in the Arctic.' *Acta Pædiatrica* 92:1255–66.

Odland, J.Ø., T. Sandanger, and E. Heimstad. 2005. *Kartlegging av miljøgifter i humane blodprøver fra Taimyr, Russland og Bodø, Norge – en pilotstudie av 'nye' miljøgifter*. Oslo: Statens forurensningstilsyn/Norwegian Pollution Control Agency (SPFO-rapport: 930/2005).

Oksa, J. 1998. 'Cooling and Neuromuscular Performance in Man.' PhD diss., University of Jyväskylä, Finland.

Oksa, J., M. Ducharme, and H. Rintamäki. 2002. 'Combined effect of repetitive work and cold on muscle function and fatigue.' *Journal of Applied Physiology* 92:354–61.

Oksa, J., H. Rintamäki, T. Mäkinen, J. Hassi, and H. Rusko. 1995. 'Cooling-induced changes in muscular performance and EMG activity of agonist and antagonist muscles.' *Aviation, Space, and Environmental Medicine* 66:26–31.

Oksa, J., H. Rintamäki, S. Rissanen, S. Rytky, U. Tolonen, and P.V. Komi. 2000. 'Stretch- and H-reflexes of the lower leg during whole-body cooling and local warming.' *Aviation, Space, and Environmental Medicine* 71:156–61.

Oksa, J., E. Sormunen, U. Koivukangas, S. Rissanen, and H. Rintamäki. 2006. 'Changes in neuromuscular function due to intermittently increased workload during repetitive work in cold conditions.' *Scandinavian Journal of Work and Environmental Health* 32:300–9.

O'Leary, C.M. 2004. 'Fetal alcohol syndrome: Diagnosis, epidemiology, and developmental outcomes.' *Journal of Paediatrics and Child Health* 40:2–7.

Olsen, O.R., A. Koch, T.G. Krause, G. Barselajsen, C.B. Christiansen, and M. Melbye. 2000. 'Population screening for HIV in Sisimiut, Greenland' (in Norwegian). *Ugeskrift for Læger* 162:4652–5.

Olsen, O.R., P. Skinhøj, K. Krogsgaard, and L. Baek. 1989. 'Hepatitis B: An endemic sexually transmitted infection in a local community in Greenland' (in Norwegian). *Ugeskrift for Læger* 151:1668–70.

Olshansky, S.J., and A.B. Ault. 1986. 'The fourth stage of the epidemiologic transition: The age of delayed degenerative diseases.' *Milbank Quarterly* 64:355–91.

Omran, A.R. 1971. 'The epidemiological transition: A theory of the epidemiology of population change.' *Milbank Memorial Fund Quarterly* 49:509–38.

O'Neil, J., M.E.K. Moffatt, R.B. Tate, and T.K. Young. 1994. 'Suicidal behaviour among Inuit in the Keewatin region, N.W.T.' In G. Pétursdottir, S.B. Sigurdsson, M.M. Karlsson, and J. Axelsson, eds., *Circumpolar Health 93*. Proceedings of the 9th International Congress on Circumpolar Health. *Arctic Medical Research* 53 (Suppl. 2):558–61.

Organization for Economic Co-operation and Development. 2006a. *OECD Health Data 2006*. Paris: OECD.

– 2006b. *OECD Economic Surveys: Russian Federation*. Paris: OECD.

O'Rourke, D.H. 2006. 'Blood groups, immunoglobulins, and genetic variation.' In D.H. Ubelaker, ed., *Handbook of North American Indians*, Vol. 3, *Environment, Origins, and Population*, 762–76. Washington, DC: Smithsonian Institution.

Orr, P., S. Mcdonald, D. Milley, and R. Brown. 2001. 'Bronchiolitis in Inuit children from a Canadian central arctic community, 1995–1996.' *International Journal of Circumpolar Health* 60:649–58.

Osler, M., and S.K. Kjær. 1996. 'Determinants of smoking behaviour in random samples of Greenlandic and Danish women 20–39 years of age.' *Arctic Medical Research* 55:62–8.

O'Sullivan, E., and M. McHardy. 2004. *The Community Well-Being (CWB) Index: Disparity in well-being between First Nations and other Canadian communities over time*. Ottawa: Indian and Northern Affairs Canada (Cat. No. R2-349/2004E).

Ousley, S.D. 1995. 'Relationships between Eskimos, Amerindians, and Aleuts: Old data, new perspectives.' *Human Biology* 67:427–58.

Pääkkönen, T. 2002. 'Cold exposure and hormonal secretion: A review.' *International Journal of Circumpolar Health* 61:265–76.

Palinkas, L.A. 2001. 'Mental and cognitive performance in the cold.' *International Journal of Circumpolar Health* 60:430–9.

Palinkas, L.A., T.M. Mäkinen, T. Pääkkönen, H. Rintamäki, J. Leppäluoto, and J. Hassi. 2005. 'Influence of seasonally adjusted exposure to cold and darkness on cognitive performance in urban circumpolar residents.' *Scandinavian Journal of Psychology* 46:39–246.

Palinkas, L.A., H.L. Reed, K.R. Reedy, N.V. Do, H.S. Case, and N.S. Finney. 2001. 'Circannual pattern of hypothalamic-pituitary-thyroid (HPT) function and mood during extended Antarctic residence.' *Psychoneuroendocrinology* 26:421–31.

Parkinson, A.J., A.A. Bell, and J.C. Butler. 1999. 'International circumpolar surveillance of infectious diseases: Monitoring community health in the Arctic.' *International Journal of Circumpolar Health* 58:222–5.

Parkinson, A.J., and J.C. Butler. 2005. 'The potential impact of climate change on infectious diseases in the Arctic.' *International Journal of Circumpolar Health* 64:478–86.

Parkinson, A.J., B.D. Gold, L. Bulkow, R.B. Wainwright, B. Swaminathan, B. Khanna, K.M. Petersen, and M.A. Fitzgerald. 2000. 'High prevalence of *Helicobacter pylori* in the Alaska native population and association with low serum ferritin levels in young adults.' *Clinical and Diagnostic Laboratory Immunology* 7:885–8.

Pars, T., M. Osler, and P. Bjerregaard. 2001. 'Contemporary use of traditional and imported food among Greenlandic Inuit.' *Arctic* 54(1):22–31.

Patz, J.A., D. Campbell-Lendrum, T. Holloway, and J.A. Foley. 2005. 'Impact of regional climate change on human health.' *Nature* 438:310–7.

Pavlov, P. and S. Indrelid. 2000. 'Human occupation in northeastern Europe during the period 35000–18000 BP. In W. Roebroeks et al., eds., *Hunters of the Golden Age: The Mid Upper Palaeolithic of Eurasia 30,000–20,000 BP*, 165–72. Leiden: Leiden University Press.

Peart, A.F., and F.P. Nagler. 1952. 'Measles in the Canadian Arctic, 1952.' *Canadian Journal of Public Health* 45:146–57.

Pedersen, C.B., and B. Zachau-Christiansen. 1986. 'Otitis media in Greenland children: Acute, chronic and secretory otitis media in three- to eight-year-olds.' *Journal of Otolaryngology* 15:332–5.

Peek-Asa, C., and C. Zwerling. 2003. 'Role of environmental interventions in injury control and prevention.' *Epidemiologic Reviews* 25:77–89.

Pego, C.M., R.F. Hill, G.W. Solomon, R.M. Chisholm, and S.E. Ivey. 1995. 'Tobacco, culture, and health among American Indians: A historical review.' *American Indian Culture and Research Journal* 19:143–64.

Pekeles, G.S., J.C. McDonald, T.W. Gyrokos, B. Alberton, J.D. MacLean, G.

Richer, and D. Juranek. 1991. 'An outbreak of congenital toxoplasmosis in northern Quebec.' In B.D. Postl, P. Gilbert, J. Goodwill, M.E.K. Moffatt, J.D. O'Neil, P.A. Sarsfield, and T.K. Young, eds., *Circumpolar Health 90*, 360–2. Winnipeg: University of Manitoba Press.

Pekeles, G., J. McDonald, R. Schreffier, and R. Allen. 1994. 'Epidemic of hepatitis A in young Inuit associated with high incidence of fulminant hepatitis and renal insufficiency.' *Arctic Medical Research* 53 (Suppl. 2):635–8.

Pekkarinen, A., H. Anttonen, and J. Hassi. 1992. 'Prevention of accidents in reindeer herding work.' *Arctic Medical Research* 51 (Suppl. 7):59–63.

Perham-Hester, K.A., H.N. Wiens, and J. Schoellhorn. 2005. *Alaska Maternal and Child Health Data Book 2004: PRAMS Edition*. Anchorage: Department of Health and Social Services.

Petersen, R. 1984. 'East Greenland before 1950.' In D. Damas, ed. *Handbook of North American Indians*. Vol. 5, *Arctic*, 622–39. Washington, DC: Smithsonian Institution.

– 1995. 'Colonialism as seen from a former colonized area.' *Arctic Anthropology* 32:118–126.

Petersen, D., U.S. Boe, and B. Persson. 2005. *Radon i Grønlandske Boliger*. Nuuk: ASIAQ Greenland Survey.

Peterson, E., A. Fenaughty, and J.E. Eberhart-Phillips. 2004. *Tobacco in the Great Land: A Portrait of Alaska's Leading Cause of Death*. Anchorage: Alaska Health and Social Services.

Phillips, D.R. 1994. 'Does epidemiological transition have utility for health planners?' *Social Science and Medicine* 38:vii–vix.

Piazza, A., P. Menozzi, and L.L. Cavalli-Sforza. 1981. 'Synthetic gene frequnecy maps of man and selective effects of climate.' *Proceedings of the National Academy of Science* 78:2638–42.

Pienimäki, T. 2002. 'Cold exposure and musculoskeletal disorders and diseases: A review.' *International Journal of Circumpolar Health* 61:173–82.

Piirtola, M., and P. Era. 2006. 'Force platform measurements as predictors of falls among older people: A review.' *Gerontology* 52:1–16.

Pika, A. and B. Prokhorov. 1994. *Neotraditionalism in the Russian North: Ethnic Revival of Indigenous Northern Peoples and National Regional Policy* (in Russian). Moscow: Institute of Economic Forecasting, Russian Academy of Sciences.

Pilcher, J., E. Nadler, and C. Busch. 2002. 'Effects of hot and cold temperature exposure on performance: A meta-analytic review.' *Ergonomics* 45:682–98.

Pivneva, E.A. 1995. 'Some aspects of reproduction system among the modern Lyapino-Sos'va Mansi population. In G. Afanasjeva, ed., *Ethno-demographic*

Peculiarities in Reproduction among the Peoples of the Russian North (in Russian), 182–224. oscow: Institute of Ethnology and Anthropology, Russian Academy of Sciences.

Poikolainen, K., S. Näyhä, and J. Hassi. 1992. 'Alcohol consumption among male reindeer herders of Lappish and Finnish origin.' *Social Science and Medicine* 35:735–8.

Poirier, S., H. Ohshima, G. de The, A. Hubert, M.C. Bourgade, and H. Bartsch 1987. 'Volatile nitrosamine levels in common foods from Tunisia, south China and Greenland, high-risk areas for nasopharyngeal carcinoma (NPC).' *International Journal of Cancer* 39:293–6.

Pollan, B. 1993. *Samiske sjamaner: Religion og helbredelse* (Sami shamans: Religion and faith healing). Gyldendal Norsk Forlag A/S.

Pollex, R.L., A.J. Hanley, B. Zinman, S.B. Harris, H.M. Khan, and R.A. Hegele. 2006. 'Metabolic syndrome in aboriginal Canadians: Prevalence and genetic associations.' *Atherosclerosis* 184:121–9.

Poppel, B., J. Kruse, G. Duhaime, and L. Abryutina. 2007. *SLiCA Results*. Anchorage: Institute of Social and Economic Research, University of Alaska Anchorage.

Pothoff, S.J., L.H. Bearinger, C.L. Skay, N. Cassuto, R.W. Blum, and M.D. Resnick. 1998. 'Dimensions of risk behaviors among American Indian youth.' *Archives of Pediatric and Adolescent Medicine* 152:157–63.

Prinz, C., S. Schwendy, and P. Voland. 2006. '*H. pylori* and gastric cancer: Shifting the global burden.' *World Journal of Gastroenterology* 12:5458–64.

Prokhorov, B. 2001. *Health of the Population of Russia in the twentieth Century* (in Russian). Moscow: MNEPU.

Proulx, J.F., S. Dery, L.P. Jette, J. Ismael, M. Libman, and W.P. De. 2002. 'Pneumonia epidemic caused by a virulent strain of *Streptococcus pneumoniae* serotype 1 in Nunavik, Quebec.' *Canada Communicable Disease Reports* 28:129–31.

Proulx, J.F., J.D. MacLean, T.W. Gyorkos, D. Leclair, A.K. Richter, B. Serhir, L. Forbes, and A.A. Gajadhar. 2002. 'Novel prevention program for trichinellosis in Inuit communities. *Clinical Infectious Diseases* 34:1508–14.

Provins, K.A., D.J. Glencross, and C.J. Cooper. 1973. 'Thermal stress and arousal.' *Ergonomics* 16:623–31.

Public Health Agency of Canada. 2006a. *Tuberculosis in Canada 2005*. Ottawa: PHAC.

– 2006b. *HIV and AIDS in Canada: Surveillance Report to Dec. 31, 2005*. Ottawa: PHAC.

Quickfall, J., and N. el-Guebaly. 2006. 'Genetics and alcoholism: How close are we to potential clinical applications?' *Canadian Journal of Psychiatry* 51:461–7.

Raab-Traub, N. 2002. 'Epstein-Barr virus in the pathogenesis of NPC.' *Seminars in Cancer Biology* 12:431–41.

Raab-Traub, N., P. Rajadurai, K. Flynn, and A.P. Lanier. 1991. 'Epstein-Barr virus infection in carcinoma of the salivary gland.' *Journal of Virology* 65:7032–6.

Raatikka, V.P., M. Rytkönen, S. Näyhä, and J. Hassi. 2007. 'Prevalence of cold-related complaints, symptoms and injuries in the general population: The FINRISK 2002 cold substudy.' *International Journal of Biometeorology* 51:441–8

Ramsey, J.D., C.L. Burford, M.Y. Beshir, and R.C. Jensen. 1983. 'Effects of workplace thermal conditions on safe work behaviour.' *Journal of Safety Research* 14:105–14.

Ray, J.G., V. Meier, M.J. Vermeulen, S. Boss, P.R. Wyatt, and D.E.C. Cole. 2002. 'Association of neural tube defects and folic acid fortification in Canada.' *Lancet* 360:2047–8.

Receveur, O., M. Boulay, and H.V. Kuhnlein. 1997. 'Decreasing traditional food use affects diet quality for adult Dene/Metis in 16 communities of the Canadian Northwest Territories.' *Journal of Nutrition* 127:2179–86.

Redding, G., R. Singleton, T. Lewis, P. Martinez, J. Butler, D. Stamey, L. Bulkow, H. Peters, J. Gove, B. Morray, and C. Jones. 2004. 'Early radiographic and clinical features associated with bronchiectasis in children.' *Pediatric Pulmonology* 37:297–304.

Reed, H.L. 1995. 'Circannual changes in thyroid hormone physiology: the role of cold environmental temperatures.' *Arctic Medical Research* 54 (Suppl. 2):9–15.

Reed, H.L., K.R. Reedy, L.A. Palinkas, N.V. Do, N.S. Finney, H.S. Case, H.J. LeMar, J. Wright, and J. Thomas. 2001. 'Impairment in cognitive and exercise performance during prolonged Antarctic residence: Effect of thyroxid supplementation in the polar triiodothyronine syndrome.' *Journal of Clinical Endocrinology and Metabolism* 86:110–6.

Reed, H.L., E.D. Silverman, K.M. Shakir, R. Dons, K.D. Burman, and J.T. O'Brian. 1990. 'Changes in serum triiodothyronine (T3) kinetics after prolonged Antarctic residence: The polar T3 syndrome.' *Journal of Clinical Endocrinology and Metabolism* 70:965–74.

Rehm, J. 1998. 'Measuring quantity, frequency and volume of drinking. *Alcoholism, Clinical and Experimental Research* 22 (Suppl. 2):4S-14S.

Rehn, B., R. Lundström, T. Nilsson, I. A. Bergdahl, C. Ahlgren, G. Sundelin,

C. From, and B. Järvholm. 2002. 'Musculoskeletal symptoms among drivers of all-terrain vehicles.' *Journal of Sound Vibration* 253:21–9.

Reid, A.H., T.G. Fanning, J.V. Hultin, and J.K. Taubenberger. 1999. 'Origin and evolution of the 1918 "Spanish" influenza virus hemagglutinin gene.' *Proceedings of the National Academy of Sciences USA* 96:1651–6.

Reijula, K., E. Larmi, J. Hassi, and M. Hannuksela. 1990. 'Respiratory symptoms and ventilatory function among Finnish reindeer herders.' *Arctic Medical Research* 49:74–80.

Retterstøl, N., Ø. Ekeberg, and L. Mehlum. 2002. *Selvmord – et personlig og samfunnsmessig problem.* Oslo: Gyldendal.

Rhoades, E.R., L.L. Reyes, and G.D. Buzzard. 1987. 'The organization of health services for Indian people.' *Public Health Reports* 102:352–6.

Richardus, J.H., W.C. Graafmans, S.P. Verloove-Vanhorick, and J.P. Mackenbach. 2003. 'Differences in perinatal mortality and suboptimal care between 10 European regions: Results of an international audit.' *British Journal of Obstetrics and Gynaecology* 110:97–105.

Ringstad, J., J. Aaseth, K. Johnsen, E. Utsi, and Y. Thomassen. 1991. 'High serum selenium concentrations in reindeer breeding Lappish men.' *Arctic Medical Research* 50:103–6.

Rink, H. 1857. *Grønland geografisk og statistisk beskrevet.* København: n.p.

Rintamäki, H. 2000. 'Predisposing factors and prevention of frostbite.' *International Journal of Circumpolar Health* 59:114–21.

– 2001. 'Human cold acclimatisation and acclimation.' *International Journal of Circumpolar Health* 60:422–9.

Rintamäki, H., S. Rissanen, T. Mäkinen, and A. Peitso. 2004. 'Finger temperatures during military field training at 0 to –29°C.' *Journal of Thermal Biology* 29:857–60.

Risica, P.M., S.O.E. Ebbesson, C.D. Schraer, E.D. Nobmann, and B.H. Caballero. 2000. 'Body fat distribution in Alaskan Eskimos of the Bering Straits region: The Alaskan Siberian Project.' *International Journal of Obesity* 24:171–9.

Rissanen, S., J. Hassi, K. Juopperi, and H. Rintamäki. 2001. 'Effects of whole body cooling on sensory perception and manual performance in subjects with Raynaud's phenomenon.' *Comparative Biochemistry and Physiology: A Molecular and Integrative Physiology* 128:749–57.

Roberts, D.F. 1953. 'Body weight, race and climate.' *American Journal of Physical Anthropology* 11:533–58.

Robinson, J.N., J.A. Regan, and E.R. Norwitz. 2001. 'The epidemiology of preterm labor.' *Seminars in Perinatology* 25:204–14.

Robitaille, N., and R. Choinière. 1985. *An Overview of Demographic and Socioe-*

conomic Conditions of the Inuit in Canada. Ottawa: Research Branch, Indian and Northern Affairs Canada.

Rode, A., and R.J. Shephard. 1994. 'The ageing of lung function: Cross-sectional and longitudinal studies of an Inuit community.' *European Respiratory Journal* 7:1653–9.

Roden, R., and T.C. Wu. 2006. 'How will HPV vaccines affect cervical cancer?' *Nature Reviews Cancer* 6:753–63.

Rosenthal, N.E., D.A. Sack, J.C. Gillin, A.J. Lewy, F. Goodwin, Y. Davenport, P.S. Mueller, D.A. Newsome, and T.A. Wehr. 1984. 'Seasonal affective disorder, a description of the syndrome and preliminary findings with light therapy.' *Archives of General Psychiatry* 41:72–80.

Rotermann, M. 2005. 'Sex, condoms and sexually transmitted diseases among young people.' *Health Reports* 16:39–45.

Rubicz, R., T.G. Schurr, P.L. Babb, and M.H. Crawford. 2003. 'Mitochondrial DNA variation and the origins of the Aleuts.' *Human Biology* 75:809–35.

Rudolph, K.M., A.J. Parkinson, A.L. Reasonover, L.R. Bulkow, D.J. Parks, and J.C. Butler. 2000. 'Serotype distribution and antimicrobial resistance patterns of invasive isolates of Streptococcus pneumoniae: Alaska, 1991–1998.' *Journal of Infectious Diseases* 182:490–6.

Ruhlen, M. 1994. *The Origin of Language: Tracing the Evolution of the Mother Tongue.* New York: John Wiley.

Runyan, C.W. 2003. 'Back to the future: Revisiting Haddon's conceptualization of injury epidemiology and prevention.' *Epidemiologic Reviews* 25:60–4.

Ruong, I. 1982. *Samerna – I historien och nutiden,* 102–3. 4th. ed. Stockholm: Bonnier Fakta.

Rutkove, S.B. 2001. 'Effects of temperature on neuromuscular electrophysiology.' *Muscle and Nerve* 24:867–82.

Ryberg, C. 1894. 'Om Erhvervs-og Befolkningsforholdene i Grønland.' *Geografisk Tidsskrift* 12:87–131.

Rytkönen, M., V.P. Raatikka, S. Näyhä, and J. Hassi. 2005. 'Cold exposure and cold related symptoms' (in Finnish). *Duodecim* 121:419–23.

Rytkönen, M., J. Ranta, J. Tuomilehto, and M. Karvonen for the SPAT Study Group and the Finnish Childhood Diabetes Registry Group. 2001. 'Bayesian analysis of geographical variation in the incidence of type 1 diabetes in Finland.' *Diabetologia* 44 (Suppl. 3):B37–B44.

Saemundsen, A.K., H. Albeck, J.P. Hansen, N.H. Nielsen, M. Anvret, W. Henle, G. Henle, K.A. Thomsen, H.K. Kristensen, and G. Klein. 1982. 'Epstein-Barr virus in nasopharyngeal and salivary gland carcinomas of Greenland Eskimoes.' *British Journal of Cancer* 46:721–8.

Saillard, J., P. Forster, N. Lynnerup, H. J. Bandelt, and S. Nørby. 2000.

'mtDNA variation among Greenland Eskimos: The edge of the Beringian expansion.' *American Journal of Human Genetics* 67:718–26.

Salo, W.L., A.C. Aufderheide, J. Buikstra, and T.A. Holcomb. 1994. 'Identification of *Mycobacterium tuberculosis* DNA in a pre-Columbian Peruvian mummy.' *Proceedings of the National Academy of Sciences USA* 91:2091–4.

Salonen, J.T. 1982. 'Socioeconomic status and risk of cancer, cerebral stroke, and death due to coronary heart disease and any disease: A longitudinal study in eastern Finland.' *Journal of Epidemiology and Community Health* 36:294–7.

Salvesen, H. 1995. 'Sami Ædnan: Four states – one nation?' In S. Tägil, ed., *Ethnicity and Nation Building in the Nordic World*, 106–43. London: Hurst.

Sammallahti, P. 1998. *The Saami Languages*. Karasjok, Norway: Sámi Instituhtta.

Sampson, P.D., A.P. Streissguth, F.L. Bookstein, and H.M. Barr. 2000. 'On categorizations in analyses of alcohol teratogenesis.' *Environmental Health Perspectives* 108 (Suppl. 3):421–8.

Sampson, P.D., A.P. Streissguth, F.L. Bookstein, R.E. Little, S.K. Clarren, P. Dehaene, J.W. Hanson, and J.M. Graham. 1997. 'Incidence of fetal alcohol syndrome and prevalence of alcohol-related neurodevelopmental disorder.' *Teratology* 56:317–26.

Santos, M. 2005. 'Alcohol-related injury deaths in the Northwest Territories (1999–2003).' *EpiNorth* 17(2):9–13.

Sargeant, A.J. 1987. 'Effect of muscle temperature on leg extension force and short-term power output in humans.' *European Journal of Applied Physiology* 56:693–8.

Schaefer, O. 1971. 'Otitis media and bottle-feeding: An epidemiological study of infant feeding habits and incidence of recurrent and chronic middle ear disease in Canadian Eskimos.' *Canadian Journal of Public Health* 62:478–89.

Schaefer, O., J.A. Hildes, L.M. Medd, and D.G. Cameron. 1975. 'The changing pattern of neoplastic disease in Canadian Eskimos.' *Canadian Medical Association Journal* 112:1399–404.

Scheer, W.D., D.A. Boudreau, G.T. Malcolm, and J.P. Middaugh. 1995. 'Apolipoprotein E and atherosclerosis in Alaska Natives.' *Atherosclerosis* 114:197–202.

Schlife, C. 1987. 'Smokeless tobacco use in rural Alaska.' *Mortality and Morbidity Weekly Report* 36:140–3.

Schnohr, C., T.I.A. Sørensen, and B.V.L. Niclasen. 2005. 'Changes since 1980 in body mass index and the prevalence of overweight among inschooling children in Nuuk, Greenland.' *International Journal of Circumpolar Health* 64:157–62.

Scholander, P.F., H.T. Hammel, K.L. Andersen, and Y. Loyning. 1958. 'Metabolic acclimation to cold in man.' *Journal of Applied Physiology* 12:1–8.

Scholander, P.F., H.T. Hammel, J.S. Hart, D.H. Le Messurier, and J. Steen. 1958. 'Cold adaptation in Australian aborigines.' *Journal of Applied Physiology* 113:211–8.

Schraer, C.D., S.O.E. Ebbesson, E. Boyko, E. Nobmann, A. Adler, and J. Cohen. 1996. 'Hypertension and diabetes among Siberian Yupik Eskimos of St. Lawrence Island, Alaska.' *Public Health Reports* 111 (Suppl. 2):51–2.

Schraer, C.D., A.M. Mayer, A.M. Vogt, J. Naylor, T.L. Brown, J. Hastie, and J. Moore. 2001. 'The Alaska Native Diabetes Program.' *International Journal of Circumpolar Health* 60:487–94.

Schreeder, M.T., T.R. Bender, B.J. McMahon, M.R. Moser, B.L. Murphy, M.J. Sheller, W.L. Heyward, D.B. Hall, and J.E. Maynard. 1983. 'Prevalence of hepatitis B in selected Alaskan Eskimo villages.' *American Journal of Epidemiology* 118:543–9.

Schumacher, C., M. Davidseon, and G. Ehrsam. 2003. 'Cardiovascular disease among Alsaka Natives: A review of the literature.' *International Journal of Circumpolar Health* 62:343–62

Schurr, T.G. 2004. 'The peopling of the New World: Perspectives from molecular anthropology.' *Annual Review of Anthropology* 33:551–83.

Schurr, T.G. and S.T. Sherry. 2004. 'Mitochondrial DNA and Y chromosome diversity and the peopling of the Americas: Evolutionary and demographic evidence.' *American Journal of Human Biology* 16:420–39.

Scott, C.L., S. Iyasu, D. Rowley D, and H.K. Atrash. 1998. 'Postneonatal mortality surveillance – United States, 1980–1994.' *Mortality and Morbidity Weekly Reports. CDC Surveillance Summaries* 47:15–30.

Segal, B., and B. Saylor. 2007. 'Social transition in the North: Comparisons of drug-taking behaviour among Alaska and Russian Natives.' *International Journal of Circumpolar Health* 66:71–6.

Senécal, S., and E. O'Sullivan. 2005. *The Well-Being of Inuit Communities in Canada*. Ottawa: Indian and Northern Affairs Canada (Cat. No. R2-419/2005E).

Shields, G.F., A.M. Schmiechen, B.L. Frazier, A. Redd, M.I. Voevoda, J.K. Reed, and R.H. Ward. 1993. 'mtDNA sequences suggest a recent evolutionary divergence for Beringian and northern North American populations.' *American Journal of Human Genetics*:549–62.

Silva, J.E. 2006. 'Thermogenic mechanisms and their hormonal regulation.' *Physiological Reviews* 86:435–64.

Silventoinen, K., J. Pankow, P. Jousilahti, G. Hu, and J. Tuomilehto. 2005. 'Educational inequalities in the metabolic syndrome and coronary heart disease among middle-aged men and women.' *International Journal of Epidemiology* 34:327–34.

Silviken, A., T. Haldorsen, and S. Kvernmo. 2006. 'Suicide among indigenous Sami in Arctic Norway, 1970–1998.' *European Journal of Epidemiology* 21:707–13.

Silviken, A., and S. Kvernmo. 2007. 'Suicide attempts among indigenous Sami adolescents and majority peers in Arctic Norway: Prevalence and associated risk factors.' *Journal of Adolescence* 30:613–26.

Simonsen, P. 1976. 'Nordkalotten igår – Fra urtid til nær fortid.' In *Nordkalotten – mulighetens land*, 27–31. Oslo: Foreningen Nordens Forbund.

Sing, C.F., and J. Davignon. 1985. 'Role of the apolipoprotein E polymorphism in determining normal plasma lipid and lipoprotein variation.' *American Journal of Human Genetics* 37:268–85.

Singleton, R., L. Hammitt, T. Hennessy, L. Bulkow, C. DeByle, A. Parkinson, T.E. Cottle, H. Peters, and J.C. Butler. 2006. 'The Alaska *Haemophilus influenzae* type b experience: Lessons in controlling a vaccine-preventable disease.' *Pediatrics* 118:e421–9.

Singleton, R.J., K.M. Petersen, J.E. Berner, E. Schulte, K. Chiu, C.M. Lilly, E.A. Hughes, L.R. Bulkow, and T.L. Nix. 1995. 'Hospitalizations for respiratory syncytial virus infection in Alaska Native children.' *Pediatric Infectious Disease Journal* 14:26–30.

Singleton, R.J., G.J. Redding, T.C. Lewis, P. Martinez, L. Bulkow, B. Morray, H. Peters, J. Gove, C. Jones, D. Stamey, D.F. Talkington, J. DeMain, J.T. Bernert, and J.C. Butler. 2003. 'Sequelae of severe respiratory syncytial virus infection in infancy and early childhood among Alaska Native children.' *Pediatrics* 112:285–90.

Sjölin R. 2004. 'Samer och samefrågor i svensk politik – En studie i ickemakt.' In P. Lantto and P. Sköld, eds., *Befolkning och Bosättning I Norr – etnicitet, identitet och gränser I historiens sken*, 237–44. Umeå: Centre for Sami Research.

Skifte, T.B. 2004. 'Tuberculosis in Greenland – still a problem to bear in mind: Development and strategy.' *International Journal of Circumpolar Health* 63 (Suppl. 2):221–4.

Skinhøj, P. 1977. 'Hepatitis and hepatitis B-antigen in Greenland. II: Occurrence and interrelation of hepatitis B associated surface, core, and 'e' antigen-antibody systems in a highly endemic area.' *American Journal of Epidemiology* 105:99–106.

Skinhøj, P., F. Mikkelsen, and F.B. Hollinger FB. 1977. 'Hepatitis A in Greenland: Importance of specific antibody testing in epidemiologic surveillance.' *American Journal of Epidemiology* 105:140–7.

Sköld, P. 1998. 'Samiska giftermålsstrategier.' *Kulturens Frontlinjer/Kulturgräns Norr* 13:31–51.

Sköld, P., and R. Kvist. 1988. 'Alkoholen och de nomadiserande samerna: Jokkmokks socken 1860–1910.' *Tidsskrift for Nordisk Alkoholforskning* 5:249–53.

Skretting, A. 1996. *Ungdom og rusmidler.* Oslo: Rusmiddeldirektoratet, Statens Institutt for Alkohol-og Narkotikaforskning.

Smith, D.G., J. Lorenz, C.K. Rolfs, R.L. Bettinger, B. Green, J. Esheleman, B. Schultz, and R. Malhi. 2000. 'Implications of the distribution of Albumin Naskapi and Albumin Mexico for New World prehistory.' *American Journal of Physical Anthropology* 111:557–72.

Snellman, A. 1998. 'Post-Soviet Russian indigenous health: The Sami people of the Kola Peninsula.' *International Journal of Circumpolar Health* 57:636–8.

Snodgrass, J.J., W.R. Leonard, L.A. Tarskaia, V.P. Alekseev, and V.G. Krivoshapkin. 2005. 'Basal metabolic rate in the Yakut (Sakha) of Siberia.' *American Journal of Human Biology* 17:155–72.

Snyder, O.B., J.J. Kelly, and A.P. Lanier. 2006. 'Prostate cancer in Alaska Native men, 1969–2003.' *International Journal of Circumpolar Health* 65:8–17.

Sobel, J., N. Tucker, A. Sulka, J. McLaughlin, and S. Maslanka. 2004. 'Food-borne botulism in the United States, 1990–2000.' *Emerging Infectious Diseases* 10:1606–11.

Soborg, C., B. Soborg, S. Pouelsen, G. Pallisgaard, S. Thybo, and J. Bauer. 2001. 'Doubling of the tuberculosis incidence in Greenland over an 8–year period (1990–1997).' *International Journal of Tuberculosis and Lung Diseases* 5:257–65.

Socialdepartementet. 2000. *Hälsa på lika villkor – nationella mål för folkhälsan – Betänkande från Nationella folkhälsokommittén.* Stockholm.

Socialstyrelsen. [various years]. *Medicinsk födelseretistering.* Stockholm [*Hälsa och Sjukdomar* 2002:3; 2003:1; 2004:3, and 2005:4].

– 2000. *Olika villkor – olika hälsa.* Stockholm.

– 2001. *Folkhålsorapport 2001.* Stockholm.

– 2003. *Socialstyrelsens föreskrifter om ändring i föreskrifterna om kompetenskrav för sjuksköterskor vid förskrivning av läkemedel.* Stockholm.

– 2005. *Folkhålsorapport 2005.* Stockholm.

– 2006. *Amning av barn fodda 2004.* Stockholm [*Hälsa och Sjukdomar* 2006:7].

Soininen, L., S. Järvinen, and E. Pukkala. 2002. 'Cancer incidence among Sami in northern Finland, 1979–1998.' *International Journal of Cancer* 100:342–6.

Solbakk, J.T., ed. 2006. *The Sámi People: A Handbook.* Karasjok: Davvi Girji OS.

Sorlie, T., and J.I. Nergoard. 2005. 'Treatment satisfaction and recovery in Saami and Norwegian patients following psychiatric hospital treatment: A comparative study.' *Transcultural Psychiatry* 42:295–316.

Sosial-og helsedepartementet. 1995. 'Risikogrupper blant samisk ungdom' In *Samisk helse-og sosialplan. Plan for helse-og sosialtjenester til den samiske befolkningen i Norge*, 197–231. Oslo.

– 1998–99. 'Levekår i samiske områder.' In: *Utjamningsmeldinga om fordeling av inntekt og levekår i Norge*, 167–8. Oslo.

Spady, D.W., ed. 1991. *Between Two Worlds: The Report of the Northwest Territories Perinatal and Infant Mortality and Morbidity Study*. Rev. ed. Edmonton: Canadian Circumpolar Institute, University of Albert.

Spein, A.R., S. Kvernmo, and H. Sexton. 2002. 'The North Norwegian Youth Study: Cigarette smoking among ethnically diverse adolescents.' *Ethnicity and Health* 7:163–79.

Spein, A.R., H. Sexton, and S. Kvernmo. 2004. 'Predictors of smoking behaviour among indigenous Sami adolescents and non-indigenous peers in north Norway.' *Scandinavian Journal of Public Health* 32:118–29.

– 2006. 'Longitudinal drinking patters in indigenous Sami and non-indigenous youth in northern Norway.' *Journal of Ethnicity in Substance Abuse* 5:103–17.

Spencer, F.A., R.J. Goldberg, R.C. Becker, and J.M. Gore. 1998. 'Seasonal distribution of acute myocardial infarction in the second national registry of myocardial infarction.' *Journal of the American College of Cardiology* 6:1226–33.

Spiller, H.A. 2004. 'Epidemiology of volatile substance abuse (VSA) cases reported to U.S. poison centers.' *American Journal of Drug and Alcohol Abuse* 30:155–65.

Sreter, S. 1988. 'The importance of social intervention in Britain's mortality decline c.1850–1914: A re-interpretation of the role of public health.' *Social History of Medicine* 1:1–38.

– 2003. 'The population health approach in historical perspective.' *American Journal of Public Health* 93:421–31.

STAKES. (various years). *Parturients, Births and Newborn Infants*. Helsinki: STAKES.

Starikovskaya, Y.B., R.I. Sukernik, T.G. Schurr, A.M. Kogelnik, and D.C. Wallace. 1998. 'mtDNA diversity in Chukchi and Siberian Eskimos: Implications for the genetic history of ancient Beringia and the peopling of the New World.' *American Journal of Human Genetics* 63:1473–91.

Statistics Canada. 1993. *Language, Tradition, Health, Lifestyle and Social Issues: 1991 Aboriginal Peoples Survey*. Ottawa: Statistics Canada.

– 2003a. *Aboriginal Peoples Survey 2001 – Initial Release – Supporting Tables.* Ottawa: Statistics Canada (Cat. No. 89-592-XIE).

– 2003b. *Aboriginal Peoples Survey 2001 – Initial Findings: Well-Being of the Non-Reserve Aboriginal Population.* Ottawa: Statistics Canada (Cat. No. 89-589-XIE).

– 2004. *Comparable Health Indicators.* Ottawa: Statistics Canada (Cat. No. 82-401-XIE).

– 2006. *Health Indicators.* Ottawa: Statistics Canada (Cat. No. 82-221-XIE).

Statistics Greenland. 2005. *Greenland in Figures, 2005.* Nuuk: Statistics Greenland.

Stein, K.P., P.K. Lange, U. Gad, and E. Wilbek. 1968. 'Tuberculosis in Greenland.' *Archives of Environmental Health* 17:501–6.

Stepanova, E.G., and E.V. Shubnikov. 1991. 'Diabetes, glucose intolerance and some risk factors of diabetes mellitus in natives and newcomers of Chukotka.' In B.D. Postl, P. Gilbert, J. Goodwill, M.E.K. Moffatt, J.D. O'Neil, P.A. Sarsfield, and T.K. Young, eds., *Circumpolar Health 90*, 413–4. Winnipeg: University of Manitoba Press.

Stevenson, M.R., L.J. Wallace, J. Harrison, J. Moller, and R.J. Smith. 1998. 'At risk in two worlds: Injury mortality among indigenous people in the U.S. and Australia, 1990–92.' *Australian and New Zealand Journal of Public Health* 22:641–4.

Stocks, J.M., N.A.S. Taylor, M.J. Tipton, and J.E. Greenleaf. 2004. 'Human physiological responses to cold exposure.' *Aviation, Space, and Environmental Medicine* 75:444–57.

Storm, H.H., and Nielsen, N.H. 1996. 'Cancer of the digestive system in circumpolar Inuit.' *Acta Oncologica* 35:553–70.

Strand, P., T.D. Selnaes, E. Boe, O. Harbitz, and A. Andersson-Sorlie. 1992. 'Chernobyl fallout: Internal doses to the Norwegian population and the effect of dietary advice.' *Health Physics* 63:385–92.

Sundhedsstyrelsen. (various years). *Fødselsregisteret.* Copenhagen.

– 1950. *Grønlandskommissionens betænkning 4.* Copenhagen. [Sundhedsstyrelsens skrivelse af 21. oktober 1948].

Svendsen, S.K. 1930. 'Om Tuberkulosen I Egedesminde Distrikt, Nordgrønland.' *Ugeskrift for Læger* 92:1225–7.

Szathmary, E.J. 1993. 'Genetics of Aboriginal North Americans.' *Evolutionary Anthropology* 1:202–20.

Szathmary, E.J.E., and N.S. Ossenberg. 1978. 'Are the biological differences between North American Indians and Eskimos truly profound?' *Current Anthropology* 19:673–701.

Tägil, S. 1995. 'Ethnic and national minorities in the Nordic nation-building process: Theoretical and conceptual premises.' In S. Tägil, ed., *Ethnicity and Nation Building in the Nordic World*, 8–29. London: Hurst.

Tambets, K., et al. 2004. 'The western and eastern roots of the Saami: The story of genetic "outliers" told by mitochondrial DNA and Y chromosomes.' *American Journal of Human Genetics* 74:661–82.

Tanner, C.E., M. Staudt, R. Adamowski, M. Lussier, S. Bertrand, and R.K. Prichard. 1987. 'Seroepidemiological study for five different zoonotic parasites in northern Quebec.' *Canadian Journal of Public Health* 78:262–6.

Taubenberger, J.K., A.H. Reid, R.M. Lourens, R. Wang, G. Jin, and T.G. Fanning. 2005. 'Characterization of the 1918 influenza virus polymerase genes.' *Nature* 437:889–93.

Taylor, N.A.S. 2006. 'Ethnic differences in thermoregulation: Genotypic versus phenotypic heat adaptation.' *Journal of Thermal Biology* 31:90–104.

Taylor, S.E., and R.L. Repetti. 1997. 'What is an unhealthy environment and how does it get under the skin?' *Annual Review of Psychology* 48:411–47.

Teichner, W.H. 1958. 'Reaction time in the cold.' *Journal of Applied Physiology* 42:54–9.

Terry, P., P. Lichtenstein, M. Feychting, A. Ahlbom, and A. Wolk. 2001. 'Fatty fish consumption and risk of prostate cancer.' *Lancet* 357:1764–6.

Thelle, D.S., and Forde, O.H. 1979. 'The cardiovascular study in Finnmark county: Coronary risk factors and the occurrence of myocardial infarction in first degree relatives and in subjects of different ethnic origin.' *American Journal of Epidemiology* 110:708–15.

Thompson, R., H. Dubowitz, D.J. English, K.B. Nooner, T. Wike, S.I. Bangdiwala, D.K. Runyan, and E.C. Briggs. 2006. 'Parents' and teachers' concordance with children's self-ratings of suicidality: Findings from a high-risk sample.' *Suicide and Life-Threatening Behavior* 36:167–81.

Thomsen, V.O., T. Lillebaek, and F. Stenz. 2004. 'Tuberculosis in Greenland: Current situation and future challenges.' *International Journal of Circumpolar Health* 63 (Suppl. 2):225–9.

Thorslund, J. 1991. 'Suicide among Inuit youth in Greenland 1977–86.' *Arctic Medical Research* (Suppl.):299–302.

Tjepkema, M. 2002. 'The health of the off-reserve Aboriginal population.' *Health Reports* 13 (Suppl.):73–88.

– 2005. 'Non-fatal injuries among Aboriginal Canadians.' *Health Reports* 16:9–22.

Togeby, L. 2002. *Grønlændere I Danmark – en overset minoritet*. Aarhus: Aarhus Universitetsforlag.

Torroni, A., T.G. Schurr, C.C. Yang, E.J.E. Szathmary, R.C. Williams, M.S. Schanfield, Troup, G.A., W.C. Knowler, D.N. Lawrence, K.M. Weiss, and

D.C. Wallace. 1992. 'Native American mitochondrial DNA analysis indicates that the Amerind and the Nadene populations were founded by two independent migrations.' *Genetics* 130:153–62.

Tough, S.C., L.W. Svenson, D.W. Johnston, and D. Schopflocher. 2001. 'Characteristics of preterm delivery and low birth weight among 113,994 infants in Alberta: 1994–1996.' *Canadian Journal of Public Health* 92:276–80.

Transport Canada. 2005. *Results of Transport Canada's September 2004 Survey of Seat Belt Use in Rural Areas of the Country.* Ottawa: Transport Canada.

Trevitch, A. 2002. 'Russie: population et espace.' *Population and Society: Informational Bulletin of Human Demography and Ecology Centre of the Institute of National Economy Forecasting* 869:1–4.

Trottier, H., and E.L. Franco. 2006. 'The epidemiology of genital human papillomavirus infection.' *Vaccine* 24 (Suppl. 1):S1–15.

Tune, C.E., P.G. Liavaag, J.L. Freeman, M.W. van den Brekel, T. Shpitzer, J.D. Kerrebijn, D. Payne, J.C. Irish, R. Ng, R.K. Cheung, and H.M. Dosch. 1999. 'Nasopharyngeal brush biopsies and detection of nasopharyngeal cancer in a high-risk population.' *Journal of the National Cancer Institute* 91:796–800.

Tveito, O.E., E. Førland, R. Heino, I. Hanssen-Bauer, H. Alexandersson, B. Dahlstrøm, A. Drebs, C. Kern-Hansen, T. Johnsson, E. Vaarby Laursen, and Y. Westman. 2000. *Nordic Temperature Maps.* Report No. 09/00 KLIMA. Oslo: Norwegian Meteorological Institute.

Tverdal, A. 1997. 'Cohort study of ethnic group and cardiovascular and total mortality over 15 years.' *Journal of Clinical Epidemiology* 50:719–23.

Ubelaker, D.H. 2006. 'Population size, contact to nadir.' In D.H. Ubelaker, ed., *Handbook of North American Indians*, Vol. 3, *Environment, Origins, and Population*, 694–701. Washington, DC: Smithsonian Institution.

United Nations Development Program. 2005. *Human Development Report, 2005.* New York: UNDP.

United States Census Bureau. 2003. *Characteristics of American Indians and Alaska Natives by Tribe and Language, 2000.* Washington, DC: U.S. Census Bureau (PHC-5).

United States Department of Health and Human Services. 1998. 'Tobacco use among U.S. racial/ethnic minority groups: A report of the Surgeon General, 1998. Executive summary.' *Tobacco Control* 7:198–209.

United States Indian Health Service. (n.d.). *Regional Differences in Indian Health, 2000–2001.* Rockville, MD: IHS, DHSS.

Utsi, E., and K.H. Bønaa. 1998. 'Koronar hjertesykdom hos samiskættende og norskættede i Finnmark.' *Tidsskrift for den Norske Laegeforening* 118:1358–62.

Vahtola, J. 1992. 'The main phases of colonization in northern Finland.' *Faravid* 16:141–51.

Vakhtin, N. 1992. *Native Peoples of the Russian Far North*. London: Minority Rights Group (Report 92/5).

Vakhtin, N. 1993. *Indigenous Population of the Extreme North of the Russian Federation* (in Russian). St Petersburg: European House Press.

Vaktskjold, A., J.A. Lebedintseva, D.S. Korotov, A.V. Tkatsjov, T.S. Podjakova, and E. Lund. 2005. 'Cancer incidence in Arkhangelskaja Oblast in north-western Russia.' *BMC Cancer* 5(1):82.

van Landingham, M.J., and C.J. Hogue. 1995. 'Birthweight-specific infant mortality risks for Native Americans and whites, United States, 1960 and 1984.' *Social Biology* 42:83–94.

van Marken Lichtenbelt, W.D, P. Schrauwen P, S. van de Kerkhove, and M.S. Westerterp-Platenga. 2002. 'Individual variation in body temperature and energy expenditure in response to mild cold.' *American Journal of Physiology (Physiology, Endocrinology and Metabolism)* 282:E1077–83.

van Marken Lichtenbelt, W.D, M.S. Westerterp-Platenga, and P. van Hoydonk. 2001. 'Individual variation in the relation between body temperature and energy expenditure in response to elevated ambient temperature.' *Physiology and Behaviour* 73:235–42.

van Ooijen, A.M., W.D. Marken Lichtenbelt, A.A. van Steenhoven, and K.R. Westerterp. 2004. 'Seasonal changes in metabolic and temperature responses to cold air in humans.' *Physiology and Behaviour* 82:545–53.

van Oostdam, J., S.G. Donaldson, M. Feeley, D. Arnold, P. Ayotte, G. Bondy, L. Chan, E. Dewaily, C.M. Furgal, H. Kuhnlein, E. Loring, G. Muckle, E. Myles, O. Receveur, B. Tracy, U. Gill, and S. Kalhok. 2005. 'Human health implications of environmental contaminants in Arctic Canada: A review.' *Science of the Total Environment* 351/352:165–246.

van Orden, K.F., S.T. Ahlers, J.R. Thomas, J.F. House, and J. Schrot. 1990. 'Moderate cold exposure shortens evoked potential latencies in humans.' *Aviation, Space and Environmental Medicine* 61:636–9.

Vaughan, W.S. 1977. 'Distraction effect of cold water on performance of high-order tasks.' *Undersea Biomedical Research* 4:103–16.

Virokannas, H. 1996. 'Thermal responses to light, moderate and heavy daily outdoor work in cold weather.' *European Journal of Applied Physiology* 72:483–9.

Vishnevsky, A.G., ed. 2001. *Population of Russia* (in Russian). Moscow: Universitet.

Vojnova, V.D., O.D. Zacharova, and L.L. Rybakovsky. 1993. 'Modern Russian North and its population.' In L.L. Rybakovsky, ed., *Social-Demographic Development of the Russian North* (in Russian), 7–25. oscow: Institute of Socioeconomical Problems of Population, Russian Academy of Sciences.

Wagner, B.M., S.A. Wong, and D.A. Jobes. 2002. 'Mental health professionals' determinations of adolescent suicide attempts.' *Suicide and Life-Threatening Behavior* 32:284–300.

Waldram, J.B., D.A. Herring, and T.K. Young. 2006. *Aboriginal Health in Canada: Historical, Cultural and Epidemiological Perspectives.* 2nd ed. Toronto: University of Toronto Press.

Wallace, D.C., K. Garrison, and W.C. Knowler. 1985. 'Dramatic founder effects in American mitochondrial DNAs.' *American Journal of Physical Anthropology* 68:149–55.

Wang, J., J.R. Burnett, S. Near, T.K. Young, B. Zinman, A.J. Hanley, P.W. Connelly, S.B. Harris, and R.A. Hegele. 2000. 'Common and rare ABCA1 variants affecting plasma HDL cholesterol.' *Arteriosclerrosis, Thrombosis and Vascular Biology* 20:1983–9.

Warren, J.A., J.E. Berner, and T. Curtis. 2005. 'Climate change and human health: Infrastructure impacts to small remote communities in the north.' *International Journal of Circumpolar Health* 64:487–97.

Wein, E.E., and M.M. Freeman. 1992. 'Inuvialuit food use and food preferences in Aklavik, Northwest Territories, Canada.' *Arctic Medical Research* 51:159–72.

Wein, E.E., M.M. Freeman, and J.C. Makus. 1996. 'Use of and preference for traditional food among the Belcher Island Inuit.' *Arctic* 49:256–64.

Weingartner, H., R.M. Cohen, D.L. Murphy, J. Martello, and C. Gerdt. 1981. 'Cognitive processes in depression.' *Archives of General Psychiatry* 38:42–7.

Welch, D.W., Y. Ishida, and K. Nagasawa. 1998. 'Thermal limits and ocean migrations of sockeye salmon (Oncorhynchus nerka): Long-term consequences of global warming.' *Canadian Journal of Fisheries and Aquatic Science* 55:937–48.

Westenberg, L., K.A. van der Klis, A. Chan, G. Dekker, and R.J. Keane. 2002. 'Aboriginal teenage pregnancies compared with non-Aboriginal in South Australia 1995–1999.' *Australian and New Zealand Journal of Obstetrics and Gynaecology* 42:187–92.

Westerlund, E.A., T. Berthelsen, and L. Berteig. 1987. 'Cesium-137 body burdens in Norwegian Lapps, 1965–1983.' *Health Physics* 52:171–7.

Westerterp-Plantenga, M.S., W.D. Marken Lichtenbelt, H. Strobbe, and P. Schrauwen. 2002. 'Energy metabolism in humans at a lowered ambient temperature.' *European Journal of Clinical Nutrition* 56:288–96.

Wexler, L., and B. Goodwin. 2006. 'Youth and adult community member beliefs about Inupiat youth suicide and its prevention.' *International Journal of Circumpolar Health* 65:448–58.

Wherret, G.J. 1945. 'Arctic survey 1: Survey of health conditions and medical and hospital services in the North West Territories.' *Canadian Journal of Economics and Political Science* 11(1):49–60.

Wichstrøm, L. 2000. 'Predictors of adolescent suicide attempts: A nationally representative longitudinal study of Norwegian adolescents.' *Journal of the American Academy of Child and Adolescent Psychiatry* 39:603–10.

Wiklund, K., L.E. Holm, and G. Eklund. 1990. 'Cancer risks in Swedish Lapps who breed reindeers.' *American Journal of Epidemiology* 132:1078–82.

Wilcox, S., C. Castro, A.C. King, R. Housemann, and R.C. Brownson. 2000. 'Determinants of leisure time physical activity in rural compared with urban older and ethnically diverse women in the United States.' *Journal of Epidemiology and Community Health* 54:667–72.

Wilson, J.F., R.L. Rausch, and F.R. Wilson. 1995. 'Alveolar hydatid disease: Review of the surgical experience in 42 cases of active disease among Alaskan Eskimos.' *Annals of Surgery* 221:315–23.

Winsa, B. 2005. 'Language policies: instruments in cultural development and well-being.' *International Journal of Circumpolar Health* 64:170–83.

Wissow, L.S., J. Walkup, A. Barlow, R. Reid, and S. Kane. 2001. 'Cluster and regional influences on suicide in a Southwestern American Indian tribe.' *Social Science and Medicine* 53:1115–24.

Witmer, J.M., M.R. Hensel, P.S. Holck, A.S. Ammerman, and J.C. Will. 2004. 'Heart disease prevention for Alaska Native women: A review of pilot study findings.' *Journal of Women's Health* 13:569–78.

Wolfe, R.J. 1982. 'Alaska's Great Sickness, 1900: An epidemic of measles and influenza in a virgin soil population.' *Proceedings of the American Philosophical Society* 126(2):91–121.

Wolsko, C., C. Lardon, G.V. Mohatt, and E. Orr. 2007. 'Stress, coping, and well-being among the Yup'ik of the Yukon-Kuskokwim delta: The role of enculturation and acculturation.' *International Journal of Circumpolar Health* 66:51–61.

Woodhouse, P.R., K.T. Khaw, and M. Plummer. 1993. 'Seasonal variation of blood pressure and its relationship to ambient temperature in an elderly population.' *Journal of Hypertension* 11:1267–74.

Woods, W., M.E.K. Moffatt, T.K. Young, J. O'Neil, R. Tate, and I. Gillespie. 1994. 'Hearing loss and otitis media in Keewatin children.' *Arctic Medical Research* 53 (Suppl. 2):693–6.

World Health Organization. 1992. *International Statistical Classification of Diseases and Related Health Conditions.* 10th rev. ed. Geneva: WHO.

– 1999. *Definition, Diagnosis and Classification of Diabetes Mellitus and its Complications: Report of a WHO Consultation.* Geneva: WHO (WHO/NCD/NCS/99.2).

– 2000. *Obesity: Preventing and Managing the Global Epidemic: Report of a WHO Consultation on Obesity.* Geneva: WHO.

– 2003a. *Climate Change and Human Health Risks and Responses*, 37. Geneva: WHO.

– 2003b. *Global Strategy for Infant and Child Feeding*. Geneva: WHO.

– Commission on Health and the Environment. 1992. *Our Planet, Our Health*. Geneva: WHO.

World Health Organization and International Society for the Prevention of Childhood Abuse and Neglect. 2006. *Preventing Child Maltreatment: A Guide for Taking Action and Generating Evidence*. Geneva: WHO.

Yip, R., P.J. Limburg, D.A. Ahlquist, H.A. Carpenter, A. O'Neill, D. Kruse, S. Stitham, B.D. Gold, E.W. Gunter, A.C. Looker, A.J. Parkinson, E.D. Nobmann, K.M. Petersen, M. Ellefson, and S. Schwartz. 1997. 'Pervasive occult gastrointestinal bleeding in an Alaska native population with prevalent iron deficiency: Role of *Helicobacter pylori* gastritis.' *Journal of the American Medical Association* 277:1135–9.

Young, A.J., and C.M. Blatteis. 1996. 'Homeostatic responses to prolonged cold exposure: Human cold acclimatization.' In M.J. Fregly and C.M. Blatteis, eds., *Handbook of Physiology*. Vol. 1, *Section 4: Environmental Physiology*, 419–38. New York: Oxford University Press.

Young, L.T., E. Hood, S. Abbey, and S. Malcolmson. 1991. 'Reasons for psychiatric referral in an Inuit population.' In B.D. Postl, P. Gilbert, J. Goodwill, M.E.K. Moffatt, J.D. O'Neil, P.A. Sarsfield, and T.K. Young, eds., *Circumpolar Health 90*, 296–8. Winnipeg: University of Manitoba Press.

Young, T.K. 1996a. 'Sociocultural and behavioural determinants of obesity among Inuit in the central Canadian Arctic.' *Social Science and Medicine* 43:1665–71.

– 1996b. 'Obesity, central fat patterning and their metabolic correlates among the Inuit of the central Canadian Arctic.' *Human Biology* 68:245–63.

– 1994. *The Health of Native Americans: Towards a Biocultural Epidemiology*. New York: Oxford University Press.

Young, T.K., P. Bjerregaard, E. Dewailly, P.M. Risica, M.E. Jørgensen, and S.E.O. Ebbesson. 2007. 'Prevalence of obesity and its metabolic correlates among the circumpolar Inuit in 3 countries.' *American Journal of Public Health* 97:691–5.

Young, T.K., D. Chateau, and M. Zhang. 2002. 'Factor analysis of ethnic variation in the multiple metabolic (insulin resistance) syndrome in three Canadian populations.' *American Journal of Human Biology* 14:649–58.

Young, T.K., J.M. Gerrard, and J.D. O'Neil. 1999. 'Plasma phospholipid fatty acids in the central Canadian Arctic: Biocultural explanations for ethnic differences.' *American Journal of Physical Anthropology* 109:9–18.

Young, T.K., M.E. Moffatt, and J.D. O'Neil. 1992. 'An epidemiological perspective of injuries in the Northwest Territories.' *Arctic Medical Research* 51 (Suppl. 7):27–36.

– 1993. 'Cardiovascular diseases in a Canadian Arctic population.' *American Journal of Public Health* 83:881–7.

Young, T.K., and Mollins, J. 1996. 'The impact of housing on health: An ecological study from the Canadian Arctic.' *Arctic Medical Research* 55:52–61.

Young, T.K., Y.P. Nikitin, E.V. Shubnikov, T.I. Astakhova, M.E.K. Moffatt, and J.D. O'Neil. 1995. 'Plasma lipids in two indigenous arctic populations with low risk for cardiovascular diseases.' *American Journal of Human Biology* 7:223–6.

Young, T.K., J. Reading, B. Elias, and J.D. O'Neil. 2000. 'Type-2 diabetes in Canada's First Nations: Status of an epidemic in progress.' *Canadian Medical Association Journal* 163:561–6.

Young T.K., C.D. Schraer, E.V. Shubnikoff, E.J.E. Szathmary, and Y.P. Nikitin. 1992. 'Prevalence of diagnosed diabetes in circumpolar indigenous populations.' *International Journal of Epidemiology* 21:730–6.

Young, T.K., E.J. Szathmary, S. Evers, and B. Wheatley. 1990. 'Geographical distribution of diabetes among the native population of Canada: A national survey.' *Social Science and Medicine* 31:129–39.

Ytterstad, B., and H. Wasmuth. 1995. 'The Harstad Injury Prevention Study: Evaluation of hospital-based injury-recording and community-based intervention for traffic injury prevention.' *Accidents Analysis and Prevention* 27:111–23.

Ytterstad, B. 2003. 'The Harstad Injury Prevention Study: A decade of community-based traffic injury prevention with emphasis on children. Postal dissemination of local injury data can be effective.' *International Journal of Circumpolar Health* 62:61–74.

Yu, M.C., and J.M. Yuan. 2002. 'Epidemiology of nasopharyngeal carcinoma.' *Seminars in Cancer Biology* 12:421–9.

Zebrowski, P.L., and R.J. Gregory. 1996. 'Inhalant use patterns among Eskimo school children in western Alaska.' *Journal of Addictive Diseases* 15:67–77.

Zegura, S.L., T.M. Karafet, L.A. Zhivotovsky, and M.F. Hammer. 2004. 'High-resolution SNPs and microsatellite haplotypes point to a single, recent entry of Native American Y chromosomes into the Americas.' *Molecular Biology and Evolution* 21:164–75.

Zimmerman, M.R., and A.C. Aufderheiden. 1984. 'The frozen family of Ytriagvik: The autopsy findings.' *Arctic Anthropology* 21:53–64.

Zorgdrager, N. 1997. *De rettferdiges strid: Kautokeino 1952.* Nesbru: Norsk Folkemuseum.

Contributors

Laura Arbour, MD, MSc, is associate professor in the Department of Medical Genetics at the University of British Columbia's Island Medical Program located in Victoria, BC. She graduated in medicine from McMaster University and trained in pediatrics and medical genetics at McGill University. She served as a consultant paediatrician in the Nunavik region of northern Quebec in the 1990s. Her clinical practice and research focuses on northern and Aboriginal health issues as they pertain to genetics, in particular the prevention of birth defects.

James Berner, MD, served as director of community health of the Alaska Native Tribal Health Consortium from 1984–2006, and is currently its senior director for Science. A graduate in medicine of the University of Oklahoma and a board certified specialist in internal medicine and pediatrics, he has practised medicine in the Alaska Native health care system since 1974. He directs the Alaska Native Traditional Food Safety Monitoring program, which assesses contaminant and micronutrient levels in pregnant women and their health effects. He has been the key national expert for the U.S. on the Human Health Advisory Group of the Arctic Monitoring and Assessment Program (AMAP) and a lead author of the 2005 Arctic Climate Impact Assessment report. In 2005 he was appointed to the National Academy of Sciences Polar Research Board.

Peter Bjerregaard, MD, PhD, is professor of Arctic health at the National Institute of Public Health in Copenhagen, affiliated with the Directorate of Health in Greenland and the University of Southern Denmark. A graduate in medicine from the University of Copenhagen, he specialized in public health and epidemiology. He worked as a district medical officer in northern Greenland and as a public health administrator in Kenya, but since the early 1990s he has concentrated on epidemiological research in Greenland as the principal investigator of several large population surveys. His current research interests include cardiovascular disease and diabetes as well as social epidemiology among the Inuit. He has published extensively on various aspects of health in Greenland, including scientific papers and the monographs *Disease Pattern in Greenland* (1991), *Living Conditions, Life Style, and Health in Greenland* (1995), *The Circumpolar Inuit* (1998, with Kue Young), and *Public Health in Greenland* (2004). He served as the president of the International Union for Circumpolar Health from 2000–3 and is currently a scientific editor of the *International Journal of Circumpolar Health*.

Michael Bruce, MD, MPH, is epidemiology team leader at the Centers for Disease Control and Prevention's Arctic Investigations Program in Alaska. He graduated in medicine and public health from Tufts University and is a specialist in both internal medicine and preventive medicine. His recent work has focused on the creation of two sentinel surveillance systems: in Alaska for detecting *Helicobacter pylori* infections and for the International Circumpolar Surveillance (ICS) network to detect invasive bacterial diseases. His current areas of interest include meningococcal disease, peptic ulcer, and gastric cancer associated with *Helicobacter pylori* infection, invasive bacterial pneumonia, avian influenza, human papillomavirus, and cervical cancer.

Jeppe Friborg, MD, PhD, is a researcher at the Department of Epidemiology Research, Statens Serum Institute, Copenhagen. He received his MD from the University of Southern Denmark and his PhD from the University of Copenhagen. His main areas of research are in head-neck cancers, particularly the Epstein-Barr virus related carcinomas, and cancer epidemiology in Arctic populations. Despite his years in research, he has maintained his clinical work and is currently undergoing specialist training in clinical oncology.

Sven Hassler, DrMedSci, is assistant professor in the Department of Nursing, Health, and Culture at the University West, Trollhättan, Sweden. He is also a researcher at the Southern Lapland Research Department in Vilhelmina, pursuing epidemiological research in the health and living conditions of the Sami population of Sweden. He received his doctorate of medical science from the Department of Public Health and Clinical Medicine at Umeå University, Sweden.

Robert Hegele, MD, is Distinguished University Professor of Medicine and Biochemistry at the University of Western Ontario, where he holds the Edith Schulich Vinet Canada Research Chair in Human Genetics and the Jacob Wolfe Distinguished Medical Research Chair. A graduate of the University of Toronto, he is a specialist in internal medicine and in endocrinology and metabolism. He completed post-doctoral research fellowships at Rockefeller University (New York) and the Howard Hughes Medical Institute (Salt Lake City). His laboratory at the Robarts Research Institute has discovered the genomic basis of ten human diseases, including Oji-Cree type 2 diabetes. He was a charter member of the advisory board for the Canadian Institute for Aboriginal Peoples' Health.

Preben Homøe, MD, DrMSc, PhD, is associate professor and consultant in otorhinolaryngology and head and neck surgery at Rigshospitalet, the University Hospital of Copenhagen. Since 1999 he has served regularly as a consultant in Greenland, and from 2001–4 he was responsible for the otolaryngology program operated jointly by the Greenland Home Rule Government and Rigshospitalet. Currently, he is chair of the Danish/Greenlandic Society for Circumpolar Health and secretary of the International Union of Circumpolar Health. He has conducted anthropological, historical, epidemiological, microbiological, and immunological research in Greenland, especially on otitis media, upper respiratory tract infections, and hearing impairment.

Urban Janlert, MD and specialist in social medicine, is professor in the Department of Public Health and Clinical Medicine, Umeå University, Sweden. His research interests are mainly in the field of social epidemiology (work deprivation, social stratification, and health). He is also active in the Swedish East European Committee with a focus on health issues within the Barents region of northern Scandinavia and European Russia.

Marit Eika Jørgensen, MD, PhD, is a clinical endocrinologist and epidemiology researcher affiliated with the Centre for Health Research in Greenland of the National Institute of Public Health and the Steno Diabetes Centre. A graduate of the University of Copenhagen, she has provided clinical services and conducted research in Greenland since the mid-1990s. Her current research focuses on diabetes, obesity, and the associated cardiovascular risk among Greenland Inuit.

Anders Koch, MD, PhD, is a senior researcher at the Department of Epidemiology Research, Statens Serum Institut, Copenhagen, and leader of its Section for Greenland Research. A graduate of the University of Copenhagen, he has conducted health research in Greenland since 1994. His has carried out and supervised clinical, sero-epidemiological, and register-based studies in Greenland on a number of infectious diseases as well as asthma, allergy, and cancer. He is a board member of the Danish/Greenlandic Society for Circumpolar Health and the International Circumpolar Surveillance System. He also conducts epidemiological studies in Denmark and drafted the National Pandemic Influenza Preparedness Plan for the Danish National Board of Health in 2005.

Andrew Kozlov, MD, PhD, DSc, is head of laboratory in the Institute of Developmental Physiology of the Russian Academy of Education in Moscow. He graduated from Perm Medical University in the Western Urals. In 1986, he became the head of the Laboratory of Medical Anthropology in the Tjumen Medical University in Western Siberia. In 1991 he founded (with G. Vershubsky) an independent ArctAn-C Innovative Laboratory. During his career he has conducted field research in different parts of Russia (Kola Peninsula, northern regions of European Russia, the Urals, Siberia, Trans-Baikal, Far East, and Chukotka), Byelorussia, and the Caucasus. A full professor from 2002, he served as chair of human ecology at the International Independent University of Ecological and Political Sciences in Moscow. He is the author of six books.

Siv Kvernmo, MD, PhD, is associate professor at the medical faculty of the University of Tromsø and chief consultant in child and adolescent psychiatry at the University Hospital of North-Norway. She has a specific research interest in epidemiology and the mental health of Sami adolescents, and in ethnocultural topics. She has been project leader/manager of several epidemiological studies on adolescent mental health and of clinical research projects in child and adolescent psychiatry.

Dmitry Lisitsyn, PhD, is senior research scientist at the Institute of Developmental Physiology, Russian Academy of Education, Moscow. He graduated from the Kazan State University, where he studied physical anthropology of ancient and modern populations of the Middle Volga and participated in archaeological and anthropological fieldwork. Since the early 1990s he has focused on the physical and cultural anthropology of Finno-Ugrian peoples of European Russia as a member of the ArctAn-C Innovative Laboratory in Moscow.

Tiina Mäkinen, PhD, is a scientist in the Institute of Health Sciences at the University of Oulu, Finland, and the editor of the *International Journal of Circumpolar Health*. Trained as a physiologist at the University of Oulu, she has conducted research on the effects of cold exposure on human health and performance related to living in northern environments. More recently, her research interests have focused on the effects of climate and climate change on human health, especially in identifying susceptible population groups and planning and implementing appropriate prevention and protection measures to mitigate the expected adverse effects of climate change.

Jon Øyvind Odland, MD, PhD, is scientific director and professor at the Centre for International Health, University of Tromsø, Norway. A medical graduate of the University of Trondheim, he qualified as an obstetrician-gynecologist and defended his doctoral thesis at the Institute of Community Medicine, University of Tromsø. His main research interests are in Arctic health problems, especially infectious diseases; contaminants and pregnancy outcomes; the development of pregnancy care programs in different cultures; the use of epidemiological methods in public health services; and global environmental health issues. He is deputy secretary of the Arctic Monitoring and Assessment Programme (AMAP) and was co-editor of its 1998 report, *Arctic Pollution Issues*, and its 2002 report, *Human Health in the Arctic*, and a contributor to several of the report's chapters.

Rebecca Pollex, MSc, is a biochemistry and phenomics research assistant with the Vascular Biology Group at the Robarts Research Institute in London, Ontario. She received her Honours BSc degree from the University of Waterloo and her MSc degree from the University of Western Ontario. Her master's thesis focused on the metabolic syndrome and diabetes complications in Aboriginal populations in Canada.

Mika Rytkönen, PhD, has previously conducted research with leading diabetes and cardiovascular epidemiologists at the National Public Health Institute of Finland. He was a member of the multidisciplinary SPAT study group at the Institute involved in developing geographic information systems and statistical methods for health research. He has also carried out research on climate-environment-health relationships.

Anne Silviken is a clinical psychologist with the Sami Psychiatric Youth Team of the Sami National Centre for Mental Health in Karasjok, Norway. The team works with adolescents and young adults with substance abuse and suicidal behaviour, and in suicide prevention. She graduated in psychology from the University of Tromsø and has been working as a clinician since 1998. In 2007, she received her PhD from the Centre for Sami Health Research of the Institute of Community Medicine, University of Tromsø, focusing on suicidal behaviour among the Sami in northern Norway.

Per Sjölander, DrMedSci, is director of the Southern Lapland Research Department in Vilhelmina, Sweden, and professor at the Centre for Musculoskeletal Research, University of Gävle. For more than two decades he has conducted sensorimotor research on pathological mechanisms of musculoskeletal pain conditions. In more recent years he has also been involved in different research projects aimed at increasing our knowledge of the health and living conditions of the Swedish Sami population.

Anna Rita Spein, MD, PhD, is a physician with the Sami National Centre for Mental Health, working with adolescents and youths manifesting substance use-related problems and suicidal behaviour. She is also affiliated with the Centre for Sami Health Research, Institute of Community Medicine at the University of Tromsø, where she defended in 2007 her doctoral thesis on substance use among ethnically diverse adolescents and youths in northern Norway. Her research and clinical interests are in Sami ethnic/cultural issues in relationship to legal and illicit substance use.

Thomas Stensgaard, MD, is district medical officer at the Primary Health Care Centre in Nuuk, Greenland. A graduate of the University of Copenhagen, he received his specialist training in family medicine in northern Sweden. Except for a few short breaks, he has been working in Greenland since 1983, when he had his first job in Scoresbysund in east Greenland. He has served for nine years as president of the Greenland Medical Association and was president of the 12th International Congress on Circumpolar Health held in Nuuk in 2003. His main interests are in health care organization, with a more recent focus on telemedicine and diabetes program planning.

Kue Young, MD, DPhil, is professor in the Department of Public Health Sciences at the University of Toronto, where he holds the endowed TransCanada Pipelines Chair. He graduated in medicine, public health, and biological anthropology from McGill University, the University of Toronto, and Oxford University, respectively. He spent much of his professional career in primary health care, public health administration, and academic research in northern Canada and developing countries. His current research focuses on the epidemiology and prevention of emerging chronic diseases in indigenous populations in the circumpolar region. He is the author of four books on the health of indigenous peoples: *Health Care and Cultural Change* (1988), *The Health of Native Americans* (1994), *Aboriginal Health in Canada* (1994, with James Waldram and Ann Herring), and *The Circumpolar Inuit* (1998, with Peter Bjerregaard); he has also written a general textbook, *Population Health* (1998). He served as president of the International Union for Circumpolar Health from 1993-6. In 2004 he founded the International Network for Circumpolar Health Research.